ART THERAPY AND THE NEUROSCIENCE OF TRAUMA

Art Therapy and the Neuroscience of Trauma, 2nd edition, lays out a unified framework of neural plasticity and resilience, and places it within a broader social context. Using a lens grounded in multicultural humility, renowned figures in art therapy have updated chapters with content that takes a systematic yet inclusive approach. New chapters and new authors offer stimulating insights into individual and community factors that drive comprehensive care.

This revitalized second edition offers an accessible and comprehensive text intended for novice and sage art therapists and students. The book also fosters a vision and a translational pathway for research that explores the protective factors of resilience and the universal impacts of psychological trauma with the systematic integration of art therapy and neuroscience.

Juliet L. King, PhD, ATR-BC, LPC, LMHC, is an associate professor in the Department of Art Therapy at the George Washington University and an adjunct associate professor in the Department of Neurology at the Indiana University School of Medicine.

Christianne E. Strang, PhD, ATR-BC, CEDS, is an assistant professor in the Department of Psychology at the University of Alabama at Birmingham, where she teaches graduate and undergraduate courses in neurobiology, behavioral neuroscience, developmental neuroscience, and creative arts therapies.

T0299896

"This innovative second edition comes at a time when understanding the transformative healing potential of neuroaesthetics is paramount. This edition delves into neuroplasticity, neuroscience-informed art therapy, and the artmaking process, illuminating the profound impact that art can have on the brain and well-being of individuals who have experienced trauma.

As the fields of art therapy and behavioural health continues to make strides in understanding the neurobiological grounds of artmaking and its many therapeutic benefits, this new edition masterfully synthesizes cutting-edge research with practical perspectives that are relevant and relatable, making it an indispensable resource.

The authors have provided an insightful understanding of how art therapy can effectively address and heal trauma at a neurological level emphasizing valuable insights on art, trauma, and the brain. Readers are provided rich case studies and techniques that will equip clinicians to deepen their understanding and enhance therapeutic outcomes across various settings. I am honored to endorse this edition and commend the authors for their continued and invaluable contributions to the field."

Lindsey D. Vance, ATR-BC, LPC, arts innovation manager in the Office of Teaching and Learning, District of Columbia Public Schools, Washington DC

"King and Strang brilliantly set new horizons in the growing and robust landscape where neuroscience meets art therapy. The first edition of this book transformed the art therapy profession. Its neuroscientific discussion supported art therapy practices that struggled for decades for validation. This second edition unpacks the most recent, groundbreaking research. Theory and evidence-based findings are intertwined effectively to explore the impact of art therapy interventions on diverse populations in novel settings. Clinicians and researchers will welcome this second edition with as much enthusiasm and gratitude as we had for the first edition."

Marygrace Berberian, PhD, LCAT, ATR-BC, LCSW, director of the New York University Graduate Art Therapy Program

"This new edition delves further into brain function, dysfunction, and amelioration by embracing state-of-the-art diagnostics and proposing integration with art therapy practice. As it is essential to understand medical diagnoses and psychological issues, it is also critical to understand neurological etiologies and their implication to refine clinical interventions.

Since the last publication, scientific fields have illuminated neuronal activity and re-generation enabling a more focused art therapy approach with complex brain injured clients. The editors and contributors provide invaluable perspectives to inform our work, enhance our treatment of trauma and optimize outcomes."

Irene Rosner David, PhD, ATR-BC, LCAT, HLM

"This new edition offers an in-depth understanding of the application of science to art therapy and the treatment of trauma. The authors build on prior concepts and forge new pathways to demonstrate effective art therapy treatment. The case examples translate theory to practice with a variety of treatment issues."

Linda Chapman, MA, retired art therapist

ART THERAPY AND THE NEUROSCIENCE OF TRAUMA

Theoretical and Practical Perspectives

Second Edition

Edited by
Juliet L. King and Christianne E. Strang

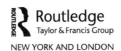

Routledge
Taylor & Francis Group

NEW YORK AND LONDON

Designed cover image: © Gina M. Baird

Second edition published 2025
by Routledge
605 Third Avenue, New York, NY 10158

and by Routledge
4 Park Square, Milton Park, Abingdon, Oxon, OX14 4RN

Routledge is an imprint of the Taylor & Francis Group, an informa business

© 2025 selection and editorial matter, Juliet L. King and Christianne E. Strang; individual chapters, the contributors.

The right of Juliet L. King and Christianne E. Strang to be identified as the authors of the editorial material, and of the authors for their individual chapters, has been asserted in accordance with sections 77 and 78 of the Copyright, Designs and Patents Act 1988.

First edition published by Routledge 2016
Classic Edition published by Routledge 2021

Library of Congress Cataloging-in-Publication Data
Names: King, Juliet L., editor. | Strang, Christianne E., editor.
Title: Art therapy and the neuroscience of trauma : theoretical and
practical perspectives / edited by Juliet L. King and Christianne E. Strang.
Description: Second edition. | New York, NY : Routledge, 2024. |
"First edition published by Routledge 2016. Classic Edition published by
Routledge 2021." | Includes bibliographical references and index. |
Identifiers: LCCN 2023059058 (print) | LCCN 2023059059 (ebook) |
ISBN 9781032380780 (hardback) | ISBN 9781032380766 (paperback) |
ISBN 9781003348207 (ebook)
Subjects: LCSH: Brain damage–Patients–Rehabilitation. | Brain–Wounds and
injuries–Patients–Rehabilitation. | Art therapy–Methodology.
Classification: LCC RC489.A72 A782 2024 (print) | LCC RC489.A72 (ebook) |
DDC 616.89/1656–dc23/eng/20240408
LC record available at https://lccn.loc.gov/2023059058
LC ebook record available at https://lccn.loc.gov/2023059059

ISBN: 978-1-032-38078-0 (hbk)
ISBN: 978-1-032-38076-6 (pbk)
ISBN: 978-1-003-34820-7 (ebk)

DOI: 10.4324/9781003348207

Typeset in New Baskerville Std
by KnowledgeWorks Global Ltd.

We dedicate this book to the timeless pioneers and unsung heroes who have laid the foundations for our important and meaningful profession. We are emboldened by a deeper understanding of science that has forever informed art therapy theory, practice, and research approaches.

CONTENTS

Acknowledgments   ix

About the Cover Image   x

Contributors   xiii

Foreword by Robert M. Pascuzzi, MD   xvi

Preface   xix

1 **INTRODUCTION**   1
   Juliet L. King and Christianne E. Strang

2 **NEUROSCIENCE CONCEPTS FOR CLINICAL PRACTICE IN
   BEHAVIORAL HEALTH AND ART THERAPY**   17
   Lukasz M. Konopka, Christianne E. Strang, and Juliet L. King

3 **USING THE EXPRESSIVE THERAPIES CONTINUUM
   AS A FRAMEWORK IN THE TREATMENT OF TRAUMA:
   INFLUENCE OF CREATIVITY ON RESILIENCE**   51
   Lisa D. Hinz and Vija B. Lusebrink

4 **THE IMAGE COMES FIRST: TREATING PREVERBAL
   TRAUMA WITH ART THERAPY**   76
   Linda Gantt and Tally Tripp

5 **PRINCIPLES OF MEMORY RECONSOLIDATION: ADVANCED
   ART THERAPY RELATIONAL NEUROSCIENCE PERSPECTIVES**   106
   Noah Hass-Cohen

6 **NEUROSCIENCE AND ART THERAPY WITH SEVERELY
   TRAUMATIZED CHILDREN: THE ART IS THE EVIDENCE**   130
   P. Gussie Klorer

7 **PRACTICAL APPLICATIONS OF NEUROSCIENCE IN
   ART THERAPY: A HOLISTIC APPROACH TO TREATING
   TRAUMA IN CHILDREN**   150
   Christopher M. Belkofer and Emily Nolan

8 **NEA CREATIVE FORCES® ADVANCES ART THERAPY
   RESEARCH WITH MILITARY-CONNECTED POPULATIONS**   166
   Gioia Chilton, Janell S. Payano Sosa, Chandler Sours Rhodes,
   and Melissa Walker

9   THE INTERPOSITIONAL ROLE OF ART THERAPY IN
    MUSEUM SETTINGS   197
    Denise Wolf, Kathryn Snyder, and Raquel Farrell-Kirk

10 VOICES

    Addressing Parkinson's Disease Symptomatology with
    Clay Manipulation   213
    Morgan Gaydos and Deborah Elkis-Abuhoff

    Applied Educational Neuroscience©   216
    Lori Desautels and Ashlee Harmon

    Neuro-Informed Art Therapy, Trauma, and Supervision
    Training Approach, Guided by the Principles of
    Adlerian Psychology   220
    Erin Rafferty-Bugher

    Storycloths   225
    Lisa Garlock

    Connecting Neuroscience to Caribbean Art Therapy
    Trauma Practice   230
    Sarah Soo Hon and Karina Donald

    Connecting the Words of Healing Through
    Amorphous Art   233
    Laura Gruce

    Short Perspective: Neurobiologically Informed Art Therapy
    Work Within the Context of Complex Socio-Political Realities 237
    Einat Metzl

    The Integration of Imagery Rehearsal Therapy and Art Therapy
    (IRT + AT) for Post-Traumatic Nightmares (PTN)   240
    Adrienne Stamper

    Redrawing Value: Gaining New Understanding of Identity
    Through Art Therapy   243
    Barbara van der Vossen

11 CONCLUSION   251
    Kerry Kruk-Borisov, Juliet L. King, and Christianne E. Strang

    Glossary   267
    Index   276

ACKNOWLEDGMENTS

King:

While editing a book and conducting psychotherapy have different immediate outcomes, they both involve interpersonal interactions, effective communication, and clear goals, all of which emerge from trusting relationships. I would like to acknowledge the contributing authors who have generously volunteered their knowledge and time with a tolerance of ambiguity and within a culture of respect. Christianne E. Strang, PhD, is a steadfast mentor and editorial partner who honors autonomy and creativity in the effective translation of scientific concepts. Her leadership empowers us to know and do better. Over the last decade, neurologist Robert Pascuzzi, MD, has consistently supported the awareness of art therapy as a medical and health-care profession, selflessly sharing his knowledge with an open-mind that illuminates compassion and transformation for all involved, most importantly the patients. The research, administrative, and editorial support provided by Georgia Baltimore is nothing short of profound, actions that are overshadowed only by her kindness and consistency. Although art therapist Michael Franklin, PhD is not directly represented in this book, his legendary wisdom is woven throughout as we, if nothing else, *lead with empathy* in collective efforts to understand and advance our work. And of course, I acknowledge my family (real and chosen) and friends who are always with me no matter where we might be, and where we might go.

Strang:

My life and work have been shaped by many extraordinary people. My parents, Dr. Eleanor Strang and my late father David M. Strang, made sure that art and creativity were aspects of everyday life and supported me in all the ways that matter. My art therapy mentors and colleagues, especially Dr. Patricia Isis, supported the development and honing of my creative and clinical skills in art therapy practice. My neuroscience mentors, Dr. Kent Keyser, Dr. Paul Gamlin, and Dr. Frank Amthor, helped me understand that there is curiosity, creativity, and wonder in science. Together they, and so many others, supported me in stepping into the unexpected beauty in the fusion of art and science.

ABOUT THE COVER IMAGE

Criss Cross and the Stained-Glass Window is part of "The Super Series," a spontaneous process painting series devoted to my work with clients who experienced extreme complex trauma and dissociative identities. When I started this painting, I wanted to convey a particular feeling of countertransference that I was experiencing. I began by using my hand and my arm as a stencil and reaching across the canvas, as though reaching out to assist someone who was stuck and/or afraid. I reached out with both arms from opposite sides of the canvas, giving the canvas the appearance of being held and sending a visual invitation of reaching out to those suffering and struggling with heavy burdens. Kind and supportive touch was one of the healthy forms of physical comfort the clients were denied and were yearning for. I wanted this gesture within the canvas to say, "I acknowledge you. Your needs are important, and I am here and present with you." I was normalizing, and demonstrating healthy boundaries, while also communicating appropriate rapport and respect for the complex parental countertransference, and transference, that is always present when healing extreme complex trauma.

Although all the layers of this painting were done spontaneously, guided by a knowing that wasn't entirely deliberate, I wanted the symbolism in the foundation of the painting to illustrate that I was attuned to the clients' needs that were often denied and masked. My act of painting this series, at every layer, confirmed something that I was feeling, responding to, and tracking that I couldn't verbalize and that symbolically was a parallel process to clinical issues that my clients were working on. One example of this is the young figure shown reaching out for support. This symbolically occurred weeks before it was verbally validated in session that a client was reaching out for resources for the first time in their lives.

I experienced sensory resonance as countertransference to my clients in and out of sessions while providing this intensive therapy. I was extremely attuned to emotions being held by the clients who were raw with pain from being trapped, for years, with unspeakable traumas. After creating layers of imagery, I would find that narratives in my paintings were playing out in parallel within the therapy sessions. The painting was a way for me to record progress as much as it also served as a way for me to keep track of complexities and changing dynamics within the therapeutic relationship. I was being guided by the clients through attunement, and through following my countertransference responses to understand complex transference and shifts within the client's internal systems. Creating art to process my clinical work is as effective for my own self-care as it is a window into my client's unspoken, but fully felt, attachment needs, developmental wounds, and transference.

The paintings in this series are alive with symbolism, color, and narrative that call my attention to my love for being an art therapist. My use of color mirrors, my understanding and acknowledgement of the incredible resilience that was taking place because of the therapy we were doing. Working with this population is the most dangerous work that I participated in as a therapist due to the constant threat of vicarious trauma and other challenges. However, working with survivors of extreme complex trauma has been the most satisfying and rewarding work of my career. I used my abilities with art's intrinsic medicine and the healing power of creativity to turn vicarious trauma into vicarious resilience. As art therapists, we have the incredible sensory medicine of art materials and the well-earned respect for the process of creating. We can use those abilities to access our own powerful medicine of expression and creation. For me, each therapy session itself was a work of art, the art created within and outside of those sessions continued the healing potential in infinite ways. Through painting I built the landscape that I was feeling and each layer mirrored back to me the healthy and supportive therapeutic partnership between client and therapist.

There is a faceless crowd protected within the shoulder of the lion figure in the painting. It exists to first acknowledge a crowd-of-hurt tucked in a place where we shoulder burdens and tensions. Looking at that part of the image further, the crowd resembles an exposed lung that naturally occurred as if covering the heart of the lion. My hand reaches to support the heart, the exposed lung, and the expectant crowd. The young female figure shares my other hand as she reaches for a pink leaf. This symbol holds specific significance to a particular case where one learned to receive and trust in emotional care for the first time, healing profound developmental and attachment traumas. The hidden messages within the images, and the layers of the painting that the viewers can't see, are a testament to the profound safety and the impact of privacy and confidentiality, also speaking a symbolic shared language that represents how intimately a therapist and client begin to know each other in their collaborative relationship.

The image of a lion's face recurred many times within this series of paintings and has multiple levels of significance to my clinical work as a symbol from my early days as a student to the present moment. Because of this it was not a surprise to see this glorious king appear in the painting; it was another energy that paid tribute to the ability to heal and for my love for both painting and my work as an art therapist. The initial gesture and stencil of my hands transformed into arms and hands of the lion figure. The narrative in the painting mirrored an expression of self and tenderness towards self that I saw taking shape for my clients who began to conceptualize love toward themselves within the process of therapy.

The mandala that forms a boundary around the lion's face is a tribute to the power, incredible strength, and the persistent will that it takes to recover and heal from extreme mental injury and traumas over the course of all developmental stages. Contrasting lines hold protective and solid boundaries that mirror the shape of the people seen in the crowd. The head of the young girl is encircled by a spiral and as she leans her head into my hand that spiral gives way to a road leading back within the deeper figure. The tree in the young male figure's head is reaching just to the boundary of the arch in the lion's body. It is reaching out towards the healing light of the stained-glass window around it. There is a knowing and symbolic attention in the details surrounding the heads of the figures of this painting that illustrate finding resources both internally and externally.

I witnessed the most incredible courage in these clients who were all ages and genders. A beautiful aspect within this painting is each character's deeply expressive face, capturing transference and authentic emotions which then become mirrored by me in the painting. Feelings once feared, internalized, forbidden, and despised now are welcomed, honored, and preserved to validate healthy feelings being expressed unconditionally. The tree that finds root and carries into the face of the young male figure reflects the neurobiology within the neural networks depicted that are also tree branches. There are strong roots on the outside of the neck that rest like a foundation of insignia symbolizing bold actions of healthy leadership taken by one of my clients though his process of recovery.

The stained-glass window within a partially visible arch carries with it themes of spiritual healing that are apparent throughout my work. It is also a tribute to sacred and devotional art that can be found existing within other art, in the way that a stained-glass window is art, as is the structure that houses it and as is the light and shadow that is cast within it. This is also true of the human brain and its incredible and miraculous capacity to use dissociation as a means of protection and survival. The painting illustrates this art-within-art perspective that is foundational in the way I work and that honors the artistry of the clients' minds, bodies, and spirits. We see a main trinity of figures in the painting that all fit and function together. The three main figures are stepping forward in the painting and there are many vehicles at play that symbolize growth and connection, such as the hands, the heads, the road, the roots, and the branches.

It is difficult to find the correct words to illustrate the incredible dimension and depth in the art we create about, and in, our clinical work. The narratives, and the processes, that I witnessed in this work were elevated with my spontaneous painting as reflection that I have been prolifically creating since I was an art therapy student decades ago. This painting is an excellent example of an explorational guide that allowed me to remain immersed in trauma humility and be emotionally regulated, which is so necessary and important in this intense clinical work. When we participate in this work, we must accept a vast and ever-changing continuum of complex countertransference that involves denial, horror, anger, and gut-wrenching grief.

Countertransference is very much a living part of the work that a therapist must be aware of, and work with, on a daily and ongoing basis. The healing power of painting, of all art-creation, is an important aspect of the therapeutic and healing processes. The images in this painting, and my ability to read my own image as my intuitive language, helped me hold space for clients to heal. There were incredible adaptive changes happening for my clients. I witnessed extreme shifts in my clients' ability to demonstrate living with empowerment, and their (?) leadership, self-care, self-compassion, and themes of spirituality began to become refuge for my clients. This painting tells that story. The frame of this archway represents a window that was opened for my clients. Symbolically passing through the initiation of our trauma work made it possible for a healing that words can't quantify. This may be why my painting, which represents incredible healing and honors the power of the therapeutic relationship, wraps its arms around this next edition of *Art Therapy, Trauma, and Neuroscience: Theoretical and Practical Perspectives*.

Gina M. Baird, LMHC, ATR-BC, ATCS

CONTRIBUTORS

Christopher M. Belkofer, Ph.D., ATR-BC, LPC, Professor, Mount Mary University, Milwaukee, WI and Psychotherapist, Lead Art Therapist, Education Consultant at Clara Healing Institute, Wauwatosa, WI, USA.

Gioia Chilton, **Ph.D., ATR-BC, CSAC**, Creative Arts Therapist, Intrepid Spirit Center, A.T. Augusta Military Medical Center, Fort Belvoir, Virginia, USA. email: gioia.c.chilton.civ@health.mil

Lori Desautels, Ph.D., Assistant Professor, College of Education, Butler University, Indianapolis, IN.

Karina Donald, Ph.D., ATR-BC, LMFT, Assistant Professor, Department of Art Education, Florida State University, Tallahassee, FL, USA.

Deborah Elkis-Abuhoff, Ph.D., LCAT, ATR-BC, BCPC, Associate Professor Art Therapy, Hofstra University, Hempstead, NY, USA.

Raquel Farrell-Kirk, M.A., ATR-BC, Owner, Creative Energy Art Therapy, Jacksonville, FL, USA.

Linda Gantt, Ph.D., ATR-BC, HLM, Co-owner of the ITR Training Institute and Help for Trauma LLC, Morgantown, West Virginia, USA.

Lisa Garlock, LCPAT, ATR-BC, ATCS, Adjunct Professor, The George Washington University, Washington DC; Art Therapist, Common Threads Project, New York, USA.

Morgan Gaydos, LCAT, ATR-BC, Creative Arts Therapist, Nassau University Medical Center; Assistant Professor Art Therapy, Hofstra University, Hempstead, NY, USA.

Laura Gruce, LCAT, ATR-BC, MS, CMBP, Art Therapist, Miami VA Medical Center, Miami, FL, USA.

Ashlee Harmon, **B.A.**, Language Arts and Social Studies Teache, Avon Community Schools, Indianapolis, IN, USA.

Noah Hass-Cohen, Psy-D, ATR-BC, Associate Professor, Couple and Family Masters and Doctoral Programs, California School of Professional Psychology at Alliant International University, Alhambra, CA, USA.

Lisa D. Hinz, Ph.D., ATR-BC, Associate professor and director of the doctoral program in art therapy psychology at Dominican University of California, San Rafael, CA, USA.

Sarah Soo Hon, Ph.D., ATR, Art Therapist, Trinidad and Tobago.

P. Gussie Klorer, Ph.D., ATR-BC, LCPC, LCSW, HLM, Professor Emeritus, Art Therapy Counseling Program, Southern Illinois University, Edwardsville, USA.

Lukasz M. Konopka, AM, PhD, ECNS, BCN, qEEG-DL, Director of Brain to Behavior Program at Duly Health and Care, Romeoville, IL, USA.

Kerry Kruk, MS, LPC, CSAC, ATR-BC, Clinician IV – Team Lead, Human Rights Coordinator at City of Virginia Beach.

Vija B. Lusebrink (1924–2022), Ph.D., ATR, HLM, Professor Emerita, Expressive Therapies, The University of Louisville, Louisville, KY, USA.

Einat Metzl, Ph.D., LMFT, ATR-BC, Associate Professor Art Therapy, Drexel University, Philadelphia, PA, USA; Associate Professor and Chair, Graduate Art Therapy Program, Bar Ilan University, Israel.

Emily Nolan, DAT, ATRL, LPC, LCAT, SEP, Professor of Practice, Department of Creative Arts Therapy, College of Visual and Performing Arts, Syracuse University, New York, USA.

Erin Rafferty-Bugher, ATR-BC, LPCC, Owner BrainsparkArt Trauma and Neuro-informed Art Therapy Services, Minneapolis, MN, USA.

Chandler Sours Rhodes, Ph.D., Service Chief Treatment and Rehabilitation, National Intrepid Center of Excellence, Walter Reed National Military Medical Center, Bethesda, MD, USA.

Kathryn Snyder, Ph.D., ATR-BC, LPC, Founding Owner & Director, Parent to Child and Spark Art Therapy, Philadelphia, PA, USA.

Janell S. Payano Sosa, Ph.D., Neuroscientist; National Intrepid Center of Excellence, Walter Reed National Military Medical Center, Bethesda, MD, USA.

Adrienne Stamper, M.A., ATR-P, Art Therapist; National Intrepid Center of Excellence, Walter Reed National Military Medical Center, Bethesda, MD, USA.

Tally Tripp (1955–2023), M.A., MSW, LCSW, LICSW, CTT, ATR-BC, Private Practice Art Therapy and Psychotherapy, Alexandria, VA, USA; Certified/Consultant Sensorimotor Psychotherapy; Certified Intensive Trauma Therapy; Certified Eye Movement Desensitization and Reprocessing EMDR; Fellow and Board Director, International Society for the Study of Trauma and Dissociation; Co-chair, International Task Force, ISSTD; Co-Founder, Creative Arts Therapies Special Interest Group, ISSTD; Director of Training, Common Threads Project.

Barbara van der Vossen, M.A., LGPC, ATR-P, Art Therapist, Psychotherapist – Terra Counseling and Consulting, Baltimore, MD, USA. Counselor – Frederick County Health Department, Frederick, MD, USA.

Melissa Walker, M.A., ATR, Healing Arts Program Coordinator, National Intrepid Center of Excellence, Walter Reed National Military Medical Center, Bethesda, MD, USA.

Denise Wolf, ATR-BC, ATCS, LPC, LPAT, Associate Clinical Professor Art Therapy and Counseling, Drexel University, Philadelphia, PA, USA.

FOREWORD

by Robert M. Pascuzzi, MD

Bringing the Science to Art Therapy

Indianapolis. January 28 (Jackson Pollock's Birthday). Neurology Clinic at the Indiana University Health Neuroscience Center. Implacable winter weather. Students and Residents learning. ALS Clinic. A 42-year-old in a crowded exam room (family and the neurology team). Story – 8 months progressive painless wasting of the right arm, lately creeping into the left. Exam – atrophy right arm and left hand. Fasciculations in all limbs. Reflexes jumpy, speech a bit slow and stiff. Normal sensation and vision. Smiles and laughs out loud as if the laughing is not his and beyond his control. Scared to death. Family on edge. Anticipation. Help us.

In this patient, the clinical evaluation is the basis for all that is about to come. Anatomy and physiology allow us to "localize" the problem. It's neurological. Upper motor neurons have their cell bodies in the cerebral cortex in the back of the frontal lobes along the "motor strip." They are malfunctioning in this patient (stiff speech, jumpy reflexes, and the uncontrolled involuntary laughter – the latter is pseudobulbar affect – some people cry without being sad, some yawn without being tired – this patient laughs). All neurologists know that just because one laughs or cries does not prove that they are happy or sad. The upper motor nerves send electrical signals down their wires or axons, through the brain, crossing over to the opposite side of the nervous system at the lower brainstem and descending into the spinal cord – eventually connecting (synapse) with the lower motor nerves having cell bodies in the anterior horn of the spinal cord. The two motor nerves are like two electrical wires hooked up in series. The lower motor nerve is under management by the upper motor nerve and sends its signal to a specific muscle. All volitional movement requires this continuum from the upper motor neuron to the lower motor neuron to the muscle. When the lower motor nerves malfunction the muscles atrophy, become floppy, and they flicker (twitching or fasciculation). This patient has a combination of upper and lower motor neuron dysfunction and a slow progressive clinical course, starting in one arm and spreading to the other – like a creeping paralysis. The diagnosis is clear. Amyotrophic lateral sclerosis (ALS, "Lou Gehrig's disease" in the United States).

Communication. The most important of core competencies in the practice of medicine. Patient informed; family aware. Why does he have it? Nobody knows. Sometimes we know (5–10% are "familial" or "genetic" and we will check his DNA). The cause for all the others is unknown. This will progress, slowly. Two to five years typical survival but 20% have a slow form. We can treat symptoms but can't stop the disease. Hope and Research. Research and Hope … inextricably intertwined. While the outlook is depressing, we could get lucky. A form of genetic ALS has proven to respond to a new treatment with a small molecule that targets a toxic defective gene (SOD-1). Essentially shuts down a damaging protein. *Science works!* Seems so simple but really so complicated and while we sound like we know nearly everything about this patient there is so much we are lacking. Stressful (horrible) news for the patient. Fear of this diagnosis and what lies ahead. Fear of the future. Can't sleep. Can't work. Family consumed. The spouse is now a "caregiver," also without sleep. Anticipation, planning, preparation, finances, meaning of it all? Fairness, why, crying, uncertainty, fear, coping, crying, surviving, and more crying. What do we do?

So, this is trauma. Just one patient on one day and a slow progressive trauma. As with much in the neurology clinic, making a diagnosis is just one step. Management is the next, and the reality is that some disorders require more than time and a pill. A slow degenerative brain or spine disease like ALS (or for that matter Parkinson's disease or Alzheimer's disease, Lewy body dementia, Huntington's disease, the list goes on) affects the patient, the family, the caregivers, the friends, and colleagues and in many cases an entire community. How do we best help all these individuals with their psychological, emotional, and existential challenges?

Physical trauma from injury (including traumatic brain injury), psychological trauma from childhood events, and situational stresses that can pile so high as to seem insurmountable, biological mechanisms from depression to anxiety, pain, physical pain, emotional pain, direct effects on the body and the mind, all the indirect effects (sleep deprivation) not to mention side effects and financial burdens of various well-intended therapeutics. Stresses can pile up without respite. A Charles Dickens metaphor from *Bleak House*, "adding new deposits to the crust of mud, sticking at those points tenaciously to the pavement, and accumulating at compound interest." Stress can do this.

Trauma is everywhere. And much like ALS there is so much known and so much we are good at doing – but so very much that has yet to be learned and resolutions to be discovered.

Science works! A few decades back it was said that neurologists were great at making diagnoses but could not really fix anything. Well, thanks to science that is no longer the case. Spinomuscular atrophy (SMA) is a progressive paralytic condition affecting newborns which in recent years has transitioned from a rapidly fatal disease of childhood to being one that is fixable with early treatment. Pompe disease was once a progressive disease of muscle and now can be held in check. Newer therapeutics for stroke and multiple sclerosis work with amazing effectiveness. **Science works.**

In the second edition of *Art Therapy and the Neuroscience of Trauma: Theoretical and Practical Perspectives*, the distinguished editors (Juliet L. King and Christianne E. Strang) have set the stage for an inevitable and essential set of steps in what may be considered the great frontier of medicine (cognition, behavior, and therapeutics). They have provided us updates on many of the enlightening topics presented in the original edition. And they have broadened the palate of perspectives and considerations by recruiting authors from diverse backgrounds (*Voices*) to provide intriguing and valuable new perspectives and approaches to trauma, neuroscience, and therapeutics. The second edition explores contemporary and scientifically sound approaches to applications of art therapy in a broader socio-cultural context. This collage of writings, updates, and perspectives could stand alone with distinction. But the editors have brought the tools of science, methodology, and investigation to this compendium. In essence, we have a framework for conducting research for the intersecting fields of neuroscience, trauma, art therapy, and related therapeutics. The "Three Tenets" (concepts of therapeutic relationship, symbolic/non-verbal communication, creative process, materials and methods) provide focus, organization, and continuity. Themes of resiliency and neuroplasticity are emphasized. Neuroanatomy, neurophysiology, and related principles of neuroscience provide the platform upon which much of the new research is fostered and tested. And as a clinician there is the goal to link the topics to therapeutics – the importance of potential applications to clinical practice. There is a realization that we are a diverse bunch here on this big blue ball – with value in exploring a wider cultural context and the limitations of methods and interventions.

More than a colorful collage of ideas and observations, the book commits to corralling and then harnessing such diverse works and establishing a framework for making scientifically sound and clinically meaningful advances in understanding, proving, and implementing – all with the final common pathway of helping people. Applying principles of scientific investigation. Testing hypotheses, seeking methodology with controls, measured outcomes, minimizing the randomness and the accidental. **Science works.** For this, and on behalf of all the professionals caring for patients with trauma, and for all our patients and their families and their communities, I congratulate and thank the Editors of *Art Therapy and the Neuroscience of Trauma: Theoretical and Practical Perspectives,* Juliet L. King and Christianne E. Strang, along with their most talented contributors, for providing us with such a valuable next step in advancing the science of art therapy.

What happens to the patient seen January 28? We have a multidisciplinary clinic for patients needing complex coordinated care. There are medications that can control/ improve symptoms, and a number of medications that may slow down the progression of paralysis, and we have investigational treatment. We also have art therapy. Years ago, in response to a towering need for help with the psychological, emotional, and existential crises faced by so many of our patients in neurology, we recognized the potential for collaboration between our academic department and professionals in art therapy. The Art Therapy in Neurology program at Indiana University (designed and implemented by this book's editor, Juliet L. King) remains an essential component to our mission of providing comprehensive services for our patients – attempting to recognize and appreciate the whole patient – and understanding that we need this collaborative effort if we really care about patient well-being. Over the years, we have looked inward and applied expertise in art therapy to wellness programing for physicians, residents, medical students, nursing, and administrators. This team has helped patients with ALS, myasthenia gravis, TBI, Parkinson Disease, Alzheimer Disease, Stroke … and the list never ends. We have been fortunate.

Jackson Pollock's birthday, January 28. He had many complex challenges, not the least of which were psychological. His own profound observations on painting tell us something of the cognitive and emotional power inherent in creating art.

"Art is coming face to face with yourself."

"Painting is self-discovery. Every good artist paints what he is."

When Jackson Pollock was asked about the randomness of dripping and splattering paint, he pointed out that there was nothing random or accidental about his paintings, "I can control the flow of paint: there is no accident." Sounds like a scientist.

Robert M. Pascuzzi MD
Professor Emeritus of Neurology
Indiana University School of Medicine
Indianapolis

PREFACE

In this second edition of *Art Therapy and the Neuroscience of Trauma: Theoretical and Practical Perspectives*, we continue a journey that transcends boundaries and invites the reader to explore the profound intersections of science, art, and healing. Edited by pragmatic visionaries deeply committed to the systematic integration of neuroscience and art therapy theory, practice, and research, our aim is to balance a depth of knowledge with critical thinking, all in service of practical applications that enhance trauma treatment and build the evidence base for the profession.

In the ever-evolving landscape of arts and health, we find ourselves both hopeful and introspective. The first edition of this text was published in 2016, and over the years we have attained a deeper understanding of the many ways that art therapy benefits those who are exposed to trauma. Recently we have seen a growing emphasis on how neuroscience informs culture, arts, and health outcomes, generating enthusiasm from policymakers, funding agencies, and advocacy groups. And amidst the flurry of discussions and discoveries, we often find ourselves asking, "Where do we stand?" "Who pilots our definitions, and who possesses the resources to explore these questions?" We are often left wondering how to navigate the shifting currents of knowledge and build on the efforts of those who have ignited the conversation for nearly a century.

Some of the answers are within the pages of this book. The contributors to this second edition have generously dedicated their time and expertise with a spirit of kindness and camaraderie.

This text captures the voices of many pioneers, and we introduce and share new minds and theories, some of which have significantly evolved since the first edition. We recognize the importance of unity and collaboration, fostering practical applications that honor a diverse worldview and necessary variance that accompanies the creative approaches to treatment.

Our aim is to enrich the profession by updating and translating knowledge of neuroscience as it informs art therapy theory, practice, and research. We remain steadfast in maintaining the integrity of the artist, art therapist, and subjective experiences of our clients, while upholding a professional definition and scope of practice that fosters innovation in the therapeutic approach. Simultaneously we provide context and clarity for how art therapy informs the broad terrain of neurosciences and strive for an accessible and shared language that captures and effectively communicates what it is that we do and how we go about doing it.

These trying times challenge us to find meaning amidst chaos, the lifeblood of art therapy. This book offers us a way forward, providing insights into the world as we experience it through our senses, shaped by culture, language, and history, and a world that is often defined by empirical evidence and experimentation. Together we navigate the divide and propel our ongoing journey toward a destination of healing and change.

Juliet L. King

CHAPTER 1

INTRODUCTION

Juliet L. King and Christianne E. Strang

We're excited to share ways in which advances in the knowledge and understanding of the practice of art therapy can be integrated with new information about the functions of the brain, body, and nervous system. This text advances the understanding of how the disciplines of art therapy and neuroscience complement one another and contribute to practical applications in the clinical treatment of trauma. This text builds on the theory and evidence base for neuro- informed art therapy practices. Our goal is to support the grounding of clinical intuition, rationales, and interventions in a deep understanding of the complexity of neurobiological mechanisms that are thought to underlie human experience and behavior.

Art therapy, neuroscience, and trauma are individually broad topics with varied definitions, multiple parameters, and seemingly limitless dimensions. We'd like to begin by identifying some of the parameters and dimensions to provide a basis for understanding the myriad, complex interactions between these topics.

1.1 ART THERAPY

In the United States, art therapy is a stand-alone profession, with identified educational requirements and defined scope of practice (AATA, 2021; ACATE, 2016). Art therapy practice falls within the scope of the creative arts therapies (Davies & Clift, 2022), with training traditionally obtained within the humanities and social science academic disciplines. Art therapy's notion of health typically follows that of the World Health Organization (WHO): "a state of complete physical, mental, and social well-being and not merely the absence of disease or infirmity" (WHO, 1948).

Art therapy is a social and human science with broad inter- and transdisciplinary roots of art and psychology and historically informed by medicine and the humanities (Gerber et al., 2012; Junge, 2016; Junge & Linesch, 1993; Vick, 2003). Art therapy capitalizes on knowledge and experience generated through the artmaking process and subsequent products. Art therapists are traditionally committed to a pluralistic worldview that contributes to its theoretical foundations (Chilton et al., 2015; Johnson & Gray, 2010; Ulman, 2001). Multiple forms of knowledge influence art therapy and are inherent in its definition: "a complex multidimensionality of intersecting theories grounded in decades of clinical evidence that attests to successful practice and intervention" (King et al., 2019, p. 149).

The same year the first edition of this text was published, *Art Therapy: The Journal of the American Art Therapy Association* released a special issue that embraced the question "Is there a need to redefine art therapy?" Authors in the issue offered critical review on the traditional binary of art as therapy v. art psychotherapy (Ulman & Dachinger, 1975), and in doing so complicated the binary, as the "dominant framework within

DOI: 10.4324/9781003348207-1

which art therapy has remained trapped is the dichotomy of art as therapy versus art psychotherapy" (Talwar, 2016, p. 116). This binary framework fails to include the perspectives of founders of color who shaped the beginning of the profession but whose contributions receive little recognition (Stepney, 2019) and thus contributed to the marginalization and disenfranchisement of art therapists of color (Potash et al., 2016). Efforts have been made to update the history and definition of the profession to an inclusive socio-cultural worldview that has been supported by the American Art Therapy Association (AATA) (see for example AATA Multicultural Bibliography, 2020). Culturally competent and culturally informed practice in art therapy (Jackson, 2020; Stepney, 2022) supports practice and research strategies that need to be flexible in honoring the complexity of each individual (Bitonte & DeSanto, 2014; Potash et al., 2016; Van Lith, 2016). Practitioner choice is typically intentional as it allows for therapist decision making that is necessarily inclusive of the client's phenomenological experience in treatment (Bowen-Salter et al., 2021; McWilliams, 2021). We look beyond the art as therapy or art as psychotherapy dichotomy to engage the holistic and embodied human that is seeking healing and support. This transition from a dichotomous view of the art therapy profession to an integrative and flexible approach aligns with our evolving understanding of creativity. This shift moves away from simple dual-factor models (right brain v. left brain; top down v. bottom up) to more intricate perspectives where multiple systems collaborate (Khalil & Demarin, 2023).

1.2 NEUROSCIENCE

While neuroscience can be defined simply as the study of the nervous system, contemporary neuroscience is considered to be an interdisciplinary science that interfaces with many disciplines such as engineering, philosophy, and medicine. Thus, there are multiple branches of modern neuroscience that can be categorized broadly and often intersect. For example, The Eunice Kennedy Shriver National Institute of Child Health and Human Development identifies areas of neuroscience as encompassing development, how the brain grows and changes; cognition, how language, thought, and memory are understood; molecular and cellular, which focuses on proteins, genes, and molecules; behavior, which examines processes underlying animal and human behavior; and clinical, the study of disease and health (*What Are Some Different Areas of Neuroscience?*, 2018). These categories are not mutually exclusive. For example, autistic spectrum disorder may be understood through developmental neuroscience, which intertwines with behavior and cognition, in the context of individual clinical goals, all of which have molecular and cellular roots. Neuroscience explains that human behavior and cognition represent inherent fundamental collections of highest levels of cerebral function (Friedman & Robbins, 2022). However, the mechanistic processes underlying complex human thought, emotion, and behavior are traditionally difficult to study. Emotions and emotional expressions are connected to brain and nervous system processes that reciprocally influence and interconnect with neuroanatomy, neurophysiology, and neurotransmitter systems (Tyng et al., 2017; Koban et al., 2021), and understanding the correspondence between neuronal organization and specific brain functions remains limited (Amaducci et al., 2002). In fact, researchers are coming to understand that most complex cognition and behavior is related to intricate patterns of brain activity and interconnections that span a number of anatomically distinct brain regions are organized into large-scale brain networks (Koban et al., 2021) and interacting systems (Khalil & Demarin, 2023).

1.3   TRAUMA

Trauma is a complicated and multidimensional phenomenon. Its impact varies widely in individuals and across cultures. Trauma is defined according to the subjective experience of the individual and type of trauma experienced. The medical definition of trauma refers to "an injury (such as a wound) to living tissue caused by an extrinsic agent, a disordered psychic or behavioral state resulting from severe mental or emotional stress or physical injury, an emotional upset" (Merriam Webster, 2018). Human responses to traumatic experiences are natural, subjective, and informed by the processes of evolution that have a biological basis. The first characterization of trauma was defined by Freud and Janet (Freud, 1962; Herman, 1992) who based postulations on the work of their mentor, Jean-Martin Charcot, commonly known as the Father of Neurology (Waraich & Shah, 2018). Charcot was instrumental in describing how the localization of physical symptoms of hysteria do not reflect the physical rules of anatomy, but rather mirror an imaginary anatomy that are the outcomes of psychic, rather than physical, trauma (Fulford et al., 2013). Over time, the Diagnostic and Statistical Manual of Mental Disorders (DSM) has transformed definitions from events that happen "outside the range of usual human experience" (APA, 1980, p. 236) to those that are now conceptualized on a continuum (Breslau & Kessler, 2001). Trauma, once labeled an anxiety disorder, is now defined in the most current version of the DSM-5-TR as trauma-and-stressor-related disorders (TSRD) (APA, 2022). Symptoms range from anxiety and depression to extremes of post-traumatic stress disorder (PTSD). Traumatic experiences underlie most mental health diagnoses, representing nearly 80% of clients in mental health clinics (Jones & Cureton, 2014; Sheffler et al., 2020; Schilling et al., 2007). The manifestations, causes, and core assumptions of trauma have been notoriously debated and creating an all-purpose definition has proved difficult due to multiple and intersecting individual and contextual factors (Suleiman, 2008; Weathers & Keane, 2007). The lack of broad definitions complicates the search for effective, generalizable approaches to the treatment of trauma. Further, since generalized approaches can also be reductionistic, clinicians and researchers seek effective approaches to healing that incorporate an individual's unique embodied experiences.

A plethora of complex human emotional responses to trauma is illuminated with the growing knowledge of genetic and biological factors that contribute to its psychological sequelae. Individual and group differences matter greatly in psychotherapy and are dependent upon factors including (but not limited to) current situation, life stage, personality, economic position, gender experience, racial and ethnic identity (McWilliams, 2021). For example, it is now well known that Adverse Childhood Experiences (ACEs), those traumatic experiences occurring during childhood and adolescence, have a significant impact on physical and mental health throughout the lifespan, yet there are multiple variables that influence a person's susceptibility to work through and heal from these earlier experiences (Felitti et al., 1998; Hughes et al., 2017).

The experiences of trauma are cumulative. The impacts of collective, historic, intergenerational, and racial traumas have been found to alter gene expression for offspring of the traumatized, significantly influencing our understanding of etiology and complicating our understanding of the most effective treatment approaches (Isobel et al., 2019; Menakem, 2017; Yehuda & Lehrner, 2018). Differentiating the etiology of trauma along with the range and variance of responses is a complicated and challenging task for clinicians that is made more difficult when considering social, cultural, and racial disparities, historical, generational, and systemic influences, along with traditional biopsychosocial approaches commonly relied upon in the Westernized medical model of mental health diagnoses (Backos, 2021; Breslau & Kessler, 2001; Jackson, 2020; Menakem, 2021; Nadal, 2018). Trauma survivors require specialized knowledge and multiple considerations from the therapist for effective treatment to take place (Briere & Scott, 2006; Jones & Cureton, 2014).

1.4   COMPLEX WICKED PROBLEMS

The understanding, impact, and treatment of psychological trauma is a *complex wicked problem* that influences biopsychosocial and spiritual domains, results in complicated sequela, and involves multiple stakeholders. The "wicked problem" is a term introduced in 1973 by Rittel and Webber to draw attention to the complexities and challenges of articulation and logic and are subject to multiple constraints of the real world. This concept has contributed to theoretical development and research methods that address challenges in complex adaptive systems such as healthcare, where problems have many causes that are associated with multiple environmental and social contexts, unpredictable outcomes, and challenges in identifying best solutions (Cleland et al., 2018; Sturmberg & Martin, 2008).

Integrating neuroscience with art therapy theory, practice, and research is also considered a complex wicked problem. Merging theories and principles from different disciplines is an inter- and transdisciplinary effort and requires a negotiation of epistemological and methodological differences. Here, an obvious problem is the persistent debate regarding the nature and definition of evidence as it relates to both practice and research in art therapy, an argument that is shared with neighboring disciplines of counseling and allied health (Cardona et al., 2009; Cook et al., 2017; Wester & McKibben, 2019; Zarbo et al., 2016). Technological constraints limit our ability to isolate and measure variables, establishing boundaries for accessible knowledge. This also applies to sharing information obtained from the rapid technological progress of recent years. To consider the intricacies that take place in the process of any therapeutic discipline through an objective lens is not only mainstream best practice but also an ethical and professional responsibility. However, despite decades of advancement in generating knowledge based on high quality evidence, the systematic translation of research findings into practice in diverse settings for frontlines clinical practice has not been achieved (Cook et al., 2004; Sussman et al., 2006).

1.5   WHY WE NEED EVIDENCE-BASED PRACTICE (EBP)

Evidence-based practice (EBP) supports clinical decision-making processes based on published systematic investigations. Its definition has expanded in the last few decades to emphasize patient voice depending on preference, clinical state, and circumstances (Cook et al., 2017; Haynes et al., 2002). A key goal of EBP is to maximize patient choice about treatment options through the application of evidence-based principles (Cook et al., 2017). This clinically useful diagnostic and treatment sensibility fosters the ability for contemporary psychotherapy theorists to recognize the challenges and potential ethical malfeasance of adhering to strict recommendations (McWilliams, 2021). Clinical reasoning should be driven by EBP in a way that allows the provider to use the best existing evidence as a starting framework for individualized treatment (Cook et al., 2017; Norman et al., 2000). In this context, research evidence, clinical expertise, patient preference, and patient culture are the building blocks of EBP (Norcross & Wampold, 2019). As we increase our understanding of the neurobiological processes that underlie human experiences and human healing, we can scaffold that understanding to expand the number of evidence-based approaches to support individuals of different ages, experiences, and cultural backgrounds.

1.6 MOVING EVIDENCE TO INTEGRATIVE PRACTICE

Healthcare entities rely heavily on evidence-based treatments when considering the funding for medical and mental healthcare provision (Cook et al., 2017). Cognitive approaches such as Prolonged Exposure Therapy and Cognitive Processing Therapy (CPT) have proven to be effective in the treatment of trauma (Friedman et al., 2009; Resick et al., 2016) and it is well known that Cognitive Behavioral Therapy (CBT) has strong evidence that supports its efficacy. Yet, these approaches are not always effective for all groups of people and additional research is needed to build a firmer evidence base (Hofmann et al., 2012; Kar, 2011). Art therapists often integrate strategies with trauma-informed best practices from neighboring professions. For example, art therapy has been used in conjunction with CPT (Campbell et al., 2016), and Acceptance and Commitment Therapy (ACT) (Backos & Mazzeo, 2017) to address symptoms of PTSD.

Art therapists often ground their approaches in practices that rely on neuroscience and interpersonal neurobiology, such as Perry's (2006) Neurosequential Model of Therapeutics, Porges's (2011) Polyvagal Theory, and Ogden and Fisher's (2015) Sensorimotor Psychotherapy. We commonly pull upon the work of Siegel (1999), van der Kolk (2014), and Schore (2012) to support and expand our approaches. Eye Movement Desensitization Reprocessing (EMDR) (Shapiro, 2002) is a common treatment for trauma and art therapists often seek to integrate collaborative approaches into their treatment strategies (Davis et al., 2022; Kolodny & Mazero, 2022; Talwar, 2007; Tripp, 2007).

The effects of art therapy, and all creative arts therapies (CATs) are thought to result from such elements as client-centered care, therapeutic alliance, safety, empathy, inclusion, and unconditional positive regard, giving rise to changes in behavior, cognition, and creative expression (Dunphy et al., 2019; Potash et al., 2016; Regev & Cohen-Yatziv, 2018). However, we are limited in our understanding of the mechanisms of such changes. A recent scoping review of studies on change factors (de Witte et al., 2021) has helped move the needle by identifying key factors that are theorized to be agents of change in the application of arts in the context of health and are specialized to the CATs: creativity, symbolism and metaphor, embodiment, and concretization (de Witte et al., 2021). These factors are termed joint *change factors*; namely, well-specified factors that are shared across all art forms and are theorized to produce therapeutic benefits in CATs.

Understanding how, and why, art therapy works and the underlying factors that account for those changes supports the growing evidence base for the profession (Czamanski-Cohen, 2021; de Witte et al., 2021) and while testing these "active ingredients" (Kapitan, 2012) typically takes place in studies of efficacy and effectiveness, art therapists have used a range of theoretical, conceptual, and methodological approaches to address the inquiry (Ball, 2002; Bosgraaf et al., 2020; Czamanski-Cohen & Weihs, 2016; Gerber et al., 2018; Gerge et al., 2019; Hinz, 2019; Lusebrink, 2004; Smith, 2016; Schnitzer et al., 2022). An understanding of the mechanisms by which art therapy exerts its effects has advanced and the profession is beginning to more accurately identify the underlying factors associated with emotion, cognition, and learning that enhance the capacities to change through psychotherapy (Czamanski-Cohen & Weihs, 2016; Kaimal, 2019; King et al., 2019; Walker et al., 2018). Central to this inquiry is artistic expression, which involves the engagement of neurological systems including the visual, cognitive, emotional, motor, perceptual, and sensory (King & Parada, 2021; Lusebrink & Hinz, 2020; Vaisvaser, 2021).

Much of the knowledge in psychotherapy is simultaneously explicit and implicit and the development of practice strategies is reliant on what is known and easily transferable, the skills and abilities of the practitioner–therapist, and the context within which the treatment takes place (Sturmberg & Martin, 2008). Art therapists, like most clinicians, tend to use skills from our preferred domain at the expense of other skills and persist with treatment approaches that may not be accurately assessing the problems we see in treatment (Gray, 2017).

1.7   KNOWLEDGE TRANSLATION

Translating and integrating knowledge from neuroscience is challenging. The first edition of this book attempted to do this and in its creation emerged the *Three Tenets*, a set of precise principles that distill the primary domains of art therapy and motivate the integration neuroscience: (1) The art-making process and the artwork itself are integral components of treatment that help to understand and elicit verbal and nonverbal communication, self-awareness and reflection within the therapeutic relationship; (2) The multi-directional processes of creativity are healing and life enhancing; (3) The materials and methods used effect self-expression, assist in emotional self-regulation, and are applied in specialized ways (King, 2016). Conceptualizing the translation of neuroscience theory, principles and evidence within these tenets guides art therapy theory, practice, and research strategies and allows for the consideration of their dynamic and overlapping nature in a necessarily phenomenological context. Neuroscience research provides an opportunity to explore and understand the mechanisms of change in therapy, with such understanding leading to increased effectiveness of art therapy interventions based on individuals within their emotional, relational, contextual, and embodied experience.

1.8   PERILS AND PROMISES OF A NEUROSCIENCE-BASED APPROACH

How do we measure the effectiveness and outcomes within an individual's embodied context? Brain and neuroscience-based approaches hold promise for understanding both individual and generalizable effects. These approaches remain limited in that correlations between regional activation and observable behavior do not necessarily reflect causality.

The function of the human brain has been described as creating predictive internal models to make meaning of situations and experiences, support homeostasis and allostasis, and anticipate and prepare for future events (Vaisvaser, 2021). While adaptive in making meaning of current situations and predicting the future, the heuristics can also be reductionistic and result in erroneous association between patterns and events. In the case of trauma, this can result in applications of old behavior patterns to new situations. In the case of neuroscience-based approaches, simplified descriptions can result in erroneous identification of mechanisms of action. Two examples are frequently found in the public understanding of neuroscience and creativity:

The first commonly held misconception, that the hemispheres of the brain function independently, with one hemisphere responsible for creativity and the other responsible for language and cognition, arose from a misinterpretation of the results of studies done on patients whose corpus callosum was surgically severed as a treatment for intractable epileptic seizures (Karolis et al., 2019). In fact, even the extent to which information is isolated to one hemisphere or the other after severing the corpus callosum remains an area of debate (Rosen, 2018). While the hemispheres of the brain do have specializations that are associated with avoiding duplication of function and increasing cognitive capacity, and even with social behavior (Rogers, 2021), high creativity is associated with bilateral activation and interhemispheric cooperation (Atchley et al., 1999; Carlsson et al., 2000). Recent data indicate that functional asymmetry in the human brain may be distributed along axes of symbolic communication, perception/action, emotion, and decision making (Karolis et al., 2019). This expanded idea of interhemispheric communication aligns well with art therapy theory and opens new avenues for research and practical applications.

A second commonly oversimplified concept is the attribution of empathy to the activity of populations or systems of mirror neurons. Mirror neurons, so called because they respond to observed movements as well as performed movements, were discovered in the 1990s during single cell-recording from the brains of awake, behaving monkeys (Heyes & Catmur, 2022). There is evidence that human mirror neurons are involved in movement recognition, selection of movement, and imitation (Mukamel et al., 2010; Kilner & Lemon, 2013) but the evidence that the human mirror neuron system underlies empathy or the ability to infer the emotions of intentions of others, while plausible, is limited (Napolitano, 2021; Heyes & Catmur, 2022). Yet, patient treatment is informed with the understanding that mechanisms for empathy, recognition of emotion, and attribution of intention exist, whether we know the exact populations of neurons or the systems that underlie those abilities.

Our understanding is moving from simplified single or dual factor models where one brain region is responsible for complex behavior to the idea that multiple factors and multiple regions interact cooperatively (Khalil & Demarin, 2023). This expanded understanding is driven in part by improvements in technology and studies that incorporate naturalistic paradigms to better understand the role of the brain and nervous system in complex behaviors (Smith, 2023).

A promising concept in neuroscience with direct application to the field of art therapy is that of brain plasticity, also termed neural plasticity or neuroplasticity. While there are subtle difference in the usage of the terms, all refer to the cellular and molecular processes that underlie learning and change and can include rewiring of the connections between individual neurons that result in changes in brain circuits and networks (Rădulescu et al., 2021). Neuroplasticity is thought to be disrupted or impaired in mood and anxiety disorders (Fuchs et al., 2004, Artin et al., 2021), and in PTSD (Nash et al., 2014). It has become evident that antidepressant treatment (Fuchs et al., 2004, Pittenger & Duman, 2008), treatment with ketamine (Wang et al., 2022), or treatment with serotonergic psychedelics (Artin et al., 2021, Vargas et al., 2023) can enhance neuroplasticity and may work to reopen critical periods for learning, making it easier to establish new neural connections (Nardou et al., 2023). These data combined with data that indicate that creativity training (Sun et al., 2016, 2020) and artistic training (Schlegel et al., 2015) are associated with neuroplastic changes in organization, activity, and connectivity in frontal, limbic, and posterior brain areas, provide a support for a potential, testable hypothesis that the positive effects of art therapy are related to changes in neuroplasticity.

1.9   NEUROSCIENCE-INFORMED ART THERAPY THEORY AND PRACTICE

The neurobiological underpinnings of trauma and often nonverbal nature of traumatic memory point to the value of the expressive and nonverbal therapies in treatment (Spiegel et al., 2006; Hass-Cohen & Findlay, 2015; Malchiodi, 2020; Gaskill & Perry, 2011; Linesch, 2013; Perry, 2014; van der Kolk, 2014). Art therapists have a long history of success when working with people who have been traumatized and over time the efficacy and effectiveness of art therapy as a *treatment of choice* (Tripp, 2016) has become more pronounced (Campbell et al., 2016; Collie et al., 2006; Gantt & Vesprini, 2017; Johnson et al., 1997; Jones et al., 2018; Lobban, 2016; Kopytin & Lebedev, 2013; Schouten et al., 2014; Spring, 2004).

Neuroscience principles have been applied when working with traumatized patients and have demonstrated that art therapy: (1) facilitates the organization and integration of traumatic memories; (2) reactivates positive emotions and serves as a vehicle for exposure and externalization of difficult content; (3) reduces heightened arousal responses; (4) enhances emotional self-efficacy and maintains a space for the exploration of self-perception and psychic integration; and (5) enhances the development of identity (Chapman et al., 2001; Chapman, 2014; Hass-Cohen et al., 2014; Hass-Cohen & Carr, 2008; King, 2016; King, 2015; Malchiodi, 2020; McNamee, 2005, 2006; Talwar, 2007; Tripp, 2007). While the mechanisms underlying the frameworks have not yet been established, they provide the beginning of the journey for understanding, analyzing, and extending the connections between art therapy, neuroscience, and trauma. In this current edition, we highlight a variety of neuroscience-informed conceptual frameworks for art therapy with associated case studies to illustrate their use in the treatment of trauma.

In Chapter 2, we provide an overview of neuroscience concepts and measurement techniques to enhance clinical understanding of the frameworks described throughout this edition. Chapter 3 addresses the Expressive Therapies Continuum in the context of the activity and connections of large-scale brain networks as a framework for resilience and the integration of traumatic memories. Chapter 4 provides a framework for the treatment of preverbal trauma within the Instinctual Trauma Response® (ITR) model, while Chapter 5 takes an in-depth look at the role of memory reconsolidation in the treatment of trauma from the art therapy relational neuroscience (ATR-N) model. Chapters 6 and 7 specifically focus on the treatment of trauma in children in the contexts of neuroscience-informed, body-based, and holistic approaches with extended case studies.

We have included several new chapters in this edition. Chapter 8 addresses the use of art therapy in the treatment of trauma for US military-connected populations. The chapter focuses on the history of art therapy and the military, current implementation, and standardized interventions in the context of the neurobiology of the trauma response, along with cultural considerations and suggestions for future reference. Chapter 9 addresses the role of museums for trauma-sensitive community engagement and provides guidelines for community-based practice of art therapy in museum settings. Finally, Chapter 10 includes the voices of practitioners in a series of case vignettes that provide a glimpse into the many ways that a neuroscience-informed perspective can be interwoven into the practice of art therapy.

Together these theories and interventions can be used to inform the treatment of trauma, and the broad and deep reference lists provide evidence for the outcomes that guide clinical practice. The therapeutic response to intervention strategies is based on evidence. There are specific procedures and protocols that have demonstrated efficacy. The efficacy may be outcomes based, even if a mechanistic understanding of how the intervention works has not been established. We are learning about the physiology and neurobiology of art making and viewing, as well as the impacts of therapy and psychotherapy on the brain and nervous system. Despite the wealth of clinical experience, promising anecdotal evidence, and empirical studies that attest to its success, the biological mechanisms that explain the value of art therapy are not yet known (King & Parada, 2021). The steps of probing and sensing prior to responding lend themselves to the process of research into new practices, applications, and information about mechanisms of change that arise from the wide range of practice and research that is included in this text. We invite you to approach the information with curiosity and openness to new paradigms that bolster the evidence for conceptual frameworks of practice.

REFERENCES

Accreditation Council for Art Therapy Education. (2016). *Art Therapy*. Commission on Accreditation of Allied Health Education Programs. https://caahep-public-site-5be3d9.webflow.io/committees-on-accreditation/art-therapy

Amaducci, L., Grassi, E., & Boller, F. (2002). Maurice Ravel and right-hemisphere musical creativity: Influence of disease on his last musical works? *European Journal of Neurology, 9*(1), 75–82. https://doi.org/10.1046/j.1468-1331.2002.00351.x

American Art Therapy Association. (2021). American Art Therapy Association. https://arttherapy.org/

American Art Therapy Association Multicultural Committee. (2020). *Selected Bibliography and Resource List.*

American Psychiatric Association. (1980). *Diagnostic and statistical manual of mental disorders* (3rd ed.). American Psychiatric Association.

American Psychiatric Association. (2022). *Diagnostic and Statistical Manual of Mental Disorders, Text Revision DSM-5-TR* (5th edition). Amer Psychiatric Pub Inc.

Artin, H., Zisook, S., & Ramanathan, D. (2021). How do serotonergic psychedelics treat depression: The potential role of neuroplasticity. *World Journal of Psychiatry, 11*(6), 201–214. https://doi.org/10.5498/wjp.v11.i6.201

Atchley, R. A., Keeney, M., & Burgess, C. (1999). Cerebral hemispheric mechanisms linking ambiguous word meaning retrieval and creativity. *Brain and Cognition, 40*(3), 479–499. https://doi.org/10.1006/brcg.1999.1080

Backos, A. (2021). *Post-traumatic Stress Disorder and Art Therapy.* Jessica Kingsley Publishers.

Backos, A., & Mazzeo, C. (2017). Group therapy and PTSD: Acceptance and commitment art therapy groups with Vietnam veterans with PTSD. In *Art Therapy with Military Populations* (pp. 165–176). Routledge. https://doi.org/10.4324/9781315669526-17

Ball, B. (2002). Moments of change in the art therapy process. *The Arts in Psychotherapy, 29*(2), 79–92. https://doi.org/10.1016/s0197-4556(02)00138-7

Bitonte, R. A., & De Santo, M. (2014). Art therapy: An underutilized, yet effective tool. *Mental Illness, 6*(1). https://doi.org/10.4081/mi.2014.5354

Bosgraaf, L., Spreen, M., Pattiselanno, K., & Hooren, S. van. (2020). Art therapy for psychosocial problems in children and adolescents: A systematic narrative review on art therapeutic means and forms of expression, therapist behavior, and supposed mechanisms of change. *Frontiers in Psychology, 11.* https://doi.org/10.3389/fpsyg.2020.584685

Bowen-Salter, H., Whitehorn, A., Pritchard, R., Kernot, J., Baker, A., Posselt, M., Price, E., Jordan-Hall, J., & Boshoff, K. (2021). Towards a description of the elements of art therapy practice for trauma: A systematic review. *International Journal of Art Therapy, 27*(1), 3–16. https://doi.org/10.1080/17454832.2021.1957959

Breslau, N., & Kessler, R. C. (2001). The stressor criterion in DSM-IV posttraumatic stress disorder: An empirical investigation. *Biological Psychiatry, 50*(9), 699–704. https://doi.org/10.1016/s0006-3223(01)01167-2

Briere, J. N., & Scott, C. (2006). *Principles of Trauma Therapy: A Guide to Symptoms, Evaluation and Treatment.* SAGE Publications, Inc.

Campbell, M., Decker, K. P., Kruk, K., & Deaver, S. P. (2016). Art therapy and cognitive processing therapy for combat-related PTSD: A randomized controlled trial. *Art Therapy, 33*(4), 169–177. https://doi.org/10.1080/07421656.2016.1226643

Cardona, J. P., Holtrop, K., Córdova, D., Jr., Escobar-Chew, A. R., Horsford, S., Tams, L., Villarruel, F. A., Villalobos, G., Dates, B., Anthony, J. C., & Fitzgerald, H. E. (2009). "Queremos aprender": Latino immigrants' call to integrate cultural adaptation with best practice knowledge in a parenting intervention. *Family Process, 48*(2), 211–231. https://doi.org/10.1111/j.1545-5300.2009.01278.x

Carlsson, I., Wendt, P. E., & Risberg, J. (2000). On the neurobiology of creativity: Differences in frontal activity between high and low creative subjects. *Neuropsychologia, 38*(6), 873–885. https://doi.org/10.1016/S0028-3932(99)00128-1

Chapman, L. (2014). *Neurobiologically informed trauma therapy with children and adolescents: Understanding mechanisms of change.* W.W. Norton & Company.

Chapman, L., Morabito, D., Ladakakos, C., Schreier, H., & Knudson, M. M. (2001). The effectiveness of art therapy interventions in reducing post traumatic stress disorder (PTSD) symptoms in pediatric trauma patients. *Art Therapy, 18*(2), 100–104. https://doi.org/10.1080/07421656.2001.10129750

Chilton, G., Gerber, N., & Scotti, V. (2015). Towards an aesthetic intersubjective paradigm for arts based research: An art therapy perspective. *UNESCO Observatory Multi-Disciplinary Journal in the Arts, 5*, 1–27.

Cleland, J. A., Patterson, F., & Hanson, M. D. (2018). Thinking of selection and widening access as complex and wicked problems. *Medical Education*, *52*(12), 1228–1239. https://doi.org/10.1111/medu.13670

Collie, K., Bottorff, J. L., & Long, B. C. (2006). A narrative view of art therapy and art making by women with breast cancer. *Journal of Health Psychology*, *11*(5), 761–775. https://doi.org/10.1177/1359105306066632

Cook, J. M., Schnurr, P. P., & Foa, E. B. (2004). Bridging the gap between posttraumatic stress disorder research and clinical practice: The example of exposure therapy. *Psychotherapy: Theory, Research, Practice, Training*, *41*, 374–387. https://doi.org/10.1037/0033-3204.41.4.374

Cook, S. C., Schwartz, A. C., & Kaslow, N. J. (2017). Evidence-based psychotherapy: Advantages and challenges. *Neurotherapeutics*, *14*(3), 537–545. https://doi.org/10.1007/s13311-017-0549-4

Czamanski-Cohen, J. (2021). Art therapy as a river with many streams: I think our time has come. *International Journal of Art Therapy*, *26*(4), 123–125. https://doi.org/10.1080/17454832.2021.1994810

Czamanski-Cohen, J., & Weihs, K. L. (2016). The bodymind model: A platform for studying the mechanisms of change induced by art therapy. *The Arts in Psychotherapy*, *51*, 63–71. https://doi.org/10.1016/j.aip.2016.08.006

Davies, C., & Clift, S. (2022). Arts and health glossary—A summary of definitions for use in research, policy and practice. *Frontiers in Psychology*, *13*. https://doi.org/10.3389/fpsyg.2022.949685

Davis, E., Fitzgerald, J., Jacobs, S., & Marchand, J. (2022). *EMDR and creative arts therapies*. Taylor & Francis.

de Witte, M., Orkibi, H., Zarate, R., Karkou, V., Sajnani, N., Malhotra, B., Ho, R. T. H., Kaimal, G., Baker, F. A., & Koch, S. C. (2021). From therapeutic factors to mechanisms of change in the creative arts therapies: A scoping review. *Frontiers in Psychology*, *12*. https://doi.org/10.3389/fpsyg.2021.678397

Dunphy, K., Baker, F. A., Dumaresq, E., Carroll-Haskins, K., Eickholt, J., Ercole, M., Kaimal, G., Meyer, K., Sajnani, N., Shamir, O. Y., & Wosch, T. (2019). Creative arts interventions to address depression in older adults: A systematic review of outcomes, processes, and mechanisms. *Frontiers in Psychology*, *9*. www.frontiersin.org/articles/10.3389/fpsyg.2018.02655

Felitti, V. J., Anda, R. F., Nordenberg, D., Williamson, D. F., Spitz, A. M., Edwards, V., Koss, M. P., & Marks, J. S. (1998). Relationship of childhood abuse and household dysfunction to many of the leading causes of death in adults. The Adverse Childhood Experiences (ACE) Study. *American Journal of Preventive Medicine*, *14*(4), 245–258. https://doi.org/10.1016/s0749-3797(98)00017-8

Freud, S. (1962). The aetiology of hysteria. In *The standard edition of the complete psychological works of Sigmund Freud: Vol. III* (pp. 187–221). Early Psycho-Analytic Publications.

Friedman, M. J., Cohen, J. A., Foa, E. B., & Keane, T. M. (2009). Integration and summary. In *Effective treatments for PTSD: Practice guidelines from the international society for traumatic stress studies* (pp. 617–642). The Guilford Press.

Friedman, N. P., & Robbins, T. W. (2022). The role of prefrontal cortex in cognitive control and executive function. *Neuropsychopharmacology*, *47*(1), Article 1. https://doi.org/10.1038/s41386-021-01132-0

Fuchs, E., Czéh, B., Kole, M. H. P., Michaelis, T., & Lucassen, P. J. (2004). Alterations of neuroplasticity in depression: The hippocampus and beyond. *European Neuropsychopharmacology*, *14*, S481–S490. https://doi.org/10.1016/j.euroneuro.2004.09.002

Fulford, K., Davies, M., Gipps, R., Graham, G., Sadler, J., Stanghellini, G., & Thornton, and T. (Eds.). (2013). *Oxford Handbook of Philosophy and Psychiatry*. Oxford University Press.

Gantt, L., & Vesprini, M. E. (2017). Using the instinctual trauma response model in a military setting. In *Art therapy with military populations: History, innovation, and applications* (pp. 147–156). Routledge/Taylor & Francis Group. https://doi.org/10.4324/9781315669526-15

Gaskill, R. L., & Perry, B. D. (2011). Child sexual abuse, traumatic experiences, and their impact on the developing brain. In *Handbook of child sexual abuse* (pp. 29–47). John Wiley & Sons, Inc. https://doi.org/10.1002/9781118094822.ch2

Gerber, N., Bryl, K., Potvin, N., & Blank, C. A. (2018). Arts-based research approaches to studying mechanisms of change in the creative arts therapies. *Frontiers in Psychology*, 9. www.frontiersin.org/articles/10.3389/fpsyg.2018.02076

Gerber, N., Templeton, E., Chilton, G., Liebman, M. C., Manders, E., & Shim, M. (2012). Art-based research as a pedagogical approach to studying intersubjectivity in the creative arts therapies. *Journal of Applied Arts & Health*, 3(1), 39–48. https://doi.org/10.1386/jaah.3.1.39_1

Gerge, A., Hawes, J., Eklöf, L., & Pedersen, I. N. (2019). Proposed mechanisms of change in the arts based psychotherapies. *Voices: A World Forum for Music Therapy*, 19(2). https://doi.org/10.15845/voices.v19i2.2564

Gray, A. E. L. (2017). Polyvagal-informed dance/movement therapy for trauma: A global perspective. *American Journal of Dance Therapy*, 39(1), 43–46. https://doi.org/10.1007/s10465-017-9254-4

Hass-Cohen, N., & Carr, R. (2008). *Art therapy and clinical neuro-science* (N. H.-C. & R. C. (eds.)). Jessica Kningsly.

Hass-Cohen, N., Clyde Findlay, J., Carr, R., & Vanderlan, J. (2014). "Check, change what you need to change and/or keep what you want": An art therapy neurobiological-based trauma protocol. *Art Therapy*, 31(2), 69–78. https://doi.org/10.1080/07421656.2014.903825

Hass-Cohen, N., & Findlay, J. C. (2015). *Art therapy and the neuroscience of relationships, creativity, and resiliency: Skills and practices* (Illustrated edition). W. W. Norton & Company.

Haynes, R. B., Devereaux, P. J., & Guyatt, G. H. (2002). Clinical expertise in the era of evidence-based medicine and patient choice. *BMJ Evidence-Based Medicine*, 7(2), 36–38.

Herman, J. L. (1992). *Trauma and recovery: The aftermath of violence—From domestic abuse to political terror*. Basic Books.

Heyes, C., & Catmur, C. (2022). What happened to mirror neurons? *Perspectives on Psychological Science*, 17(1), 153–168. https://doi.org/10.1177/1745691621990638

Hinz, L. D. (2019). *Expressive therapies continuum a framework for using art in therapy* (2nd ed.). Routledge. https://doi.org/10.4324/9780429299339

Hofmann, S. G., Asnaani, A., Vonk, I. J., Sawyer, A. T., & Fang, A. (2012). The efficacy of cognitive behavioral therapy: A review of meta-analyses. *Cognitive Therapy and Research*, 36, 427–440.

Hughes, K., Bellis, M. A., Hardcastle, K. A., Sethi, D., Butchart, A., Mikton, C., Jones, L., & Dunne, M. P. (2017). The effect of multiple adverse childhood experiences on health: A systematic review and meta-analysis. *The Lancet. Public Health*, 2(8), e356–e366. https://doi.org/10.1016/S2468-2667(17)30118-4

Isobel, S., Goodyear, M., Furness, T., & Foster, K. (2019). Preventing intergenerational trauma transmission: A critical interpretive synthesis. *Journal of Clinical Nursing*, 28(7–8), 1100–1113. https://doi.org/10.1111/jocn.14735

Jackson, L. (2020). *Cultural Humility in Art Therapy*. Jessica Kingsley Publishers.

Johnson, B., & Gray, R. (2010). A history of philosophical and theoretical issues for mixed methods research. In *SAGE handbook of mixed methods in social & behavioral research*. SAGE Publications, Inc. https://doi.org/10.4135/9781506335193

Johnson, D. R., Lubin, H., Rosenheck, R., Fontana, A., Southwick, S., & Charney, D. (1997). The impact of the homecoming reception on the development of posttraumatic stress disorder. The West Haven Homecoming Stress Scale (WHHSS). *Journal of Traumatic Stress*, 10(2), 259–277. https://doi.org/10.1002/jts.2490100207

Jones, J. P., Walker, M. S., Masino Drass, J., & Kaimal, G. (2018). Art therapy interventions for active duty military service members with post-traumatic stress disorder and traumatic brain injury. *International Journal of Art Therapy*, 23(2), 70–85. https://doi.org/10.1080/17454832.2017.1388263

Jones, L. K., & Cureton, J. L. (2014). Trauma redefined in the DSM-5: Rationale and implications for counseling practice. *The Professional Counselor*, 4(3), 257–271. https://doi.org/10.15241/lkj.4.3.257

Junge, M. B. (2016). History of art therapy. In *The Wiley handbook of art therapy* (pp. 7–16). Wiley Blackwell.

Junge, M. B., & Linesch, D. (1993). Our own voices: New paradigms for art therapy research. *The Arts in Psychotherapy*, 20, 61–67. https://doi.org/10.1016/0197-4556(93)90032-W

Kaimal, G. (2019). Adaptive response theory: An evolutionary framework for clinical research in art therapy. *Art Therapy*, *36*(4), 215–219. https://doi.org/10.1080/07421656.2019.1667670

Kapitan, L. (2012). Does art therapy work? Identifying the active ingredients of art therapy efficacy. *Art Therapy*, *29*(2), 48–49. https://doi.org/10.1080/07421656.2012.684292

Kar, N. (2011). Cognitive behavioral therapy for the treatment of post-traumatic stress disorder: A review. *Neuropsychiatric Disease and Treatment*, 167. https://doi.org/10.2147/ndt.s10389

Karolis, V. R., Corbetta, M., & Thiebaut de Schotten, M. (2019). The architecture of functional lateralisation and its relationship to callosal connectivity in the human brain. *Nature Communications*, *10*(1), Article 1. https://doi.org/10.1038/s41467-019-09344-1

Khalil, R., & Demarin, V. (2023). Creative therapy in health and disease: Inner vision. *CNS Neuroscience & Therapeutics*. https://onlinelibrary.wiley.com/doi/full/10.1111/cns.14266

Kilner, J. M., & Lemon, R. N. (2013). What we know currently about mirror neurons. *Current Biology*, *23*(23), R1057–R1062. https://doi.org/10.1016/j.cub.2013.10.051

King, J. L. (2015). Art therapy: A brain based profession. In *The Wiley handbook of art therapy* (pp. 77–89). John Wiley & Sons, Ltd. https://doi.org/10.1002/9781118306543.ch8

King, J. L. (2016). *Art therapy, trauma, and neuroscience: Theoretical and practical perspectives*. Routledge. https://content.taylorfrancis.com/books/download?dac=C2014-0-34034-1&isbn=9781315733494&format=googlePreviewPdf

King, J. L., Kaimal, G., Konopka, L., Belkofer, C., & Strang, C. E. (2019). Practical applications of neuroscience-informed art therapy. *Art Therapy*, *36*(3), 149–156. https://doi.org/10.1080/07421656.2019.1649549

King, J., & Parada, F. (2021). Using mobile brain/body imaging to advance research in arts, health, and related therapeutics. *The European Journal of Neuroscience*, *54*(12), 8364–8380. https://doi.org/10.1111/ejn.15313

Koban, L., Gianaros, P. J., Kober, H., & Wager, T. D. (2021). The self in context: Brain systems linking mental and physical health. *Nature Reviews Neuroscience*, *22*(5), Article 5. https://doi.org/10.1038/s41583-021-00446-8

Kolodny, P., & Mazero, S. (2022). The interweave of internal family systems, EMDR, and art therapy. In *EMDR and creative arts therapies*. Routledge.

Kopytin, A., & Lebedev, A. (2013). Humor, self-attitude, emotions, and cognitions in group art therapy with war veterans. *Art Therapy*, *30*(1), 20–29. https://doi.org/10.1080/07421656.2013.757758

Linesch, D. G. (2013). *Art therapy with families in crisis: Overcoming resistance through nonverbal expression*. Routledge.

Lobban, J. (2016). Factors that influence engagement in an inpatient art therapy group for veterans with post traumatic stress disorder. *International Journal of Art Therapy*, *21*(1), 15–22. https://doi.org/10.1080/17454832.2015.1124899

Lusebrink, V. B. (2004). Art therapy and the brain: An attempt to understand the underlying processes of art expression in therapy. *Art Therapy*, *21*(3), 125–135. https://doi.org/10.1080/07421656.2004.10129496

Lusebrink, V. B., & Hinz, L. D. (2020). Cognitive and symbolic aspects of art therapy and similarities with large scale brain networks. *Art Therapy*, *37*(3), 113–122. https://doi.org/10.1080/07421656.2019.1691869

Malchiodi, C. A. (2020). *Trauma and expressive arts therapy: Brain, body, and imagination in the healing process*. Guilford Publications. https://play.google.com/store/books/details?id=PVnPDwAAQBAJ

McNamee, C. M. (2005). Bilateral art: Integrating art therapy, family therapy, and neuroscience. *Contemporary Family Therapy*, *27*(4), 545–557. https://doi.org/10.1007/s10591-005-8241-y

McNamee, C. M. (2006). Experiences with bilateral art: A retrospective study. *Art Therapy*, *23*(1), 7–13. https://doi.org/10.1080/07421656.2006.10129526

McWilliams, N. (2021). Diagnosis and Its discontents: Reflections on our current dilemma. *Psychoanalytic Inquiry*, *41*(8), 565–579. https://doi.org/10.1080/07351690.2021.1983395

Menakem, R. (2017). *My grandmother's hands: Racialized trauma and the pathway to mending our hearts and bodies* (First Edition, Later Printing). Central Recovery Press.

Menakem, R. (2021). *My grandmother's hands: Racialized trauma and the pathway to mending our hearts and bodies*. Penguin UK.

Merriam Webster. (2018). *Trauma*. Dictionary. www.merriam-webster.com/dictionary/trauma

Mukamel, R., Ekstrom, A. D., Kaplan, J., Iacoboni, M., & Fried, I. (2010). Single-neuron responses in humans during execution and observation of actions. *Current Biology, 20*(8), 750–756. https://doi.org/10.1016/j.cub.2010.02.045

Nadal, K. L. (2018). *Microaggressions and traumatic stress: Theory, research, and clinical treatment*. American Psychological Association. https://doi.org/10.1037/0000073-000

Napolitano, A. (2021). Study casts new light on mirror neurons. *Nature Italy*. https://doi.org/10.1038/d43978-021-00101-x

Nardou, R., Sawyer, E., Song, Y. J., Wilkinson, M., Padovan-Hernandez, Y., de Deus, J. L., Wright, N., Lama, C., Faltin, S., Goff, L. A., Stein-O'Brien, G. L., & Dölen, G. (2023). Psychedelics reopen the social reward learning critical period. *Nature*, 1–9. https://doi.org/10.1038/s41586-023-06204-3

Nash, M., Galatzer-Levy, I., Krystal, J. H., Duman, R., & Neumeister, A. (2014). Neurocircuitry and neuroplasticity in PTSD. In *Handbook of PTSD: Science and practice* (2nd edition) (pp. 251–274). The Guilford Press.

Norcross, J., & Wampold, B. (2019). Relationships and responsiveness in the psychological treatment of trauma: The tragedy of the APA clinical practice guideline. *Psychotherapy, 56*(3), 391–399. http://dx.doi.org/10.1037/pst0000228

Norman, P., Conner, M., & Bell, R. (2000). The theory of planned behaviour and exercise: Evidence for the moderating role of past behaviour. *British Journal of Health Psychology, 5*(3), 249–261. https://doi.org/10.1348/135910700168892

Ogden, P., & Fisher, J. (2015). *Sensorimotor psychotherapy: Interventions for trauma and attachment (Norton series on interpersonal neurobiology*. WW Norton & Company.

Perry, B. D. (2006). Applying principles of neurodevelopment to clinical work with maltreated and traumatized children: The neurosequential model of therapeutics. In N. B. Webb (Ed.), *Working with traumatized youth in child welfare* (pp. 27–52). The Guilford Press.

Perry, B. D. (2014). *Creative interventions with traumatized children*. Guilford Publications.

Pittenger, C., & Duman, R. S. (2008). Stress, depression, and neuroplasticity: A convergence of mechanisms. *Neuropsychopharmacology, 33*(1), Article 1. https://doi.org/10.1038/sj.npp.1301574

Porges, S. W. (2011). *The polyvagal theory: Neurophysiological foundations of emotions, attachment, communication, and self-regulation* (1st edition). W. W. Norton & Company.

Potash, J., Burnie, M., Pearson, R., & Ramirez, W. (2016). Restoring Wisconsin Art Therapy Association in art therapy history: Implications for professional definition and inclusivity. *Art Therapy, 33*(2), 99–102. https://doi.org/10.1080/07421656.2016.1163994

Rădulescu, I., Drăgoi, A. M., Trifu, S. C., & Cristea, M. B. (2021). Neuroplasticity and depression: Rewiring the brain's networks through pharmacological therapy (Review). *Experimental and Therapeutic Medicine, 22*(4), 1–8. https://doi.org/10.3892/etm.2021.10565

Regev, D., & Cohen-Yatziv, L. (2018). Effectiveness of art therapy with adult clients in 2018—What progress has been made? *Frontiers in Psychology, 9*(1531). https://doi.org/10.3389/fpsyg.2018.01531

Resick, P. A., Monson, C. M., & Chard, K. M. (2016). *Cognitive processing therapy for PTSD: A comprehensive manual*. Guilford Publications.

Rittel, H. W. J., & Webber, M. M. (1973). Dilemmas in a general theory of planning. *Policy Sciences, 4*(2), 155–169. https://doi.org/10.1007/BF01405730

Rogers, L. J. (2021). Brain lateralization and cognitive capacity. *Animals : An Open Access Journal from MDPI, 11*(7), 1996. https://doi.org/10.3390/ani11071996

Rosen, V. (2018). One brain. Two minds? Many questions. *Journal of Undergraduate Neuroscience Education, 16*(2), R48–R50.

Schilling, E. A., Aseltine, R. H., & Gore, S. (2007). Adverse childhood experiences and mental health in young adults: A longitudinal survey. *BMC Public Health*, 7(1). https://doi.org/10.1186/1471-2458-7-30

Schlegel, A., Alexander, P., Fogelson, S. V., Li, X., Lu, Z., Kohler, P. J., Riley, E., Tse, P. U., & Meng, M. (2015). The artist emerges: Visual art learning alters neural structure and function. *NeuroImage*, 105, 440–451. https://doi.org/10.1016/j.neuroimage.2014.11.014

Schnitzer, G., Holttum, S., & Huet, V. (2022). "My heart on this bit of paper": A grounded theory of the mechanisms of change in art therapy for military veterans. *Journal of Affective Disorders*, 297, 327–337. https://doi.org/10.1016/j.jad.2021.10.049

Schore, A. N. (2012). *The science of the art of psychotherapy* (Norton series on interpersonal neurobiology). WW Norton & Company.

Schouten, K. A., Niet, G. J. de, Knipscheer, J. W., Kleber, R. J., & Hutschemaekers, G. J. M. (2014). The effectiveness of art therapy in the treatment of traumatized adults: A systematic review on art therapy and trauma. *Trauma, Violence, Abuse*, 16(2), 220–228. https://doi.org/10.1177/1524838014555032

Shapiro, F. (Ed.). (2002). *EMDR as an integrative psychotherapy approach: Experts of diverse orientations explore the paradigm prism.* American Psychological Association. https://doi.org/10.1037/10512-000

Sheffler, J. L., Stanley, I., & Sachs-Ericsson, N. (2020). ACEs and mental health outcomes. In *Adverse Childhood Experiences* (pp. 47–69). Elsevier. https://doi.org/10.1016/b978-0-12-816065-7.00004-5

Siegel, D. (1999). *The developing mind: Toward a neurobiology of interpersonal experience.* Guilford.

Smith, A. (2016). A literature review of the therapeutic mechanisms of art therapy for veterans with post-traumatic stress disorder. *International Journal of Art Therapy*, 21(2), 66–74. https://doi.org/10.1080/17454832.2016.1170055

Smith, K. (2023). Lab mice go wild: Making experiments more natural in order to decode the brain. *Nature*, 618(7965), 448–450. https://doi.org/10.1038/d41586-023-01926-w

Spiegel, D., Malchiodi, C., Backos, A., & Collie, K. (2006). Art therapy for combat-related PTSD: Recommendations for research and practice. *Art Therapy*, 23(4), 157–164. https://doi.org/10.1080/07421656.2006.10129335

Spring, D. (2004). Thirty-year study links neuroscience, specific trauma, PTSD, image conversion, and language translation. *Art Therapy*, 21(4), 200–209. https://doi.org/10.1080/07421656.2004.10129690

Stepney, S. A. (2019). Visionary architects of color in art therapy: Georgette Powell, Cliff Joseph, Lucille Venture, and Charles Anderson. *Art Therapy*, 36(3), 115–121. https://doi.org/10.1080/07421656.2019.1649545

Stepney, S. A. (2022). Multicultural and diversity perspectives in art therapy: Transforming image into substance. In M. Rastogi, R. P. Feldwisch, M. Pate, & J. Scarce (Eds.), *Foundations of Art Therapy* (pp. 81–122). Academic Press. https://doi.org/10.1016/B978-0-12-824308-4.00010-7

Sturmberg, J. P., & Martin, C. M. (2008). Knowing – in medicine. *Journal of Evaluation in Clinical Practice*, 14(5), 767–770. https://doi.org/10.1111/j.1365-2753.2008.01011.x

Suleiman, S. R. (2008). Judith Herman and contemporary trauma theory. *Women's Studies Quarterly*, 36(1/2), 276–281.

Sun, J., Chen, Q., Zhang, Q., Li, Y., Li, H., Wei, D., Yang, W., & Qiu, J. (2016). Training your brain to be more creative: Brain functional and structural changes induced by divergent thinking training. *Human Brain Mapping*, 37(10), 3375–3387. https://doi.org/10.1002/hbm.23246

Sun, J., Zhang, Q., Li, Y., Meng, J., Chen, Q., Yang, W., Wei, D., & Qiu, J. (2020). Plasticity of the resting-state brain: Static and dynamic functional connectivity change induced by divergent thinking training. *Brain Imaging and Behavior*, 14(5), 1498–1506. https://doi.org/10.1007/s11682-019-00077-9

Sussman, S., Valente, T. W., Rohrbach, L. A., Skara, S., & Ann Pentz, M. (2006). Translation in the health professions: Converting science into action. *Evaluation & the Health Professions*, 29(1), 7–32. https://doi.org/10.1177/0163278705284441

Talwar, S. (2007). Accessing traumatic memory through art making: An art therapy trauma protocol (ATTP). *The Arts in Psychotherapy, 34*(1), 22–35. https://doi.org/10.1016/j.aip.2006.09.001

Talwar, S. (2016). Is there a need to redefine art therapy? *Art Therapy, 33*(3), 116–118. https://doi.org/10.1080/07421656.2016.1202001

Tripp, T. (2007). A short term therapy approach to processing trauma: Art therapy and bilateral stimulation. *Art Therapy, 24*(4), 176–183. https://doi.org/10.1080/07421656.2007.10129476

Tripp, T. (2016). A body-based bilateral art protocol for reprocessing trauma. In *Art therapy, trauma, and neuroscience: Theoretical and practical perspectives* (pp. 173–194). Routledge.

Tyng, C. M., Amin, H. U., Saad, M. N. M., & Malik, A. S. (2017). The influences of emotion on learning and memory. *Frontiers in Psychology, 8.* www.frontiersin.org/articles/10.3389/fpsyg.2017.01454

Ulman, E. (2001). Art therapy: Problems of definition. *American Journal Of Art Therapy, 40*(1). www.proquest.com/docview/199281748

Ulman, E., & Dachinger, P. (1975). *Art therapy in theory and practice.* Schocken Books.

Vaisvaser, S. (2021). The embodied-enactive-interactive brain: Bridging neuroscience and creative arts therapies. *Frontiers in Psychology, 12.* www.frontiersin.org/articles/10.3389/fpsyg.2021.634079

van der Kolk, B. (2014). *The body keeps the score: Brain, mind, and body in the healing of trauma* (Reprint edition). Penguin Publishing Group.

Van Lith, T. (2016). Art therapy in mental health: A systematic review of approaches and practices. *The Arts in Psychotherapy, 47,* 9–22. https://doi.org/10.1016/j.aip.2015.09.003

Vargas, M. V., Dunlap, L. E., Dong, C., Carter, S. J., Tombari, R. J., Jami, S. A., Cameron, L. P., Patel, S. D., Hennessey, J. J., Saeger, H. N., McCorvy, J. D., Gray, J. A., Tian, L., & Olson, D. E. (2023). Psychedelics promote neuroplasticity through the activation of intracellular 5-HT2A receptors. *Science, 379*(6633), 700–706. https://doi.org/10.1126/science.adf0435

Vick, R. M. (2003). A brief history of art therapy. *Handbook of Art Therapy,* 5–15.

Walker, M. S., Stamper, A. M., Nathan, D. E., & Riedy, G. (2018). Art therapy and underlying fMRI brain patterns in military TBI: A case series. *International Journal of Art Therapy, 23*(4), 180–187. https://doi.org/10.1080/17454832.2018.1473453

Wang, Y.-T., Zhang, N.-N., Liu, L.-J., Jiang, H., Hu, D., Wang, Z.-Z., Chen, N.-H., & Zhang, Y. (2022). Glutamatergic receptor and neuroplasticity in depression: Implications for ketamine and rapastinel as the rapid-acting antidepressants. *Biochemical and Biophysical Research Communications, 594,* 46–56. https://doi.org/10.1016/j.bbrc.2022.01.024

Waraich, M., & Shah, S. (2018). The life and work of Jean-Martin Charcot (1825–1893): "The Napoleon of Neuroses." *Journal of the Intensive Care Society, 19*(1), 48–49. https://doi.org/10.1177/1751143717709420

Weathers, F. W., & Keane, T. M. (2007). The Criterion A problem revisited: Controversies and challenges in defining and measuring psychological trauma. *Journal of Traumatic Stress, 20*(2), 107–121. https://doi.org/10.1002/jts.20210

Wester, K., & McKibben, B. (2019). Integrating mixed methods approaches in counseling outcome research. *Counseling Outcome Research and Evaluation, 10*(1), 1–11. https://doi.org/10.1080/21501378.2018.1531239

What are some different areas of neuroscience? (2018, October 1). Eunice Kennedy Shriver National Institute of Child Health and Human Development. www.nichd.nih.gov/health/topics/neuro/conditioninfo/areas

World Health Organization. (1948). *Constitution of the World Health Organization.* www.who.int/about/governance/constitution

Yehuda, R., & Lehrner, A. (2018). Intergenerational transmission of trauma effects: Putative role of epigenetic mechanisms. *World Psychiatry, 17*(3), 243–257. https://doi.org/10.1002/wps.20568

Zarbo, C., Tasca, G. A., Cattafi, F., & Compare, A. (2016). Integrative psychotherapy works. *Frontiers in Psychology, 6,* 2021. https://doi.org/10.3389/fpsyg.2015.02021

CHAPTER 2

NEUROSCIENCE CONCEPTS FOR CLINICAL PRACTICE IN BEHAVIORAL HEALTH AND ART THERAPY

Lukasz M. Konopka, Christianne E. Strang, and Juliet L. King

2.1   INTRODUCTION

This chapter proposes a functional, anatomical, and neurophysiological schema to enhance the way clinicians think about their patients' lifelong neural plasticity. To that end, the chapter presents recent neuroscientific data on the cellular mechanisms regarding traumatic memories, genetics, behavior, assessment, and brain networks. In the section on brain networks, we challenge the idea of brain centers and summarize how brain complexity and identifiable networks influence health and pathology. Together, these data provide a conceptual template to help clinicians understand and implement tools that can be incorporated into the diagnostic process and identify optimal data-driven therapies that include standard interventions as well as art therapy. To exemplify this multimodal neuroscientific approach, the chapter will include clinical cases that illustrate how logical, defendable, scientific research, diagnosis, and treatment can encourage a common clinical language accessible across diagnostic and therapeutic silos. As communication and collaboration between art therapy and related disciplines improve, art therapy is more accurately defined as a valuable, substantiated therapy within the standard therapeutic armamentarium.

2.2   BRAIN CELLULAR PROCESSES: OVERVIEW

Structure

A hundred billion neurons compose the human brain, an organ comprising functional neuronal units and electrical networks that integrate many divergent sensory, cognitive, emotional, and behavioral systems through activity patterns that are coded by action potentials. Structures include the outer cortical layer, also known as gray matter, and subcortical regions that combine gray and white matter such as the thalamus and the basal ganglia. White matter is composed of myelinated axons. Within the gray matter, individual neuronal morphologies range from simple bipolar neurons to extensive and complex pyramidal cells.

Cellular Function

All neurons receive input from their dendrites. The dendrites are specialized to respond to chemical signals called neurotransmitters. Each neuron's elaborate dendritic projections respond to various neurotransmitters that stimulate numerous specialized receptors. Dendritic structures look like trees with branching, dendritic

DOI: 10.4324/9781003348207-2

arbors that integrate 10,000 (for simple bipolar morphologies) to 100,000 functional informational inputs (for pyramidal cells). As such, the dendrites' integrated inputs cause the generation and propagation of action potentials down the axon, the output portion of the cell.

An action potential is an "all or none" electrical event within a neuron caused when electrical signals from dendritic inputs reach a threshold of membrane depolarization. For an action potential to occur, the cell must compute the numerous excitatory and inhibitory inputs that are integrated in the cell body, the soma. Because an action potential begins only with sufficient depolarization and because dendritic synaptic potentials lose amplitude as they travel towards the soma, the input closest to the soma has the strongest influence on the synaptic signals, i.e., the closer the input, the greater the impact on excitation or inhibition of the neuron. Action potential generation is uncertain without multiple synchronous inputs because synchronous inputs are summed together and increase the probability of reaching the critical threshold. For example, if a single input stimulates a cell, the input must have a greater excitatory amplitude to fire an action potential than when two or three smaller independent inputs converge on the same soma (Dan & Poo, 2004). After stimulation, synchronous dendritic inputs can also serve to strengthen those synapses and increase the neuron's probability of firing an action potential. This process, called summation, also contributes to neural plasticity through the modification of synapses.

2.3   NEUROPLASTICITY AND LEARNING

In 1973, Dr. Konorski defined neuroplasticity as the dynamic neuronal response to environmental and intrinsic stimuli that gradually alters cellular structure and function (Thomas et al., 1994). Repetition causes neural remodeling throughout the brain. At the cellular level, synaptic plasticity is seen when receptors adjust their responses to neurotransmitters. Other molecules also influence synaptic efficiency and modify neuronal networks by enhancing or pruning synaptic contacts, another aspect of neuronal plasticity. For example, the brain's proteins regulate neuronal growth, maintenance, and survival, which in turn, seem to affect various brain-related disorders, such as schizophrenia, bipolar illness, and autism-spectrum disorders (Holtzman & Mobley, 1994; Martinowich et al., 2007).

Repeated cellular summation exemplifies neural plasticity and implies that cellular learning occurs most efficiently with converging multi-sensory input. From the standpoint of human behavior, this process can be understood as memory establishment. For instance, when we learn using only one sensory modality, such as vision, it takes more time and effort to master a task and form a memory; however, if we have learned using two modalities, such as vision and audition, the converging sensory information will expedite our learning. Initially, the brain requires significant metabolic resources to make novel behaviors routine, but, as the brain adapts, efficient networks develop that require less effort to engage and complete the behavior (Grabner et al., 2006).

Often, when individuals find learning difficult, they become frustrated and abandon their efforts, but just as new exercise produces sore muscles and few initial rewards, repeated training increases muscle strength and requires less effort and greater satisfaction. At first, when the brain is learning novel tasks, it requires multiple networks, but eventually, it trims superfluous networks, focuses its activity, and optimizes its performance by creating the most efficient pathway. For example, we can measure how exercise yields remarkable, quantifiable, structural brain changes that positively affect our motoric equilibrium (Lewis et al., 2009). One of the best examples is learning to ride a bicycle, a task that initially requires significant brain effort, but, over time, becomes simple and intuitive. Although most of us have learned to ride a bike, we would find it nearly impossible to describe the individual steps that led to our success because our learning resulted from numerous conscious and unconscious structural and biochemical changes.

2.4   COMMUNICATION WITHIN THE BRAIN

The human brain is hierarchically organized into well-defined developmental and functional networks that interact and provide a conceptual framework for the brain's anatomical and functional connections. Our brain has many interactive networks, and studies of their relationships contribute to understanding their functioning as multi-leveled and interactive systems (Bassett & Sporns, 2017).

First, through neuroimaging, we see clustered, closely interrelated neurons combine to form local networks and create functional modules. Smaller modules act within larger modules that seem to arrange into functional subsystems (He & Evans, 2010). Our brains engage different networks to process emotions and cognitions, yet these networks are interactive, overlapping, and dynamic (Bullmore & Sporns, 2009; Pessoa, 2018; Power et al., 2011). For example, looking at a piece of artwork activates the visual system, which may connect with memory, emotional, and reward systems to create an opinion about the artwork. Broadly speaking, we could say that the brain oscillates between enhanced and decreased connectivity determined by the person's engagement with the artwork. Here, the viewer may express an observable behavior, such as deciding whether the artwork is appealing, and engaging the language-production systems that express an opinion about the artwork. Rather than specific brain centers, as conceptualized in the past, the brain's dynamic hierarchical order engages functional hubs and networks (King & Chatterjee, 2024). Defining the brain, as a system of dynamic integrated functional networks, guides our understanding of how the brain operates. When we understand normal, expected, and predictable brain functions, we more clearly characterize individuals with behavioral pathologies. This framework helps to conceptualize the central nervous system as a hierarchical system of integrated networks rather than brain centers devoted to specific functions.

2.5   SENSORY NETWORKS

We can divide the basic sensory networks into olfaction, vision, audition, and somatosensory, existing within larger networks that integrate specific sensory processes. Sensory networks involve well-defined neuroanatomical pathways, which primarily process sensory information. Olfaction is unique in that its anatomical projections do not involve subcortical sensory structures, but directly influence the limbic system. As such, olfaction often evokes significant emotional responses including memories. The visual processing network uses the primary visual cortex, located in the mid occipital lobe, and associated adjacent higher order visual processing areas. The primary visual cortex receives and interprets information from the retina of the eye. Then, the information is broadly distributed and interpreted as images and associated with memory, emotion, language, and other senses (Kandel et al., 2021). The cortical auditory network includes the superior temporal gyrus and contains the primary and secondary auditory and associated areas. The sensorimotor system includes the primary somatosensory area in the most anterior region of the parietal cortex, which receives sensory information from the hands, feet, and body. It communicates with the secondary somatosensory cortex and posterior parietal regions that integrate bodily information with visual and auditory information (Yao et al., 2020). These integrated systems prepare for behavioral responses by communicating with the frontal cortex and motor areas. Consequently, past limbic experiences collaborate, activate, and integrate ongoing sensory systems to evoke fear-responses. For example, patients, with Vietnam-era military PTSD, experience fear and flashbacks to conditioned triggers, such as smell, sound, images, and sensory memories, e.g., rain or humidity.

Thus, conceptualizing how the brain processes sensory information and makes decisions provides a simple way to understand the subconscious and conscious integration of responses. First, discernible sensory inputs, such as vision, audition, sensation, or olfaction, are converted into electrical signals. Then, specified sensory pathways acknowledge these signals and, eventually, integrate them into unique perceptual signals. The sensory pathways connect to the brain's parietal lobes, located posterior to the central sulci and dedicated to integrating multisensory input. As the parietal lobes integrate sensory input, they communicate with another large brain region, the frontal lobes, which include areas that control movement and behavioral choices, generate or inhibit actions, and continually manage how we relate to and interact with the environment (see Figure 2.1).

Both excessive connection and disconnection within and between brain regions and networks leads to significant consequences. Epilepsy exemplifies acute extreme connectivity, hyper-synchronicity, and enhanced interregional communication often in both brain hemispheres (Lehnertz et al., 2009; Lieb et al., 1987), resulting in behavioral aberrations such as grand mal or subclinical seizures. Chronic hyper-synchronization also occurs in degenerative diseases, such as Parkinson's disease (Kühn et al., 2006; Stoffers et al., 2008). Conversely, children who have agenesis of the corpus callosum, a birth defect where the nerve bundle connecting the two brain hemispheres is missing or partially missing, lack interhemispheric communication, as demonstrated by deficits in electroencephalographic (EEG) coherence (Koeda et al., 1995) and anatomical magnetic resonance imaging (MRI) (Hofman et al., 2020). These patients present with clinical features that can include intellectual deficits, behavioral anomalies, and seizures (Hofman et al., 2020). Broadly speaking, these examples illuminate that too much or too little communication between the brain regions often alters function and results in behavioral challenges.

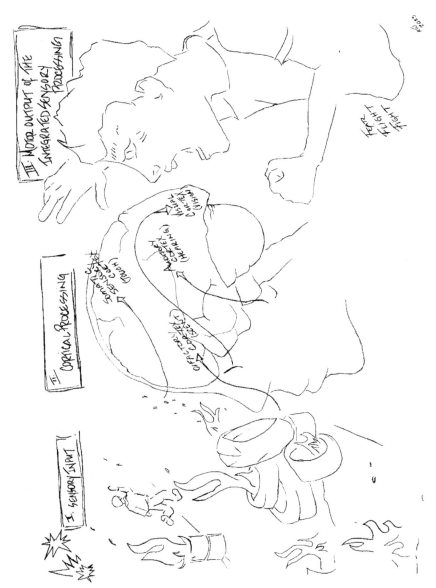

FIGURE 2.1 Simplified description for how sensory input engages cortical processing and influences motor output

2.6   LARGE-SCALE BRAIN NETWORKS

Complex behaviors, cognitions, and decisions appear to be mediated by large-scale networks. Noninvasive neuroimaging technology has advanced the understanding of network activities and communication. This knowledge helps clarify the many neuronal interactions within and across brain regions (Uddin et al., 2019). (See the imaging methods section.). Of particular interest and importance to art therapists are three large-scale brain networks (LSBN) relevant to creativity and aesthetics: the default mode network (DMN), the central executive network (CEN), also known as the executive control network, and the salience network (SN). In general, it can be understood that the DMN is active when people focus on internal mental states, such as when daydreaming. The CEN is involved in working memory and problem solving, and the SN assists in switching neural activity between the DMN and CEN, while attending to behaviorally relevant tasks (King & Chatterjee, 2024). The attention network is also considered a core brain network that is involved with voluntary attention and orientation to the environment.

2.7   THE DEFAULT MODE NETWORK

The DMN, discovered by Raichle et al. (2001), is a resting state network that continues to mature through early adulthood (Sherman et al., 2014). The DMN is active in peaceful relaxed states and is inactive when a person is performing goal-directed tasks or processing sensory information regarding a particular activity. Thus, this network engages during daydreaming and introspection, evaluating the past or the future, processing personal experiences and autobiographical memories or considering the perspective of another (Fair et al., 2008; Kim, 2012). This default network involves distributed cortical structures including the medial, lateral prefrontal cortex, and the parietal and temporal cortices; it includes functional connections to the thalamus, amygdala, and basal ganglia (Alves et al., 2019; Qin & Northoff, 2011).

Data suggest that the DMN may be dysregulated in neurodegenerative disorders, such as Alzheimer's type dementia (Binnewijzend et al., 2012; Greicius et al., 2004) and frontal temporal dementia subtypes (Seeley et al., 2009). DMN dysregulation may also play a role in depression (Zhou et al., 2020), with changes in connectivity across multiple areas, including subcortical structures such as the amygdala, the anterior and posterior cingulate cortices, and the parietal regions (Anand et al., 2005; Veer et al., 2010). Together, these studies show resting state network mapping may more clearly characterize underlying network pathologies for more precisely diagnosing and treating various disorders using neuromodulatory techniques, e.g., transcranial magnetic stimulation of the left dorsolateral prefrontal cortex in major depression.

2.8   CENTRAL EXECUTIVE NETWORK

The CEN appears to engage during cognitive tasks that require externally driven processes, e.g., active attention, working memory, rule-based problem solving, and decision making within the context of goal-directed behaviors (Aron, 2007; Curtis & D'Esposito, 2003; Koechlin & Summerfield, 2007). The CEN is also involved in maintaining and manipulating information in working memory (D'Esposito, 2007; Menon & D'Esposito, 2022). The brain regions primarily involved include the frontal, frontoparietal, dorsolateral prefrontal, anterior cingulate, and posterior parietal areas (Shen et al., 2019). The CEN also filters relevant and irrelevant stimuli to provide cognitive control for activating and discerning important vs unimportant information. Its goal is the amplification of the relevant and the elimination of distracting, inconsequential stimuli (Vossel et al., 2014). Generally, when the CEN is activated during cognitive tasks, the DMN is inhibited. This may indicate that, while engaged in specific cognitive tasks requiring focused attention, the brain needs to suppress unrelated thought processes (Sridharan et al., 2008); however, during a cognitive task that may need interaction with internally focused processes, such as traumatic memory processing and recall, the two systems may temporarily couple to retrieve needed autobiographical data (Andrews-Hanna et al., 2014).

2.9   THE SALIENCE NETWORK

As the name implies, the salience network (SN) is critically important for capturing physiologically and cognitively important "salient" events. This network facilitates emotions by filtering or triggering interoceptive and autonomic stimuli (Menon & Uddin, 2010; Seeley, 2019; Seeley et al., 2007) and alerting other brain networks for when to generate appropriate or dysfunctional behavioral responses. Anatomically, the salience network incorporates various structures such as the cortical regions that include the temporopolar cortex, anterior insula, anterior cingulate, and subcortical structures, for example, the amygdala, ventral striato-pallidum, thalamus, hypothalamus, periaqueductal gray, substantia nigra and the autonomic nervous system (Menon & Uddin, 2010; Seeley, 2019).

It appears the network's key role is identifying the most relevant stimuli, which manages and guides behavioral choices for reestablishing homeostasis (Lovero et al., 2009; Menon & Uddin, 2010; Seeley et al., 2007). The most recent data show distinct hippocampal neuronal populations that develop memory traces (Shpokayte et al., 2022) and provide evidence for positive and negative memories that may be differentially modulated by therapeutic approaches and shifting of cognitive schemas.

2.10   ATTENTION NETWORKS

To successfully connect and interact with the environment, one must closely attend to presenting stimuli and generate an appropriate response. Recent studies have discovered attentional brain networks that initiate and maintain alert states by orienting the organism towards specific sensory input. In addition to the CEN, these include the alerting network and the orienting network (Markett et al., 2022; Petersen & Posner, 2012), which influence our ability to avoid danger, learn from experience, and facilitate the completion of tasks. The alerting system focuses the brain, orients sensory input, and informs executive control, so it can respond appropriately to presenting stimuli (Sadaghiani & D'Esposito, 2015).

The dorsal attention network, the orienting system, also called the frontoparietal network focuses the brain toward the stimulus and shifts brain resources depending upon the quality and location of the stimulus/trigger. Attentional network abnormalities significantly impact many brain pathologies such as injury, stroke, schizophrenia, and attention deficit disorder. For example, in people with schizophrenia, sustained attention measures may predict the patient's response to antipsychotic medications (Cohen et al., 1998), and in children diagnosed with ADHD, imaging studies indicate abnormalities in attentional networks (Silk et al., 2019).

Neural networks, vulnerable to genetic and environmental influences, are typically sensitive to various abnormalities and, clinically, may be seen as disease states and behaviors that drive intervention strategies in varying settings and under different demands. Network integrity relies on efficient communication between networks and can be studied by network connectivity, which helps us explain and understand the impact of traumatic events on an individual's biology. Integrated brain networks arise from the function of and connection between the 100 billion human brain neurons. When we attempt to systematically investigate the cellular mechanisms behind networks, we find they are difficult to study, yet progress has been made that illuminates the connections between brain processes and behavior. A particularly relevant area is the recall and processing of traumatic memories.

2.11   TRAUMATIC MEMORY

Effects on memory may be influenced by the age at which a trauma occurs. For example, some individuals with clinically demonstrable trauma may have limited memory of their traumatic experiences, particularly when the trauma occurred in youth. Since childhood memories may not be well established or, at least, readily recalled, children may be disadvantaged by the lack of traumatic memory access, which could normally detect and alert a child to the potential for re-exposure and repeated trauma. If a trauma is repeated, and if the trauma remains unprocessed, the DMN development can be biased (Fair et al., 2008). These data are supported by animal studies that show a significant difference between recent and old fearful memories. Presumably related to memory consolidation, more distant memories appear to be more complexly represented in the brain, showing broadly distributed activated brain regions, including circuits involving the hippocampus and anterior cingulate (Makino et al., 2019).

In clinical practice, these studies are important for conceptualizing the involved brain regions. It is well known that trauma influences the processing and reconsolidation of memories. In patients with post-traumatic stress syndrome (PTSS), the anterior cingulate, part of the DMN, shows prominent engagement and influence of the hippocampus. Post-traumatic stress may be viewed as the cortex's top-down control of the hippocampus, which may influence retrieval and storage of contextual memories. Trauma also influences hippocampal size, which is significantly decreased in patients with untreated PTSS, who often present with memory difficulties (Bremner et al., 2003). One may suppose that altered interaction between the anterior cingulate and hippocampus may explain why patients with PTSS often have significantly fragmented memories. Although PTSS exemplifies traumatic memories associated with one specific event, the complex clinical presentation, and the delayed symptom onset for some PTSS patients, does not seem to support this simplistic explanation (Smid & Kleber, 2009).

Brain imaging helps to support the presence and complexity of cellular and network interactions that form traumatic memories and explains some of the complex clinical observations found in traumatized patients. Using neuroimaging, within a diagnostic category, to assess human brain circuits and evaluate PTSS patients deepens our understanding of diverse patient populations and becomes critical to clinical work (Konopka et al., 2020; Poprawski et al., 2007).

After exposure to severe stressors, PTSS symptoms seem to reflect stress-induced changes in neurobiological systems and/or an inadequate neurobiological adaptation. Identifying the links between neurobiological changes and specific features that constitute PTSS is relevant. For example, neuroimaging data illuminates altered learning mechanisms, sensitization to stress and arousal, and how these changes reflect preexisting vulnerability factors, such as genetic variability, sex differences, and developmental exposure to stress. From here, important hypotheses can be derived for developing novel strategies that identify at-risk subjects, promote resilience, and help devise targets for the prevention or treatment of PTSS. These assumptions support the value of nonverbal therapies, such as art therapy, for helping patients cope with implicit traumatic memories not readily available to verbal expression.

2.12 TRAUMATIC BRAIN INJURY

Worldwide, Traumatic Brain Injury (TBI) is the foremost cause of mortality and morbidity and often results in a cascade of cognitive, behavioral, and functional difficulties with widely variable clinical presentation (Devi et al., 2020). The consequences of brain injury depend upon the injury type, location, and often present with attentional difficulties. For example, when researchers evaluated pediatric patients with various brain injuries, the data showed that their clinical presentations depended upon their ability to recruit attentional networks and correlated with attentional deficits, particularly when there were increased system demands (Strazzer et al., 2015).

Although we presume an overt difference between psychological trauma and physical brain trauma, the etiologic abnormalities seem to involve similar neurobiological systems and produce overlapping clinical syndromes. This is important because it can be difficult to tease out where and how symptoms emerge. For example, TBI and PTSS frequently co-occur in patients who have experienced either motor vehicle accidents or military combat (Scholten et al., 2017; Walker et al., 2018). The difficulty of disambiguating the effects of TBI and PTSS complicates treatment strategies so that clinicians are challenged to disentangle the contributing co-morbidities along with individual differences (King & Chatterjee, 2024).

Scientific data and clinical experience clearly indicate that, after trauma, the brain encodes traumatic memories that may remain over a lifetime. Consequently, to normalize a traumatic event, the brain adapts to promote survival, restore behavioral equilibrium, and compartmentalize memories. One can easily understand why traumatic memories result in challenging behaviors. In PTSS patients, these behaviors may include excessive sensitivity to internal and external stimuli, "triggers," that may disrupt attentional networks, including the SN and the DMN (Sripada et al., 2012), and interfere with recalling important aspects of the trauma resulting from underlying cellular memory formation.

Trigger sensitivities affect how one interacts with the environment, resulting in behavioral symptoms such as avoidant behaviors, sound sensitivity, discomfort with converging sensory stimulation, and fear of uncomfortable, unknown, and unpredictable situations. Consequently, attaining an optimal life experience is very challenging for traumatized individuals.

Recent electrophysiological studies into cellular mechanisms influencing traumatic and non-traumatic memories reported that amygdala and prefrontal cortex activation, in both traumatic and non-traumatic events, led to the establishment of memories (Toropova et al., 2021). Their findings indicated that stimulus intensity was the most influential variable in distinguishing between non-traumatic and traumatic memories. After traumatic memories were formed, recalling those memories was also associated with greater cellular responses. These data show that the greater the electrical physiological stimulus, the greater the cellular activation that led to memory establishment. Another animal study showed that traumatic memory may involve the activation of specific inhibitory neurotransmitter receptors (non-synaptic GABA receptors) that shift cortical to subcortical processing of the fear-associated memories (Jovasevic et al., 2015). These data may provide a basis for hypothesizing why traumatic memory may be difficult to access by normal memory activation pathways and may require specific activation patterns, such as the connections between visual pathways and emotional and memory networks that connect voluntary and autonomic behavior systems (Kandel, 2001). In treating patients with PTSS, it is important to engage these various processes through various therapeutic approaches that may include art making.

2.13   HEMISPHERIC SPECIALIZATION

Anatomical human brain asymmetry can be observed as early as 29–31 weeks of gestation. As the child develops, factors such as gender, hormonal exposure, and genetic predispositions influence brain development and future adaptability to life (Toga & Thompson, 2003). Initial cerebral asymmetry studies identified significant anatomical differences between the posterior auditory cortex's planum temporale of the left and right hemispheres (Geschwind & Levitsky, 1968). Additionally, the right hemisphere appears larger than the left hemisphere and has a lower white matter to gray matter ratio (Shapleske et al., 1999).

These anatomical and functional hemispheric asymmetries impact cognition, emotion, and the control of behavior (Ocklenburg & Gunturkun, 2012). We have learned much about hemispheric specialization from patients who have undergone surgery that separates the two hemispheres to restrict the spread of seizures. After surgery, these *split-brain* patients became models for testing how each hemisphere processes sensory information without sharing interhemispheric data. Since the right hemisphere does not produce speech, when images were presented to the right hemisphere, patients could not name the objects (Levy & Trevarthen, 1977).

Research also showed that the right hemisphere is particularly sensitive to facial recognition presented to the left visual field (Turk et al., 2002; Yovel et al., 2008).

Due to the brain's inherent plasticity and its environmental adaptation, including pathology, the concept of pure hemispheric specialization has given way to understanding that while some processes are lateralized, integrated functioning and network activation entails bilateral involvement. For example, neuroscientists have discovered that, for most people, the left hemisphere controls right-sided movements and plays a special role in language comprehension and production (Hebb & Ojemann, 2013; Scheibel, 2017). Conversely, the right hemisphere controls movement on the left side and specializes in perception, emotional recognition, and the nonverbal information synthesis of music (Morton, 2020; Peretz & Zatorre, 2005). Handedness and spatial skills are also lateralized (Morton, 2020).

We must guard against simplifying our understanding of brain function. While different brains share the same basic organizational patterns, there are also unique individual differences that make them more distinct than similar or more relative than absolute. This perspective fits quite well into our earlier paradigm that addressed the brain's considerable neuroplasticity, particularly when the brain encounters psychological challenges and/or physical injury.

Advanced neuroimaging has helped us evaluate the brain's structure and function, and it has simultaneously heightened our need to understand functional asymmetries in the bilateral brain, e.g., the laterality of functional nodes or processing styles that correlate with anatomical asymmetries (Morton, 2020). Other evidence suggests that even neurotransmitters and receptors are asymmetrically distributed (Andersen & Teicher, 2000; Fink et al., 2009; Fitzgerald, 2012; Fritzsche, 2003; Iseki et al., 2009), which may result in variable medication effects on hemispheric function and impact patients taking psychotropic medications. It is important to emphasize that brain asymmetries do not indicate left-brain and right-brain dichotomies.

In healthy individuals, intact interhemispheric connections and communication result in integrated perceptual, emotional, and cognitive experiences; nevertheless, anatomy and information processing differ between the hemispheres. For example, the right ear excels in dichotically presented speech, and the left ear has the advantage in perceiving melodies (Kimura, 1967). Moreover in right-handers, somatosensory lateralization results in better tactile shape recognition with the left hand and superior letter identification using the right hand (Finlayson & Reitan, 1976; Gibson & Bryden, 1983). These examples demonstrate cortical specialization that relates directly to sensory processing. While most clinicians will not work with individuals that have undergone split-brain procedures, understanding the different processing styles may impact clinical approaches. For example, the location of a stroke or TBI may have differential impacts on a patient's ability to recognize or respond to emotional cues or comprehend complex explanations.

2.14   CASE STUDIES

The following section demonstrates how we can use quantitative EEG (qEEG) and other imaging techniques to understand individual patient's clinical presentations.

Allison

Allison, a struggling, 22-year-old woman with a complex clinical picture, had a long-standing history of serious anxiety and depression that started in childhood and had not improved for any sustained period. In addition, she described heightened autonomic arousal, such as increased heart rate, rapid breathing, muscle tension, poor temperature control, and dysregulated sleep. Allison also experienced feeling overwhelmed, helpless, apathetic, and unmotivated. Several times, she attempted suicide. In adolescence, Allison coped by disordered eating and self-injurious behaviors, including binging, purging, over-exercising, restriction, diuretics, and cutting. After struggling with these behaviors for several years, she was given a litany of diagnostic labels including Generalized Anxiety Disorder, Panic Disorder, Major Depressive Disorder, Persistent Depressive Disorder, Eating Disorder NOS, and Personality Disorder NOS.

Clinicians assessed Allison with neurobehavioral and neurophysiological measures that revealed problems with language production, sustained attention, planning, and problem solving. Her qEEG results indicated significant frontal lobe dysregulation with paroxysmal activities (see Figure 2.2). Paroxysms are abrupt electrophysiological bursts (Zimmerman & Konopka, 2013). In Allison's case, the paroxysmal activity likely took her brain "off-line," prevented complete thoughts, and disrupted her attention and executive function (Aarts et al., 1984). As her paroxysmal events increased, she experienced increased emotional and physiological stress (Konopka & Zimmerman, 2014). As seen in her auditory and visual evoked potentials, sensory processing measures, Allison could process and receive information, but lacked sustained attention because her cognition was impaired by her disrupted attentional networks.

LORETA, a type of QEEG, demonstrated that Allison had statistically significant, focal, electrophysiological abnormalities in her left mesial temporal lobe, a region that impacts emotion, language, and verbal memory. (See Figure 2.3.)

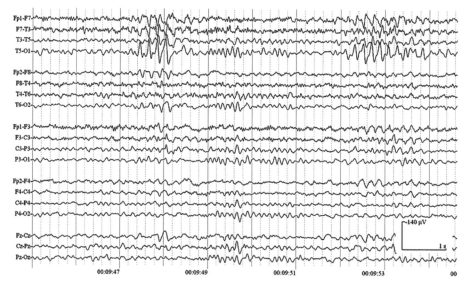

FIGURE 2.2 qEEG results recorded with eyes open: Paroxysmal discharges in the left frontal lobe. At other times, this pattern was also seen in the right hemisphere.

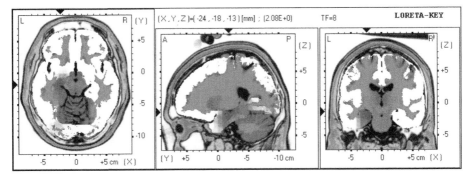

FIGURE 2.3 LORETA, qEEG alpha-1 excess, left hippocampal/parahippocampal. The shaded area identifies the brain regions where there is a statistically significant electrophysiological abnormality.

These data led Allison's clinicians to change the design of Allison's therapy. They learned that Allison could only manage small quantities of information, particularly when the topic was emotionally charged, which caused significant left hemispheric dysregulation and impacted her perceptions and verbal expression. Therefore, Allison's therapeutic sessions included short cognitive exchanges, with immediate feedback, and other nonverbal interventions, such as art therapy.

Art therapy is a well-established therapy that facilitates nonverbal emotional expression and therapeutic communication (King, 2016). Allison was referred to our program for art therapy because of her neurological dysregulation and subsequent behaviors and symptoms. We hoped that art therapy would help engage her left hemisphere and give her a tool for describing her emotions. The qEEG data and Allison's behavioral presentation were important to the treatment plan. Fortunately, she felt comfortable participating in art therapy, which allowed her to focus and extend her attention. We hoped that, eventually, she could apply her increased attentiveness to enhance her verbal processing and manage her emotions. Allison was discharged to a lower level of care with significantly improved symptoms.

Daniel

Daniel, a 24-year-old man, was referred after his first serious suicide attempt. Growing up, Daniel had difficulty with fine motor movement, speech development, writing, and struggled with a longstanding history of severe depression. He also perceived himself as a victim of parental neglect inside the home and bullying outside the home. To manage his depression and anxiety, Daniel used substances such as alcohol and marijuana. Daniel presented with rigid thinking and obsessive-compulsive behaviors. Daniel's previous treatment included adult outpatient and inpatient interventions with a diagnosis of Major Depressive Disorder, Autistic Disorder, Acute Stress Disorder, Generalized Anxiety Disorder, Alcohol Abuse, Cannabis Abuse, and Personality Disorder NOS.

A detailed clinical interview revealed that Daniel had several incidents of potentially serious head trauma, including falling downstairs at age two, hitting his head, and losing consciousness. In middle school, he was hit on the head while playing soccer. Neuropsychological testing indicated that Daniel had slow reaction time, poor planning skills, limited cognitive flexibility, and limbic dysregulation. The EEG revealed abnormalities in the sensory/motor cortex, the dorsal cingulate, and right insular regions and correlated with many of Daniel's symptoms and converged with his nuclear imaging (positron emission tomography, PET) (see Figure 2.4 and 2.5) (Kennedy et al., 2001).

In addition to functional abnormalities, the MRI's structural images also revealed an unexpected finding – a 3.5 cm posterior fossa cyst compressing the vermis of the cerebellum. The cerebellum, particularly the vermis, is increasingly recognized for its role in regulating emotions, higher-order cognition, and movement (Schmahmann, 2004). The cyst was direct objective data that provided significance to Daniel's complex clinical and psychiatric presentation (Heath et al., 1979). Since cysts are generally non-symptomatic and often develop early in childhood, the brain adapts to the tissue loss caused by the cyst, but in Daniel's case, we can surmise that because of its location, the cyst caused neural tissue loss that affected his early motor coordination and language development. Consequently, neurology followed Daniel to ensure the stability of the cyst. Despite his initial resistance, Daniel was also referred to our art therapy program to learn how to freely engage his motor skills using multiple art media. Daniel preferred simple media that provided optimal control such as pencil drawing. Interestingly, his behavior in art therapy was very similar to his behavior in

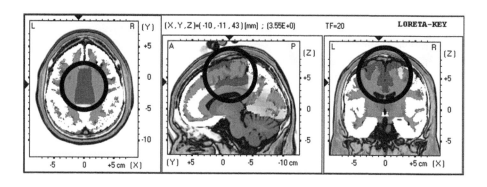

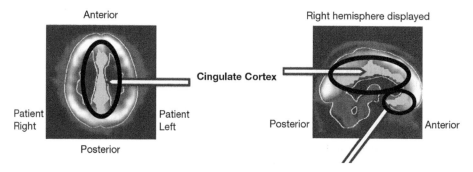

FIGURE 2.4 qEEG, excess beta, sensorimotor and dorsal cingulate regions (top right arrow) and PET, dorsal cingulate and sub-colossal regions (bottom right arrow).

Anterior

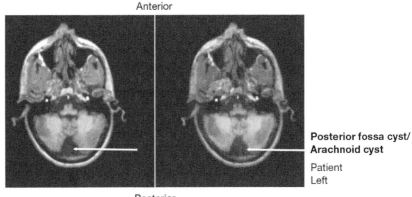

Posterior fossa cyst/
Arachnoid cyst

Patient
Right

Patient
Left

Posterior

FIGURE 2.5 MRI and PET images showing structural and functional abnormality of the medial cerebellum, the vermis (MRI, 3.5 mm arachnoid cyst); T1-MRI image on the left; co-registered, MRI and PET images on the right

psychotherapy, i.e., he would seize on an idea and struggle to extend the concept beyond his immediate experience. He strongly resisted flexible thinking, indicating that such thoughts created significant anxiety. We recognized that our suggestions to try novel approaches increased his anxiety, which increased his rigid thinking. Thus, his therapy began to focus on managing his chronic and acute anxiety and included creative writing to foster his cognitive flexibility (Gonçalves & Perrone-McGovern, 2014). For Daniel, progress was slow, but he saw a clear positive therapeutic impact. His treatment intensity decreased, and he began working in the community.

2.15   DEVELOPING A PERSON-CENTERED APPROACH/ HOLISTIC/WHOLE PERSON CARE

When we combine multimodality imaging with a detailed clinical history, subjective symptoms, clinical observation, and objective neurobehavioral assessment, we can define a patient's unique strengths and weaknesses and gain greater understanding of the person. This is the person-centered, diagnostic approach (Braš et al., 2011). Person-centered diagnostic medicine seeks more precise and effective treatments by incorporating neuroimaging within the psychological and neuropsychological paradigms. Consequently, person-centered medicine frequently confronts opposition from traditional practitioners who have received insufficient training from traditional training programs and misunderstand the relevance of objective data such as neuropsychological testing and neuroimaging. Despite this resistance, the person-centered diagnostic approach is gaining recognition.

Scientific studies that compare control groups to specific diagnostic categories often give clinicians an insufficient understanding of disorders and result in potentially generalized assumptions about a given diagnostic group, but when we carefully evaluate well-studied neurobiological disorders, such as schizophrenia, we realize the data are highly variable, as if it was collected from biologically heterogeneous populations. For example, we often accept that some individuals with schizophrenia have enlarged brain ventricles and others do not (Kašpárek et al., 2007). Despite the obvious anatomical heterogeneity, we often combine these two patient groups into one entity as though they were the same. We do this because most studies define clinical populations based solely upon symptoms, without the use of biological markers such as imaging data. It would be more useful if we defined patients based on their diagnosis as well as their objective biological findings (Kašpárek et al., 2007).

Clinicians who use the brain-to-behavior approach and assess behavioral disorders using their neurobiological underpinnings realize that individuals have significantly diverse neurobiological mechanisms that characterize their disorder, as such, any patient may defy the diagnostic categories represented in the literature.

Another current objective tool is genetic mapping that facilitates how we characterize patient groups, improves therapeutic efficacy, and potentially enhances our understanding of individual patients (Hamilton et al., 2013). In the clinic, if we combine clinical and objective imaging data, neurobehavioral evaluations, and genetic mapping, i.e., compare standardized data to well-defined normative populations, we can create personalized biological and behavioral treatments tailored to each individual patient. By using standardized approaches and sharing clinical data with facilities using electronic medical records and properly trained clinicians, we can move the field of mental health in a very new direction.

Besides informing clinicians and enhancing treatment efficacy, information generated by objective data benefits patients and their families. When we understand brain function and its relationship to behavior, we have a powerful tool for characterizing the way patients perceive their world. This type of evaluation gives the clinician, the patient, and their family a window from which to view how the patient incorporates sensory perceptions, cognitions, and emotions and on how they integrate them into their personal experience. For example, a student who has learned to compensate for unidentified visual or auditory difficulties may fail when cognitive or emotional demands are increased. As a result, he/she may experience chronic stress and exhibit aberrant adaptive behaviors. In the face of increased demand, the patient's failure may be unrelated to willingness to study, laziness, lack of interest, or motivation but rather inability to appropriately process specific information. Depending on the circumstances, when individuals experience repeated failures and are unaware of their deficits, they may develop anxiety, decreased self-worth, and, if unmanaged, depression. This process may eventually lead to dysregulation within the family system and cause conflicts, blame, distrust, and potential aggression.

In many cases, when young people face chronic stressors, they tend to reject their families and turn to their peers for support, and peers often support and utilize behaviors that acutely change an individual's state of mind and give only temporary relief. Often these behaviors focus on alcohol, illicit drug use, and eventual physical self-harm. When patients have such histories, it is important to understand the potential causes of their behaviors and symptoms. Once we identify the root causes, we can start rehabilitation and cognitive restructuring (Cicerone et al., 2011). Cognitive restructuring includes therapies such as individualized pharmacological interventions, cognitive training that capitalizes on the patient's strengths, in-depth psychotherapy that focuses on root symptoms, biofeedback, neurofeedback, family therapy, and less-structured treatments such as integrated treatments that include art therapy. These therapeutic approaches can be clearly guided by a careful person-centered approach that incorporates data from all available sources (Bryant et al., 2007).

2.16 SUMMARY

This chapter provides background for how neurons act within neuronal networks and how their interactions shape behavior. Current neuroscientific data informs us about the specificity of sensory information processing and data integration and how patients utilize these processes to initiate and sustain behaviors. Despite the brain's highly specialized neuronal circuits, we know that there are no absolutes for brain function; brain function is as unique as individuals. Clearly, the brain is a highly malleable organ capable of learning throughout our life span, but learning requires functioning distinct efficient neuronal networks. The brain establishes network dominance and plasticity by altering its structure and function in response to demands.

Newly developed neuroimaging techniques are available to clinicians and researchers and can identify and measure these changes in a living brain. Through careful study, we can observe the brain as it changes in response to maturation. By understanding maturation, we begin to appreciate brain development, particularly in early adulthood when the brain attempts to optimize its performance via increases in myelination and selective decreases in neuronal populations. We are beginning to recognize that each person develops differently through different brain processes that depend on genetics, gender, and environment. We know that genetic mutations may cause neuromodulation that results in abnormal connections and leads to aberrant, inefficient brain activity and behaviors. In addition, environmental factors, such as stress, greatly impact brain development, maturation, and the expression of vulnerabilities. Clearly, the brain's plasticity can be a double-edged sword.

With our current multimodal tools, integrated knowledge, and principles of neuromodulation, we can develop and optimize individualized therapies that help stabilize behavior and provide optimal opportunity for each patient. These therapies are predicated on our understanding the variables that underlie dysfunction. Therefore, to discover the best therapeutic course for each patient, we must prioritize our therapeutic approaches and continually evaluate the efficacy of our interventions. When we combine multimodality imaging with a detailed clinical history, subjective symptoms, clinical observation, and objective neurobehavioral assessment, we can define a patient's unique strengths and weaknesses and gain greater understanding of the person. This is the person-centered, diagnostic approach (Zimmerman et al., 2011). With this new approach in mind, we need to focus on training clinicians to have a familiarity of the whole human person, including the biology, physiology, and the ability to correlate this knowledge to behaviors. Only then can we move forward in developing and utilizing the full range of complementary or adjunct therapies. This includes art therapy, a new field that is increasingly accepted (Konopka, 2014), validated by scientific methods, and supported by subjective and objective data (Konopka et al., 2020).

The Effects of Trauma on Brain Development

Childhood brain development is critical for determining how well adult brain networks will interact and process data, i.e., *think*. During brain development, very complex, precisely organized processes cause neuronal migration into cortical and subcortical layers and the formation of appropriately connected brain regions (Hatten, 1990; Sidman & Rakic, 1973). Although we have an incomplete understanding of these developmental mechanisms, we know that developing neurons require precise biochemical and electrical inputs to ensure proper connections and functioning. At first, non-neuronal cells, glial cells, guide the individual neuronal migration. As the neocortex develops from the brain's gray matter, cells migrate to and differentiate into six distinct strata. Once the cells reach their terminus, complex dendritic connections with incoming axon projections develop in response to electrical and biochemical signals. Minutes after an axon matches with its target, the axon initiates communication, releases neurotransmitters that interact with the target's receptors, and develops fully functional synapses (Toni et al., 1999; Vicario-Abejón et al., 1998). Within the complex communication networks, chemical and electrical signals further define their roles (Heffner et al., 1990; Tessier-Lavigne & Goodman, 1996). Initially, although many neurons will die, many brain regions will have excess neurons and neuronal contacts. So, for its survival, the neuron must participate in synaptic activity and avail itself of trophic factors (proteins that support the cell's life), i.e., neurons compete for their place in the final network. As such, the network's efficiency determines the ideal neuronal numbers; excess cells will experience natural cell death or apoptosis (Paolicelli et al., 2011). This pruning allows the more active cells to develop well-defined connections based on a specific brain region's functionality. Throughout development and in addition to their initial target connections, synapses are often refined during well-defined windows of organ maturation. These critical developmental windows have been well studied in electrophysiological studies of vision, audition, and sensation, which show requirement for both intrinsic and extrinsic activity for proper development (Gogtay et al., 2004). Although these developmental stages begin before birth, cortical gray matter growth and neuronal circuit establishment are most pronounced during the early postnatal period and depend on external environmental interactions (Lohmann & Kessels, 2014), while high plasticity continues through childhood and adolescence (Tau & Peterson, 2010). Even when we consider sex-differences in brain volume, changes include progressively increased white matter volume (Lenroot & Giedd, 2006) with parallel changes in gray matter volume and density (Gennatas et al., 2017) that may reflect myelination and refinement of synapses (Gennatas et al., 2017; Lenroot & Giedd, 2006). Although recent data indicated that brain network maturation parallels maturation of brain structure and cognitive development (Le et al., 2020; Woodburn et al., 2021), various forces may drive individual differences including genetics, hormones, maturation rate, environment, gender expectations, and preferred cognitive strategies (Peper et al., 2007; Thompson et al., 2001). Through plasticity, factors such as unique personal experience, neuroplasticity, and given vulnerabilities, come together with environmental forces to influence individual development.

Because the brain adapts to its environment, brain structure is always highly responsive and readily modified by various environmental forces and genetic vulnerabilities. Significant stress can be such a factor, and each developing organism is variably vulnerable to stressors. If brain development and network organization experience severe disruption, the networks will yield to substantial cognitive and emotional dysregulation. For example, when individuals are significantly deprived of environmental input, they develop varied and significant developmental impairments. Early childhood trauma can cause neurotransmitter, hormonal, and brain circuit dysregulation in cognitive and emotional processes, which may create depression, anxiety, and PTSS (De Bellis & Zisk, 2014). Early childhood trauma correlates with alterations of the frontal cortex, cingulate, amygdala, and hippocampal gray matter (Eluvathingal et al., 2006; Jeong et al., 2021; Mehta et al., 2009), and connectivity of the corpus callosum (Eluvathingal et al., 2006; Mehta et al., 2009). These data are consistent with other studies showing that adult PTSS patients have decreased hippocampal volumes as well as decreased function (Bremner et al., 2003). Neurodevelopment is a critical process, which defines an individual's future abilities and potentials to function in adult life. Some brain dysfunctions and shortcomings may be ameliorated through therapeutic interventions.

Human Brain Imaging Methods

Besides scientific and clinical importance, there is tremendous privilege and excitement connected to exploring the live human brain. In 1924, Dr. Hans Berger, the father of clinical electroencephalography, successfully used EEG to record physiologically meaningful electrical signals from the human scalp and attempted to understand its various electrophysiological signals (Gloor, 1994). With consistent repeatable studies, he correlated observable clinical findings to the brain's potential functional mechanisms, that were verified by postmortem analyses. Although other early attempts to investigate the living human brain and correlate function with structure were driven by emerging x-ray techniques, without post-acquisition x-ray (Gawler et al., 1976), x-rays showed brain tissue as homogeneous matter. So, when clinicians wondered whether a case required surgical intervention, they were forced to use pneumoencephalography, a risky visualization technique that injected an air bolus into the cerebrospinal space (Chiro, 1964) to catch a potential glimpse of pathology. Today, computed tomography (CT) is a popular x-ray technique that uses multiple brain images enhanced by mathematical computer programs. CT is commonly used as the first step for evaluating brain injury, but CT's limited image quality and radiation exposure limits its repeated use. Now, some researchers are asking whether chronic abnormal behavior could be correlated with and explained by substantial variations in brain structure and, therefore, justify the use of objective imaging technologies for evaluating severe psychiatric disorders (Mulert & Shenton, 2014; Poprawski et al., 2007; Wahlund et al., 1992). Functional and structural imaging modalities can be used to correlate the patient's brain activity to behavior and other imaging modalities (Konopka et al., 2020; Thatcher et al., 1989). Numerous discoveries have refined our understanding of behavior by identifying the biological underpinnings for behavioral disorders. Clinical researchers published such data on patients with PTSD (Vermetten et al., 2003) and bipolar illness (Yucel et al., 2007). This section provides a short overview of techniques used to measure and image brain structure and function.

EEG

Electroencephalography (EEG) records real-time electrophysiological signals obtained from the scalp via electrodes and can be used to measure cortical and subcortical brain activity (Daly et al., 2019). Brain activity is measured as oscillations (waves) and characterized as the frequency of the oscillations (measured in Hertz, Hz, cycles per second) with specific frequencies reflecting different levels of brain activity (Figure 2.6). For instance, depending on a patient's age, electrophysiological patterns show distinct transitions from wakefulness to sleep (Carrier et al., 2001), and theta and alpha change during working memory processes (Klimesch, 1999). Gamma frequencies synchronize in consciousness and during attention (Lutz et al., 2002; Vidal et al., 2006). We can visualize EEG in 3-D by use of low-resolution brain electromagnetic tomography (LORETA). Thus, 3-D EEG data can be combined with other functional and structural imaging methods and used to identify neuronal firing frequencies that provide information about function and connectivity. Brain regions communicate through synchronizations

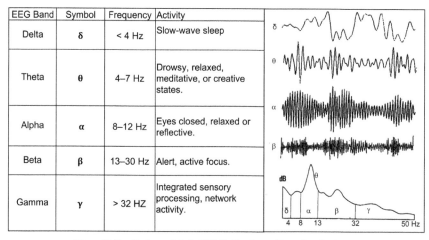

EEG Band	Symbol	Frequency	Activity
Delta	δ	< 4 Hz	Slow-wave sleep
Theta	θ	4–7 Hz	Drowsy, relaxed, meditative, or creative states.
Alpha	α	8–12 Hz	Eyes closed, relaxed or reflective.
Beta	β	13–30 Hz	Alert, active focus.
Gamma	γ	> 32 HZ	Integrated sensory processing, network activity.

Image modified from "Analyse spectrale d'un EEG.jpg" by Pierre Raymond Esteve, licensed under CC BY-SA 4.0.

FIGURE 2.6 Neuroimaging frequency bands. Image modified from "Analyse spectrale d'un EEG.jpg" by Pierre Raymond Esteve, licensed under CC BY-SA 4.0

and desynchronizations that reflect functional connectivity. Synchronized slow frequencies, such as delta, theta, and alpha-1, mostly support distant communication across brain regions. Short distance communications are primarily dependent on higher beta frequencies (von Stein et al., 2000).

While patients perform specified tasks during a qEEG, evoked potentials reveal the brain's response to those tasks. During the recording, the task's components and timing are precisely marked for analysis. Averaging numerous responses differentiates random brain activity from the signal generated from purposeful tasks. Evoked potentials can be used to record the activities of sensory systems and cognition. Of greatest interest is the evaluation of cognitive evoked potentials, which are either visual or auditory with positivity at 300 ms, the P300. The P300 reflects how well the patient sustains attention during a task specifically oriented to an infrequent stimulus (Polich & Kok, 1995). A significant body of literature supports the use of these tools for evaluating cognition (Polich & Corey-Bloom, 2005). Clinical evoked potentials enhance our understanding of a patient's electrophysiological capacity to process information. They are very powerful, especially when correlated with other tests that engage similar networks. The differences between auditory and visual evoked potential results may correlate with behavioral findings. This information may indicate that an individual prefers learning in one specific modality (Konopka et al., 2020). Consequently, we can modify the patient's learning paradigm to adopt novel strategies that eliminate the learning bias (Duffy, 2005).

Quantitative EEG

Quantitative EEG (qEEG) expands traditional EEG methods by post-acquisition processing and statistical analyses that allows clinicians to compare an individual's cortical EEG patterns to those of age-matched controls in a normative database (Prichep, 2005). qEEG is a relatively inexpensive, readily available, noninvasive, reproducible, simple, stable, and flexible technique, but it requires significant training to optimize its use. The encephalographer must evaluate signal validity, identify specific focally abnormal EEG patterns and events, and analyze and interpret the statistical data to understand their significance in order to make suggestions for treatment or additional assessment. Furthermore, qEEG data are very sensitive to artifacts that can be easily misinterpreted by individuals who are not well versed in this technology. It is crucial that the interpreter understand the difference between the expected EEG patterns of various brain states and artifacts generated by movements such as eye blinks, swallowing, yawning, generalized muscle tension around the face and neck, and states of drowsiness. In some individuals, electrocardiogram artifacts can be clearly seen in the EEG signal and may be misinterpreted as a brain event. In addition, before the data are interpreted and submitted for statistical analysis, the clinician must be aware of the patient's medications and state of alertness. Poor sleep may impact the outcomes.

To help determine the anatomical regions active during qEEG recordings, we can combine qEEG with other imaging modalities, such as structural (MRI) and functional (PET) imaging (see below). By using independent imaging methods, we can better interpret how deviations converge across modalities and, by doing so, focus on specific abnormal brain structures and how they relate to behavior. Then, we can surmise the specific cortical and sub-cortical brain networks that produce specific findings reflected in aberrant behaviors (Chennamchetty et al., 2009; Poprawski et al., 2007). With converging independent imaging data, we can prioritize and correlate the identified brain regions to functional networks, link them to clinical symptoms, and use the data to guide us in the development of data-driven interventions (Boutros et al., 2008; Konopka et al., 2020).

Extensions of qEEG technology include electrical source localization using LORETA (Konopka & Poprawski, 2008) which allows identification of the anatomical source of electrical activity, extraction of statistically significant abnormal EEG activity, and mapping of the activity on a standardized MRI atlas (Pascual-Marqui, 1997). qEEG is also used to develop discriminant functions that characterize the electrical patterns found within specific patient populations. One example of such a function is the mild traumatic brain index (mTBI) developed by Robert Thatcher (Thatcher et al., 1989). mTBI, a commercial qEEG method using available statistical techniques to compare a patient's EEG patterns to the patterns within the database of individuals, who have had verifiable traumatic brain injuries, discerns the likelihood that the patient suffered traumatic brain injury and the severity of their injury. Because imaging methods, such as CT and MRI, often miss deficits that are primarily functional (Andreasen, 1988; Hollister & Boutros, 1991), mTBI gives clinicians an objective way to evaluate patients who complain of cognitive deficits, mood dysregulation, loss of function and who, according to standardized structural imaging, lack clear evidence of injury. Although clinically, discriminant function mTBI analysis, in parallel with other clinical and neurobehavioral data, can support or call into question the possibility of malingering (Thatcher et al., 1998), variables, such as medications or illicit drugs, may produce false negative or positive results. Thus, when interpreting functional imaging data, we must consider the patient's medication status (Konopka & Zimmerman, 2014). In summary, when compared to normal controls and a well-defined patient population, qEEG can inform us about abnormal brain activity. Combining structural and functional imaging can also highlight possible structural deficits underlying neuronal dysregulation and may elucidate potential contributing factors of specific impairments or symptoms. It remains critical that EEG, qEEG research, and clinical activities must utilize highly trained, skilled professionals with a thorough understanding of clinical neurophysiology, pharmacology, and behavior.

Magnetic Resonance Imaging

Magnetic resonance imaging (MRI) provides high resolution anatomical images of the brain's gray matter, white matter, and cerebrospinal fluid, without the exposure to x-ray radiation associated with CT scanning. Therefore, clinicians can easily recognize the brain's different structures, measure the brain's total volume relative to individual structures, and assess whether the structural integrity and volume are appropriate for age and gender. Consequently, one can objectively identify the structural differences that may inform us about cognitive and/or emotional difficulty and enhance clinical understanding of disorders. In addition, after therapeutic intervention, volumetric brain imaging can aid in evaluating therapeutic effectiveness and impact on brain regions by showing tissue volume recovery (de Lange et al., 2008).

Blood-oxygen level dependent MRI

In addition to structural brain imaging, MRI principles can be used for various functional imaging techniques. One such technique, blood-oxygen level dependent (BOLD) MRI, correlates brain blood flow and changes in blood oxygenation as an indirect measure of increases in regional neuronal activity. For example, a technique like evoked potentials, BOLD-MRI allows one to compare the brain's resting activity to its activity during specific tasks. These studies have begun to identify specific interpretive brain regions and advance our understanding of the brain deficits related to symptoms. Despite its strengths, BOLD-MRI wrestles with data acquisition because a patient must engage in a mental task while restricted and lying motionless within the MRI camera. This limits BOLD-MRI for use in compliant patients, who are not suffering from overwhelming emotional dysregulation. This technique is also disadvantaged by its neurobiological underpinnings: this method measures the blood-flow changes that occur as the result of neuronal electrical activity, and neuronal electrical activity is generally measured in milliseconds, while blood perfusion changes are 1000 times slower. Therefore, BOLD is an indirect measure of neuronal activity unlike evoked potentials (Schridde et al., 2007). Despite these shortcomings, research using the resting state BOLD paradigm resulted in significant advances and discovery of functioning networks, e.g., the default mode network (DMN). Currently, this is not a clinically used method.

MRI Spectroscopy and Diffusion Tensor Imaging (DTI)

Magnetic resonance can also detect the brain's biochemical make-up (Kato et al., 1991) with a technique called MRI spectroscopy (MRS) that uses magnetic fields to identify the unique characteristics of specific molecules. Since molecules have unique profiles, this method can image a specific regional focus, evaluate its biochemical make-up, clarify the integrity or pathology of a given brain area, and track its neuroplasticity. For instance, after patients received surgery for a seizure disorder, the MRS showed recovery of the contralateral hippocampal tissue (Vermathen et al., 2002). MRS can also elucidate existing abnormalities and effectively track specific biochemical changes that occur because of therapy and provide evidence for interpretating therapeutic efficacy (Renshaw et al., 1992). Nevertheless, because the current MRS methods lack standardization and data processing, spectroscopy has limited clinical use.

Another magnetic resonance technique, Diffusion Tensor Imaging (DTI), evaluates the water molecules within axons and identifies the integrity of primary myelinated axonal brain pathways that connect brain regions (Assaf & Pasternak, 2007). This method combined with evoked potentials provides a better understanding of network's structural and functional relationships.

Single photon computed tomography (SPECT) and positron emission tomography (PET)

Two other functional imaging methods, single photon computed tomography (SPECT) and positron emission tomography (PET), use specialized cameras to view specific radioactive tracer molecules, such as neurotransmitter molecules with radioactive tags. The tracer is injected into a patient's vein, tracked while it circulates through all the body's organs, and then imaged. Specific tracers are chosen depending on whether they are being used to evaluate the brain's glucose metabolism, oxygen utilization, blood flow, or the abundance or absence of specific cellular receptor-types and proteins related to the patient's symptoms. For example, patients who have substance addictions may have more dysregulated dopamine receptors than controls (Volkow et al., 1993). Also, competitive binding studies can unveil the available receptors in a specified brain region to help evaluate the effects of medication (Farde et al., 1995) or image beta amyloid proteins in dementia. Nevertheless, nuclear medicine studies are complicated because they require specialized personnel and equipment and small doses of radiation. Furthermore, the half-life of radioactive tracers dictate the study design and determine the time of administration and scanning. Although radiation exposure is ethically debatable for scientific inquiry, these techniques are clearly appropriate diagnostic tools that help select the best therapeutic methods for many medical conditions (Henderson et al., 2020).

Magnetoencephalography

A less common method that records magnetic fields from the brain's surface is called magnetoencephalography (MEG) (Kim & Davis, 2021). Although MEG exploits the neuronal electrical properties that generate magnetic fields undistorted by biological tissues, such as bone, this technique requires expensive instrumentation and a specialized electrically insulated environment. Also, as with MRI, the patient must remain very still during the recording. Although much of the current MEG data show that MEG results are very similar to EEG (Cohen & Cuffin, 1983) and that the two techniques often complement each other, the cost of equipment and maintenance and the restrictive patient recording positions make MEG practical only in research settings (Henson et al., 2009).

Summary

There is significant need to objectively evaluate patients' ability to process information in different domains and to objectively evaluate brain function using measures standardized in non-pathological populations with precisely defined ages, gender, education, and established cross-cultural norms. Ideally, the tools used in such an endeavor would be easily administered, reliable for evaluations, and readily accessible to clinicians and researchers.

With recently advanced computational power and the availability of commercial software, a new positive trend has developed in behavioral testing that taps into specific brain networks and allows for computer-based behavioral evaluations supported by imaging studies that can reflect the function of underlying brain networks. This approach allows clinicians and researchers to evaluate and track a patient's progress or decline with noninvasive readily available scientifically validated measures (Hampshire et al., 2012). The strength of these tools lies in their ability to provide standardized clinical protocols, continuously collect data, adjust to the novel demands of clinical practice, and provide automated data analysis directly to clinicians. This provides practitioners, from all behavioral health disciplines, a chance to probe brain function with noninvasive, objective, neurocognitive behavioral tools, and consequently, familiarize themselves with the neuroscientific basis of behavior, develop more specific treatment methods, and evaluate the efficacy of their therapeutics.

REFERENCES

Aarts, J. H. P., Binne, C. D., Smit, A. M., & Wilkins, A. J. (1984). Selective cognitive impairment during focal and generalized epileptiform EEG activity. *Brain*, *107*(1), 293–308. https://doi.org/10.1093/brain/107.1.293

Alves, P. N., Foulon, C., Karolis, V., Bzdok, D., Margulies, D. S., Volle, E., & Thiebaut de Schotten, M. (2019). An improved neuroanatomical model of the default-mode network reconciles previous neuroimaging and neuropathological findings. *Communications Biology*, *2*(1), Article 1. https://doi.org/10.1038/s42003-019-0611-3

Anand, A., Li, Y., Wang, Y., Wu, J., Gao, S., Bukhari, L., Mathews, V., Kalnin, A., & Lowe, M. (2005). Activity and connectivity of brain mood regulating circuit in depression: A functional magnetic resonance study. *Biological Psychiatry*, *57*, 1079–1088. https://doi.org/10.1016/j.biopsych.2005.02.021

Andersen, S. L., & Teicher, M. H. (2000). Sex differences in dopamine receptors and their relevance to ADHD. *Neuroscience and Biobehavioral Reviews*, *24*(1), 137–141. https://doi.org/10.1016/s0149-7634(99)00044-5

Andreasen, N. C. (1988). Brain imaging: Applications in psychiatry. *Science*, *239*(4846), 1381–1388. https://doi.org/10.1126/science.3279509

Andrews-Hanna, J. R., Smallwood, J., & Spreng, R. N. (2014). The default network and self-generated thought: Component processes, dynamic control, and clinical relevance. *Annals of the New York Academy of Sciences*, *1316*, 29–52. https://doi.org/10.1111/nyas.12360

Aron, A. R. (2007). The neural basis of inhibition in cognitive control. *The Neuroscientist: A Review Journal Bringing Neurobiology, Neurology and Psychiatry*, *13*(3), 214–228. https://doi.org/10.1177/1073858407299288

Assaf, Y., & Pasternak, O. (2007). Diffusion tensor imaging (DTI)-based white matter mapping in brain research: A review. *Journal of Molecular Neuroscience*, *34*(1), 51–61. https://doi.org/10.1007/s12031-007-0029-0

Bassett, D. S., & Sporns, O. (2017). Network neuroscience. *Nature Neuroscience*, *20*(3), Article 3. https://doi.org/10.1038/nn.4502

Binnewijzend, M. A. A., Schoonheim, M. M., Sanz-Arigita, E., Wink, A. M., van der Flier, W. M., Tol-boom, N., Adriaanse, S. M., Damoiseaux, J. S., Scheltens, P., van Berckel, B. N. M., & Barkhof, F. (2012). Resting-state fMRI changes in Alzheimer's disease and mild cognitive impairment. *Neurobiology of Aging, 33*(9), 2018–2028. https://doi.org/10.1016/j.neurobiolaging.2011.07.003

Boutros, N. N., Thatcher, R. W., & Galderisi, S. (2008). *Electrodiagnostic techniques in neuropsychiatry.* In S. C. Yudofsky & R. E. Hales (Eds.), *The American Psychiatric Publishing textbook of neuropsychiatry and behavioral neurosciences* (5th ed., pp. 189–213). American Psychiatric Publishing.

Braš, M., Dorđević, V., Milunović, V., Brajković, L., Miličić, D., & Konopka, L. (2011). Person-centered medicine versus personalized medicine: Is it just a sophism? A view from chronic pain management. *Psychiatria Danubina, 23*(3), 246–250.

Bremner, J. D., Vythilingam, M., Vermetten, E., Southwick, S. M., McGlashan, T., Nazeer, A., Khan, S., Vaccarino, L. V., Soufer, R., Garg, P. K., Ng, C. K., Staib, L. H., Duncan, J. S., & Charney, D. S. (2003). MRI and PET study of deficits in hippocampal structure and function in women with childhood sexual abuse and posttraumatic stress disorder. *American Journal of Psychiatry, 160*(5), 924–932. https://doi.org/10.1176/appi.ajp.160.5.924

Bryant, R. A., Felmingham, K., Kemp, A., Das, P., Hughes, G., Peduto, A., & Williams, L. (2007). Amygdala and ventral anterior cingulate activation predicts treatment response to cognitive behaviour therapy for post-traumatic stress disorder. *Psychological Medicine, 38*(4), 555–561. https://doi.org/10.1017/s0033291707002231

Bullmore, E., & Sporns, O. (2009). Complex brain networks: Graph theoretical analysis of structural and functional systems. *Nature Reviews Neuroscience, 10*(3), 186–198. https://doi.org/10.1038/nrn2575

Carrier, J., Land, S., Buysse, D. J., Kupfer, D. J., & Monk, T. H. (2001). The effects of age and gender on sleep EEG power spectral density in the middle years of life (ages 20–60 years old). *Psychophysiology, 38*(2), 232–242.

Chennamchetty, V. N., Poprawski, T. J., Crayton, J. W., Hamilton, E. A., & Konopka, L. M. (2009). Compulsive hoarding in an older adult with aggression, delusions and memory loss: A multi-modality neuroimaging study. *Activitas Nervosa Superior, 51*(1), 6–11. https://doi.org/10.1007/bf03379920

Chiro, G. D. (1964). New Radiographic and Isotopic Procedures in Neurological Diagnosis. *JAMA, 188*(6). https://doi.org/10.1001/jama.1964.03060320046011

Cicerone, K. D., Langenbahn, D. M., Braden, C., Malec, J. F., Kalmar, K., Fraas, M., Felicetti, T., Laatsch, L., Harley, J. P., Bergquist, T., Azulay, J., Cantor, J., & Ashman, T. (2011). Evidence-based cognitive rehabilitation: Updated review of the literature from 2003 through 2008. *Archives of Physical Medicine and Rehabilitation, 92*(4), 519–530. https://doi.org/10.1016/j.apmr.2010.11.015

Cohen, D., & Cuffin, B. N. (1983). Demonstration of useful differences between magnetoencephalo-gram and electroencephalogram. *Electroencephalography and Clinical Neurophysiology, 56*(1), 38–51. https://doi.org/10.1016/0013-4694(83)90005-6

Cohen, R. M., Nordahl, T. E., Semple, W. E., Andreason, P., & Pickar, D. (1998). Abnormalities in the distributed network of sustained attention predict neuroleptic treatment response in schizo-phrenia. *Neuropsychopharmacology, 19*, 36–47. https://doi.org/10.1016/S0893-133X(97)00201-7

Curtis, C. E., & D'Esposito, M. (2003). Persistent activity in the prefrontal cortex during work-ing memory. *Trends in Cognitive Sciences, 7*(9), 415–423. https://doi.org/10.1016/S1364-6613(03)00197-9

D'Esposito, M. (2007). From cognitive to neural models of working memory. *Philosophical Trans-actions of the Royal Society of London. Series B, Biological Sciences, 362*(1481), 761–772. https://doi.org/10.1098/rstb.2007.2086

Daly, I., Williams, D., Hwang, F., Kirke, A., Miranda, E. R., & Nasuto, S. J. (2019). Electroencephalogra-phy reflects the activity of sub-cortical brain regions during approach-withdrawal behaviour while listening to music. *Scientific Reports, 9*(1), Article 1. https://doi.org/10.1038/s41598-019-45105-2

Dan, Y., & Poo, M. (2004). Spike timing-dependent plasticity of neural circuits. *Neuron, 44*(1), 23–30. https://doi.org/10.1016/j.neuron.2004.09.007

De Bellis, M. D., & Zisk, A. B. (2014). The biological effects of childhood trauma. *Child and Adolescent Psychiatric Clinics of North America, 23*(2), 185–222. https://doi.org/10.1016/j.chc.2014.01.002

de Lange, F. P., Koers, A., Kalkman, J. S., Bleijenberg, G., Hagoort, P., van der Meer, J. W. M., & Toni, I. (2008). Increase in prefrontal cortical volume following cognitive behavioural therapy in patients with chronic fatigue syndrome. *Brain: A Journal of Neurology, 131*(Pt 8), 2172–2180. https://doi.org/10.1093/brain/awn140

Devi, Y., Khan, S., Rana, P., Dhandapani, M., Ghai, S., Gopichandran, L., Dhandapani, S., & Deepak. (2020). Cognitive, behavioral, and functional impairments among traumatic brain injury survivors: Impact on caregiver burden. *Journal of Neurosciences in Rural Practice, 11*(4), 629–635. https://doi.org/10.1055/s-0040-1716777

Eluvathingal, T. J., Chugani, H. T., Behen, M. E., Juhász, C., Muzik, O., Maqbool, M., Chugani, D. C., & Makki, M. (2006). Abnormal brain connectivity in children after early severe socioemotional deprivation: A diffusion tensor imaging study. *Pediatrics, 117*(6), 2093–2100. https://doi.org/10.1542/peds.2005-1727

Fair, D. A., Cohen, A. L., Dosenbach, N. U. F., Church, J. A., Miezin, F. M., Barch, D. M., Raichle, M. E., Petersen, S. E., & Schlaggar, B. L. (2008). The maturing architecture of the brain's default network. *Proceedings of the National Academy of Sciences of the United States of America, 105*(10), 4028–4032. https://doi.org/10.1073/pnas.0800376105

Farde, L., Nyberg, S., Oxenstierna, G., Nakashima, Y., Halldin, C., & Ericcson, B. (1995). Positron emission tomography studies on D2 and 5-HT2 receptor binding in risperidone-treated schizophrenic patients. *Journal of Clinical Psychopharmacology, 15*, 19S–23S. https://doi.org/10.1097/00004714-199502001-00004

Fink, M., Wadsak, W., Savli, M., Stein, P., Moser, U., Hahn, A., Mien, L.-K., Kletter, K., Mitterhauser, M., Kasper, S., & Lanzenberger, R. (2009). Lateralization of the serotonin-1A receptor distribution in language areas revealed by PET. *NeuroImage, 45*(2), 598–605. https://doi.org/10.1016/j.neuroimage.2008.11.033

Finlayson, M. A. J., & Reitan, R. M. (1976). Handedness in relation to measures of motor and tactile-perceptual functions in normal children. *Perceptual and Motor Skills, 43*(2), 475–481. https://doi.org/10.2466/pms.1976.43.2.475

Fitzgerald, P. J. (2012). Whose side are you on: Does serotonin preferentially activate the right hemisphere and norepinephrine the left? *Medical Hypotheses, 79*(2), 250–254. https://doi.org/10.1016/j.mehy.2012.05.001

Fritzsche, M. (2003). The origin of brain asymmetry and its psychotic reversal. *Medical Hypotheses, 60*(4), 468–480. https://doi.org/10.1016/s0306-9877(02)00376-6

Gawler, J., Boulay, G. H. D., Bull, J. W., & Marshall, J. (1976). Computerized tomography (the EMI Scanner): A comparison with pneumoencephalography and ventriculography. *Journal of Neurology, Neurosurgery and Psychiatry, 39*(3), 203–211. https://doi.org/10.1136/jnnp.39.3.203

Gennatas, E. D., Avants, B. B., Wolf, D. H., Satterthwaite, T. D., Ruparel, K., Ciric, R., Hakonarson, H., Gur, R. E., & Gur, R. C. (2017). Age-related effects and sex differences in gray matter density, volume, mass, and cortical thickness from childhood to young adulthood. *Journal of Neuroscience, 37*(20), 5065–5073. https://doi.org/10.1523/JNEUROSCI.3550-16.2017

Geschwind, N., & Levitsky, W. (1968). Human brain: Left–right asymmetries in temporal speech region. *Science, 161*(3837), 186–187. https://doi.org/10.1126/science.161.3837.186

Gibson, C., & Bryden, M. P. (1983). Dichhaptic recognition of shapes and letters in children. *Canadian Journal of Psychology/Revue Canadienne de Psychologie, 37*(1), 132–143. https://doi.org/10.1037/h0080693

Gloor, P. (1994). Berger lecture. Is Berger's dream coming true? *Electroencephalography and Clinical Neurophysiology, 90*(4), 253–266. https://doi.org/10.1016/0013-4694(94)90143-0

Gogtay, N., Giedd, J. N., Lusk, L., Hayashi, K. M., Greenstein, D., Vaituzis, A. C., Nugent, T. F., Herman, D. H., Clasen, L. S., Toga, A. W., Rapoport, J. L., & Thompson, P. M. (2004). Dynamic mapping of human cortical development during childhood through early adulthood. *Proceedings of the National Academy of Sciences, 101*(21), 8174–8179. https://doi.org/10.1073/pnas.0402680101

Gonçalves, Ó. F., & Perrone-McGovern, K. M. (2014). A neuroscience agenda for counseling psychology research. *Journal of Counseling Psychology, 61*(4), 507–512. https://doi.org/10.1037/cou0000026

Grabner, R. H., Neubauer, A. C., & Stern, E. (2006). Superior performance and neural efficiency: The impact of intelligence and expertise. *Brain Research Bulletin, 69*(4), 422–439. https://doi.org/10.1016/j.brainresbull.2006.02.009

Greicius, M. D., Srivastava, G., Reiss, A. L., & Menon, V. (2004). Default-mode network activity distinguishes Alzheimer's disease from healthy aging: Evidence from functional MRI. *Proceedings of the National Academy of Sciences of the United States of America, 101*(13), 4637–4642. https://doi.org/10.1073/pnas.0308627101

Hamilton, D. V., Konopka, C. J., & Konopka, L. M. (2013). *Integrating pharmacogenomic and functional neurophysiological analyses: Homozygous COMT genotypes and associated quantitative electroencephalographic findings*. 9th Congress of the International Neuropsychiatric Association, Chicago, IL, USA.

Hampshire, A., Highfield, R. R., Parkin, B. L., & Owen, A. M. (2012). Fractionating human intelligence. *Neuron, 76*(6), 1225–1237. https://doi.org/10.1016/j.neuron.2012.06.022

Hatten, M. E. (1990). Riding the glial monorail: A common mechanism for glialguided neuronal migration in different regions of the developing mammalian brain. *Trends in Neurosciences, 13*(5), 179–184. https://doi.org/10.1016/0166-2236(90)90044-b

He, Y., & Evans, A. (2010). Graph theoretical modeling of brain connectivity. *Current Opinion in Neurology, 23*(4), 341–350. https://doi.org/10.1097/wco.0b013e32833aa567

Heath, R. G., Franklin, D. E., & Shraberg, D. (1979). Gross pathology of the cerebellum in patients diagnosed and treated as functional psychiatric disorders. *The Journal of Nervous and Mental Disease, 167*(10), 585–592. https://doi.org/10.1097/00005053-197910000-00001

Hebb, A. O., & Ojemann, G. A. (2013). The thalamus and language revisited. *Brain and Language, 126*(1), 99–108. https://doi.org/10.1016/j.bandl.2012.06.010

Heffner, C. D., Lumsden, A. G. S., & O'Leary, D. D. M. (1990). Target control of collateral extension and directional axon growth in the mammalian brain. *Science, 247*(4939), 217–220. https://doi.org/10.1126/science.2294603

Henderson, T. A., van Lierop, M. J., McLean, M., Uszler, J. M., Thornton, J. F., Siow, Y.-H., Pavel, D. G., Cardaci, J., & Cohen, P. (2020). Functional neuroimaging in psychiatry—aiding in diagnosis and guiding treatment: What the American Psychiatric Association does not know. *Frontiers in Psychiatry, 11*. www.frontiersin.org/articles/10.3389/fpsyt.2020.00276

Henson, R. N., Mouchlianitis, E., & Friston, K. J. (2009). MEG and EEG data fusion: Simultaneous localisation of face-evoked responses. *NeuroImage, 47*(2), 581–589. https://doi.org/10.1016/j.neuroimage.2009.04.063

Hofman, J., Hutny, M., Sztuba, K., & Paprocka, J. (2020). Corpus callosum agenesis: An insight into the etiology and spectrum of symptoms. *Brain Sciences, 10*(9), 625. https://doi.org/10.3390/brainsci10090625

Hollister, L. E., & Boutros, N. (1991). Clinical use of CT and MR scans in psychiatric patients. *Journal of Psychiatry and Neuroscience, 16*(4), 194–198.

Holtzman, D. M., & Mobley, W. C. (1994). Neurotrophic factors and neurologic disease. *Western Journal of Medicine, 161*(3), 246–254.

Iseki, K., Ikeda, A., Kihara, T., Kawamoto, Y., Mezaki, T., Hanakawa, T., Hashikawa, K., Fukuyama, H., & Shibasaki, H. (2009). Impairment of the cortical GABAergic inhibitory system in catatonic stupor: A case report with neuroimaging. *Epileptic Disorders, 11*(2), 126–131. https://doi.org/10.1684/epd.2009.0257

Jeong, H. J., Durham, E. L., Moore, T. M., Dupont, R. M., McDowell, M., Cardenas-Iniguez, C., Micciche, E. T., Berman, M. G., Lahey, B. B., & Kaczkurkin, A. N. (2021). The association between latent trauma and brain structure in children. *Translational Psychiatry, 11*(1), Article 1. https://doi.org/10.1038/s41398-021-01357-z

Jovasevic, V., Corcoran, K. A., Leaderbrand, K., Yamawaki, N., Guedea, A. L., Chen, H. J., Shepherd, G. M. G., & Radulovic, J. (2015). GABAergic mechanisms regulated by miR-33 encode state-dependent fear. *Nature Neuroscience*, *18*(9), Article 9. https://doi.org/10.1038/nn.4084

Kandel, E. R. (2001). The molecular biology of memory storage: A dialogue between genes and synapses. *Science*, *294*(5544), 1030–1038. https://doi.org/10.1126/science.1067020

Kandel, E. R., Koester, J. D., Mack, S. H., & Siegelbaum, S. A. (2021). *Principles of Neural Science, 6e* (6th ed.). McGraw Hill. https://neurology.mhmedical.com/book.aspx?bookID=3024

Kašpárek, T., Přikryl, R., Mikl, M., Schwarz, D., Češková, E., & Krupa, P. (2007). Prefrontal but not temporal grey matter changes in males with first-episode schizophrenia. *Progress in Neuro-Psychopharmacology and Biological Psychiatry*, *31*(1), 151–157. https://doi.org/10.1016/j.pnpbp.2006.08.011

Kato, T., Shioiri, T., Takahashi, S., & Inubushi, T. (1991). Measurement of brain phosphoinositide metabolism in bipolar patients using in vivo 31P-MRS. *Journal of Affective Disorders*, *22*(4), 185–190. https://doi.org/10.1016/0165-0327(91)90064-y

Kennedy, S. H., Evans, K. R., Krüger, S., Mayberg, H. S., Meyer, J. H., McCann, S., Arifuzzman, A. I., Houle, S., & Vaccarino, F. J. (2001). Changes in regional brain glucose metabolism measured with positron emission tomography after paroxetine treatment of major depression. *American Journal of Psychiatry*, *158*(6), 899–905. https://doi.org/10.1176/appi.ajp.158.6.899

Kim, H. (2012). A dual-subsystem model of the brain's default network: Self-referential processing, memory retrieval processes, and autobiographical memory retrieval. *NeuroImage*, *61*, 966–977. https://doi.org/10.1016/j.neuroimage.2012.03.025

Kim, J. A., & Davis, K. D. (2021). Magnetoencephalography: Physics, techniques, and applications in the basic and clinical neurosciences. *Journal of Neurophysiology*, *125*(3), 938–956. https://doi.org/10.1152/jn.00530.2020

Kimura, D. (1967). Functional asymmetry of the brain in dichotic listening. *Cortex*, *3*(2), 163–178. https://doi.org/10.1016/s0010-9452(67)80010-8

King, J. (2016). *Art therapy and palliative care*. PowerPoint presentation. https://scholarworks.iupui.edu/handle/1805/13689

King, J. L., & Chattterjee, A. (2024). Art therapy, psychology, and neuroscience: A timely convergence. In R. Fleming (Ed.), *Music and Mind*. Viking Books.

Klimesch, W. (1999). EEG alpha and theta oscillations reflect cognitive and memory performance: A review and analysis. *Brain Research Reviews*, *29*(2–3), 169–195. https://doi.org/10.1016/s0165-0173(98)00056-3

Koechlin, E., & Summerfield, C. (2007). An information theoretical approach to prefrontal executive function. *Trends in Cognitive Sciences*, *11*(6), 229–235. https://doi.org/10.1016/j.tics.2007.04.005

Koeda, T., Knyazeva, M., Njiokiktjien, C., Jonkman, E. J., Sonneville, L. D., & Vildavsky, V. (1995). The EEG in acallosal children. Coherence values in the resting state: Left hemisphere compensatory mechanism? *Electroencephalography and Clinical Neurophysiology*, *95*(6), 397–407. https://doi.org/10.1016/0013-4694(95)00171-9

Konopka, L. M. (2014). Where art meets neuroscience: A new horizon of art therapy. *Croatian Medical Journal*, *55*(1), 73–74. https://doi.org/10.3325/cmj.2014.55.73

Konopka, L. M., & Poprawski, T. J. (2008). Quantitative EEG studies of attention disorders and mood disorders in children. In *Sleep and psychiatric disorders in children and adolescents* (pp. 309–320). CRC Press.

Konopka, L. M., & Zimmerman, E. M. (2014). Neurofeedback and psychopharmacology. In *Clinical Neurotherapy* (pp. 55–84). Elsevier. https://doi.org/10.1016/b978-0-12-396988-0.00003-9

Konopka, L. M., Glowacki, A., Konopka, C. J., & Wuest, R. (2020). Objective assessments in diagnoses and treatment: A proposed change in paradigm. *Clinical EEG and Neuroscience*, *52*(2), 90–97. https://doi.org/10.1177/1550059420983998

Konopka, L. M., Glowacki, A., Konopka, C. J., & Wuest, R. (2020). Objective assessments in diagnoses and treatment: A proposed change in paradigm. *Clinical EEG and Neuroscience*, *52*(2), 90–97. https://doi.org/10.1177/1550059420983998

Kühn, A. A., Kupsch, A., Schneider, G.-H., & Brown, P. (2006). Reduction in subthalamic 8-35\ hspace1emHz oscillatory activity correlates with clinical improvement in Parkinson's disease. *European Journal of Neuroscience, 23*(7), 1956–1960. https://doi.org/10.1111/j.1460-9568.2006.04717.x

Le, T. M., Huang, A. S., O'Rawe, J., & Leung, H.-C. (2020). Functional neural network configuration in late childhood varies by age and cognitive state. *Developmental Cognitive Neuroscience, 45*, 100862. https://doi.org/10.1016/j.dcn.2020.100862

Lehnertz, K., Bialonski, S., Horstmann, M.-T., Krug, D., Rothkegel, A., Staniek, M., & Wagner, T. (2009). Synchronization phenomena in human epileptic brain networks. *Journal of Neuroscience Methods, 183*(1), 42–48. https://doi.org/10.1016/j.jneumeth.2009.05.015

Lenroot, R. K., & Giedd, J. N. (2006). Brain development in children and adolescents: Insights from anatomical magnetic resonance imaging. *Neuroscience & Biobehavioral Reviews, 30*(6), 718–729. https://doi.org/10.1016/j.neubiorev.2006.06.001

Levy, J., & Trevarthen, C. (1977). Perceptual, semantic and phonetic aspects of elementary language processes in split-brain patients. *Brain, 100*(1), 105–118. https://doi.org/10.1093/brain/100.1.105

Lewis, C. M., Baldassarre, A., Committeri, G., Romani, G. L., & Corbetta, M. (2009). Learning sculpts the spontaneous activity of the resting human brain. *Proceedings of the National Academy of Sciences, 106*(41), 17558–17563. https://doi.org/10.1073/pnas.0902455106

Lieb, J. P., Hoque, K., Skomer, C. E., & Song, X.-W. (1987). Inter-hemispheric propagation of human mesial temporal lobe seizures: A coherence/phase analysis. *Electroencephalography and Clinical Neurophysiology, 67*(2), 101–119. https://doi.org/10.1016/0013-4694(87)90033-2

Lohmann, C., & Kessels, H. W. (2014). The developmental stages of synaptic plasticity. *The Journal of Physiology, 592*(Pt 1), 13–31. https://doi.org/10.1113/jphysiol.2012.235119

Lovero, K. L., Simmons, A. N., Aron, J. L., & Paulus, M. P. (2009). Anterior insular cortex anticipates impending stimulus significance. *NeuroImage, 45*(3), 976–983. https://doi.org/10.1016/j.neuroimage.2008.12.070

Lutz, A., Lachaux, J.-P., Martinerie, J., & Varela, F. J. (2002). Guiding the study of brain dynamics by using first-person data: Synchrony patterns correlate with ongoing conscious states during a simple visual task. *Proceedings of the National Academy of Sciences, 99*(3), 1586–1591. https://doi.org/10.1073/pnas.032658199

Makino, Y., Polygalov, D., Bolaños, F., Benucci, A., & McHugh, T. J. (2019). Physiological signature of memory age in the prefrontal-hippocampal circuit. *Cell Reports, 29*(12), 3835–3846.e5. https://doi.org/10.1016/j.celrep.2019.11.075

Markett, S., Nothdurfter, D., Focsa, A., Reuter, M., & Jawinski, P. (2022). Attention networks and the intrinsic network structure of the human brain. *Human Brain Mapping, 43*(4), 1431–1448. https://doi.org/10.1002/hbm.25734

Martinowich, K., Manji, H., & Lu, B. (2007). New insights into BDNF function in depression and anxiety. *Nature Neuroscience, 10*(9), 1089–1093. https://doi.org/10.1038/nn1971

Mehta, M. A., Golembo, N. I., Nosarti, C., Colvert, E., Mota, A., Williams, S. C. R., Rutter, M., & Sonuga-Barke, E. J. S. (2009). Amygdala, hippocampal and corpus callosum size following severe early institutional deprivation: The English and Romanian Adoptees Study Pilot. *Journal of Child Psychology and Psychiatry, 50*(8), 943–951. https://doi.org/10.1111/j.1469-7610.2009.02084.x

Menon, V., & D'Esposito, M. (2022). The role of PFC networks in cognitive control and executive function. *Neuropsychopharmacology, 47*(1), Article 1. https://doi.org/10.1038/s41386-021-01152-w

Menon, V., & Uddin, L. Q. (2010). Saliency, switching, attention and control: A network model of insula function. *Brain Structure & Function, 214*(5–6), 655–667. https://doi.org/10.1007/s00429-010-0262-0

Morton, B. E. (2020). Brain executive laterality and hemisity. *Personality Neuroscience, 3*, e10. https://doi.org/10.1017/pen.2020.6

Mulert, C., & Shenton, M. E. (Eds.) (2014). *MRI in Psychiatry*. Springer Berlin Heidelberg. https://doi.org/10.1007/978-3-642-54542-9

Ocklenburg, S., & Gunturkun, O. (2012). Hemispheric asymmetries: The comparative view. *Frontiers in Psychology, 3*. www.frontiersin.org/articles/10.3389/fpsyg.2012.00005

Paolicelli, R. C., Bolasco, G., Pagani, F., Maggi, L., Scianni, M., Panzanelli, P., Giustetto, M., Ferreira, T. A., Guiducci, E., Dumas, L., Ragozzino, D., & Gross, C. T. (2011). Synaptic pruning by microglia is necessary for normal brain development. *Science, 333*(6048), 1456–1458. https://doi.org/10.1126/science.1202529

Pascual-Marqui, R. (1997). Low resolution brain electromagnetic tomography (LORETA). *Electroencephalography and Clinical Neurophysiology, 103*(1), 25–26. https://doi.org/10.1016/s0013-4694(97)88020-4

Peper, J. S., Brouwer, R. M., Boomsma, D. I., Kahn, R. S., & Pol, H. E. H. (2007). Genetic influences on human brain structure: A review of brain imaging studies in twins. *Human Brain Mapping, 28*(6), 464–473. https://doi.org/10.1002/hbm.20398

Peretz, I., & Zatorre, R. J. (2005). Brain organization for music processing. *Annual Review of Psychology, 56*(1), 89–114. https://doi.org/10.1146/annurev.psych.56.091103.070225

Pessoa, L. (2018). Understanding emotion with brain networks. *Current Opinion in Behavioral Sciences, 19*, 19–25. https://doi.org/10.1016/j.cobeha.2017.09.005

Petersen, S. E., & Posner, M. I. (2012). The attention system of the human brain: 20 years after. *Annual Review of Neuroscience, 35*, 73–89. https://doi.org/10.1146/annurev-neuro-062111-150525

Polich, J., & Corey-Bloom, J. (2005). Alzheimer's disease and P300: Review and evaluation of task and modality. *Current Alzheimer Research, 2*(5), 515–525. https://doi.org/10.2174/15672050577493214

Polich, J., & Kok, A. (1995). Cognitive and biological determinants of P300: An integrative review. *Biological Psychology, 41*(2), 103–146. https://doi.org/10.1016/0301-0511(95)05130-9

Poprawski, T. J., Pluzyczka, A. N., Park, Y., Chennamchetty, V. N., Halaris, A., Crayton, J. W., & Konopka, L. M. (2007). Multimodality imaging in a depressed patient with violent behavior and temporal lobe seizures. *Clinical EEG and Neuroscience, 38*(3), 175–179. https://doi.org/10.1177/155005940703800316

Poprawski, T. J., Pluzyczka, A. N., Park, Y., Chennamchetty, V. N., Halaris, A., Crayton, J. W., & Konopka, L. M. (2007). Multimodality imaging in a depressed patient with violent behavior and temporal lobe seizures. *Clinical EEG and Neuroscience, 38*(3), 175–179. https://doi.org/10.1177/155005940703800316

Power, J. D., Cohen, A. L., Nelson, S. M., Wig, G. S., Barnes, K. A., Church, J. A., Vogel, A. C., Laumann, T. O., Miezin, F. M., Schlaggar, B. L., & Petersen, S. E. (2011). Functional network organization of the human brain. *Neuron, 72*(4), 665–678. https://doi.org/10.1016/j.neuron.2011.09.006

Prichep, L. S. (2005). Use of Normative databases and statistical methods in demonstrating clinical utility of QEEG: Importance and cautions. *Clinical EEG and Neuroscience, 36*(2), 82–87. https://doi.org/10.1177/155005940503600207

Qin, P., & Northoff, G. (2011). How is our self related to midline regions and the default-mode network? *NeuroImage, 57*(3), 1221–1233. https://doi.org/10.1016/j.neuroimage.2011.05.028

Raichle, M. E., MacLeod, A. M., Snyder, A. Z., Powers, W. J., Gusnard, D. A., & Shulman, G. L. (2001). A default mode of brain function. *Proceedings of the National Academy of Sciences, 98*(2), 676–682. https://doi.org/10.1073/pnas.98.2.676

Renshaw, P. F., Guimaraes, A. R., Fava, M., Rosenbaum, J. F., Pearlman, J. D., Flood, J. G., Puopolo, P. R., Clancy, K., & Gonzalez, R. G. (1992). Accumulation of fluoxetine and norfluoxetine in human brain during therapeutic administration. *The American Journal of Psychiatry, 149*(11), 1592–1594. https://doi.org/10.1176/ajp.149.11.1592

Sadaghiani, S., & D'Esposito, M. (2015). Functional characterization of the cingulo-opercular network in the maintenance of tonic alertness. *Cerebral Cortex, 25*(9), 2763–2773. https://doi.org/10.1093/cercor/bhu072

Scheibel, A. B. (2017). Some structural and developmental correlates of human speech. In *Brain maturation and cognitive development* (pp. 345–354). Routledge. https://doi.org/10.4324/9781315082028-13

Schmahmann, J. D. (2004). Disorders of the cerebellum: Ataxia, dysmetria of thought, and the cerebellar cognitive affective syndrome. *The Journal of Neuropsychiatry and Clinical Neurosciences, 16*(3), 367–378. https://doi.org/10.1176/jnp.16.3.367

Scholten, J., Vasterling, J. J., & Grimes, J. B. (2017). Traumatic brain injury clinical practice guidelines and best practices from the VA state of the art conference. *Brain Injury, 31*(9), 1246–1251. https://doi.org/10.1080/02699052.2016.1274780

Schridde, U., Khubchandani, M., Motelow, J. E., Sanganahalli, B. G., Hyder, F., & Blumenfeld, H. (2007). Negative BOLD with large increases in neuronal activity. *Cerebral Cortex, 18*(8), 1814–1827. https://doi.org/10.1093/cercor/bhm208

Seeley, W. W. (2019). The salience network: A neural system for perceiving and responding to homeostatic demands. *Journal of Neuroscience, 39*(50), 9878–9882. https://doi.org/10.1523/JNEUROSCI.1138-17.2019

Seeley, W. W., Crawford, R. K., Zhou, J., Miller, B. L., & Greicius, M. D. (2009). Neurodegenerative diseases target large-scale human brain networks. *Neuron, 62*(1), 42–52. https://doi.org/10.1016/j.neuron.2009.03.024

Seeley, W. W., Menon, V., Schatzberg, A. F., Keller, J., Glover, G. H., Kenna, H., Reiss, A. L., & Greicius, M. D. (2007). Dissociable intrinsic connectivity networks for salience processing and executive control. *The Journal of Neuroscience: The Official Journal of the Society for Neuroscience, 27*(9), 2349–2356. https://doi.org/10.1523/JNEUROSCI.5587-06.2007

Shapleske, J., Rossell, S. L., Woodruff, P. W. R., & David, A. S. (1999). The planum temporale: A systematic, quantitative review of its structural, functional and clinical significance. *Brain Research Reviews, 29*(1), 26–49. https://doi.org/10.1016/s0165-0173(98)00047-2

Shen, K., Welton, T., Lyon, M., McCorkindale, A. N., Sutherland, G. T., Burnham, S., Fripp, J., Martins, R., & Grieve, S. M. (2019). Structural core of the executive control network: A high angular resolution diffusion MRI study. *Human Brain Mapping, 41*(5), 1226–1236. https://doi.org/10.1002/hbm.24870

Sherman, L. E., Rudie, J. D., Pfeifer, J. H., Masten, C. L., McNealy, K., & Dapretto, M. (2014). Development of the default mode and central executive networks across early adolescence: A longitudinal study. *Developmental Cognitive Neuroscience, 10*, 148–159. https://doi.org/10.1016/j.dcn.2014.08.002

Shpokayte, M., McKissick, O., Guan, X., Yuan, B., Rahsepar, B., Fernandez, F. R., Ruesch, E., Grella, S. L., White, J. A., Liu, X. S., & Ramirez, S. (2022). Hippocampal cells segregate positive and negative engrams. *Communications Biology, 5*(1), Article 1. https://doi.org/10.1038/s42003-022-03906-8

Sidman, R. L., & Rakic, P. (1973). Neuronal migration, with special reference to developing human brain: A review. *Brain Research, 62*(1), 1–35. https://doi.org/10.1016/0006-8993(73)90617-3

Silk, T. J., Malpas, C. B., Beare, R., Efron, D., Anderson, V., Hazell, P., Jongeling, B., Nicholson, J. M., & Sciberras, E. (2019). A network analysis approach to ADHD symptoms: More than the sum of its parts. *PloS One, 14*(1), e0211053. https://doi.org/10.1371/journal.pone.0211053

Smid, G. E., & Kleber, R. (2009). Delayed posttraumatic stress disorder: Systematic review, meta-analysis, and metaregression analysis of prospective studies. *Journal of Clinical Psychiatry.* www.academia.edu/13371773/Delayed_Posttraumatic_Stress_Disorder_Systematic_Review_Meta_Analysis_and_Metaregression_Analysis_of_Prospective_Studies

Sridharan, D., Levitin, D. J., & Menon, V. (2008). A critical role for the right fronto-insular cortex in switching between central-executive and default-mode networks. *Proceedings of the National Academy of Sciences of the United States of America, 105*(34), 12569–12574. https://doi.org/10.1073/pnas.0800005105

Sripada, R. K., King, A. P., Welsh, R. C., Garfinkel, S. N., Wang, X., Sripada, C. S., & Liberzon, I. (2012). Neural dysregulation in posttraumatic stress disorder: Evidence for disrupted equilibrium between salience and default mode brain networks. *Psychosomatic Medicine, 74*(9), 904–911. https://doi.org/10.1097/PSY.0b013e318273bf33

Stoffers, D., Bosboom, J. L. W., Deijen, J. B., Wolters, E. C., Stam, C. J., & Berendse, H. W. (2008). Increased cortico-cortical functional connectivity in early-stage Parkinson's disease: An MEG study. *NeuroImage, 41*(2), 212–222. https://doi.org/10.1016/j.neuroimage.2008.02.027

Strazzer, S., Rocca, M. A., Molteni, E., Meo, E. D., Recla, M., Valsasina, P., Arrigoni, F., Galbiati, S., Bardoni, A., & Filippi, M. (2015). Altered recruitment of the attention network is associated with disability and cognitive impairment in pediatric patients with acquired brain injury. *Neural Plasticity, 2015*. https://doi.org/10.1155/2015/104282

Tau, G. Z., & Peterson, B. S. (2010). Normal development of brain circuits. *Neuropsychopharmacology, 35*(1), 147–168. https://doi.org/10.1038/npp.2009.115

Tessier-Lavigne, M., & Goodman, C. S. (1996). The molecular biology of axon guidance. *Science, 274*(5290), 1123–1133. https://doi.org/10.1126/science.274.5290.1123

Thatcher, R. W., Walker, R. A., Gerson, I., & Geisler, F. H. (1989). EEG discriminant analyses of mild head trauma. *Electroencephalography and Clinical Neurophysiology, 73*(2), 94–106. https://doi.org/10.1016/0013-4694(89)90188-0

Thomas, K. L., Laroche, S., Errington, M. L., Bliss, T. V. P., & Hunt, S. P. (1994). Spatial and temporal changes in signal transduction pathways during LTP. *Neuron, 13*(3), 737–745. https://doi.org/10.1016/0896-6273(94)90040-x

Thompson, P. M., Cannon, T. D., Narr, K. L., Erp, T. van, Poutanen, V.-P., Huttunen, M., Lönnqvist, J., Standertskjöld-Nordenstam, C.-G., Kaprio, J., Khaledy, M., Dail, R., Zoumalan, C. I., & Toga, A. W. (2001). Genetic influences on brain structure. *Nature Neuroscience, 4*(12), 1253–1258. https://doi.org/10.1038/nn758

Toga, A. W., & Thompson, P. M. (2003). Mapping brain asymmetry. *Nature Reviews Neuroscience, 4*(1), Article 1. https://doi.org/10.1038/nrn1009

Toni, N., Buchs, P.-A., Nikonenko, I., Bron, C. R., & Muller, D. (1999). LTP promotes formation of multiple spine synapses between a single axon terminal and a dendrite. *Nature, 402*(6760), 421–425. https://doi.org/10.1038/46574

Toropova, K. A., Ivashkina, O. I., Ivanova, A. A., Konovalova, E. V., Dolgov, O. N., & Anokhin, K. V. (2021). Long-term changes in spontaneous behavior and c-fos expression in the brain in mice in the resting state in a model of post-traumatic stress disorder. *Neuroscience and Behavioral Physiology, 51*(5), 629–638. https://doi.org/10.1007/s11055-021-01116-z

Turk, D. J., Heatherton, T. F., Kelley, W. M., Funnell, M. G., Gazzaniga, M. S., & Macrae, C. N. (2002). Mike or me? Self-recognition in a split-brain patient. *Nature Neuroscience, 5*(9), 841–842. https://doi.org/10.1038/nn907

Uddin, L. Q., Yeo, B. T. T., & Spreng, R. N. (2019). Towards a universal taxonomy of macro-scale functional human brain networks. *Brain Topography, 32*(6), 926–942. https://doi.org/10.1007/s10548-019-00744-6

Veer, I. M., Beckmann, C. F., van Tol, M.-J., Ferrarini, L., Milles, J., Veltman, D. J., Aleman, A., van Buchem, M. A., van der Wee, N. J., & Rombouts, S. A. R. B. (2010). Whole brain resting-state analysis reveals decreased functional connectivity in major depression. *Frontiers in Systems Neuroscience, 4*, 41. https://doi.org/10.3389/fnsys.2010.00041

Vermathen, P., Ende, G., Laxer, K. D., Walker, J. A., Knowlton, R. C., Barbaro, N. M., Matson, G. B., & Weiner, M. W. (2002). Temporal lobectomy for epilepsy: Recovery of the contralateral hippocampus measured by 1H MRS. *Neurology, 59*(4), 633–636. https://doi.org/10.1212/wnl.59.4.633

Vermetten, E., Vythilingam, M., Southwick, S. M., Charney, D. S., & Bremner, J. D. (2003). Long-term treatment with paroxetine increases verbal declarative memory and hippocampal volume in posttraumatic stress disorder. *Biological Psychiatry, 54*(7), 693–702. https://doi.org/10.1016/s0006-3223(03)00634-6

Vicario-Abejón, C., Collin, C., McKay, R. D. G., & Segal, M. (1998). Neurotrophins induce formation of functional excitatory and inhibitory synapses between cultured hippocampal neurons. *The Journal of Neuroscience, 18*(18), 7256–7271. https://doi.org/10.1523/jneurosci.18-18-07256.1998

Vidal, J. R., Chaumon, M., O'Regan, J. K., & Tallon-Baudry, C. (2006). Visual grouping and the focusing of attention induce gamma-band oscillations at different frequencies in human magnetoencephalogram signals. *Journal of Cognitive Neuroscience, 18*(11), 1850–1862. https://doi.org/10.1162/jocn.2006.18.11.1850

Volkow, N. D., Fowler, J. S., Wang, G.-J., Hitzemann, R., Logan, J., Schlyer, D. J., Dewey, S. L., & Wolf, A. P. (1993). Decreased dopamine D2 receptor availability is associated with reduced frontal metabolism in cocaine abusers. *Synapse, 14*(2), 169–177. https://doi.org/10.1002/syn.890140210

von Stein, A., Chiang, C., & König, P. (2000). Top-down processing mediated by interareal syn-chronization. *Proceedings of the National Academy of Sciences, 97*(26), 14748–14753. https://doi.org/10.1073/pnas.97.26.14748

Vossel, S., Geng, J. J., & Fink, G. R. (2014). Dorsal and ventral attention systems: Distinct neural cir-cuits but collaborative roles. *The Neuroscientist: A Review Journal Bringing Neurobiology, Neurology and Psychiatry, 20*(2), 150–159. https://doi.org/10.1177/1073858413494269

Wahlund, L.-O., Agartz, I., Sääf, J., Wetterberg, L., & Marions, O. (1992). MRI in psychiatry: 731 cases. *Psychiatry Research: Neuroimaging, 45*(2), 139–140. https://doi.org/10.1016/0925-4927(92)90007-q

Walker, M. S., Stamper, A. M., Nathan, D. E., & Riedy, G. (2018). Art therapy and underlying fMRI brain patterns in military TBI: A case series. *International Journal of Art Therapy, 23*(4), 180–187. https://doi.org/10.1080/17454832.2018.1473453

Woodburn, M., Bricken, C. L., Wu, Z., Li, G., Wang, L., Lin, W., Sheridan, M. A., & Cohen, J. R. (2021). The maturation and cognitive relevance of structural brain network organization from early infancy to childhood. *NeuroImage, 238*, 118232. https://doi.org/10.1016/j.neuroimage.2021.118232

Yao, J. D., Gimoto, J., Constantinople, C. M., & Sanes, D. H. (2020). Parietal cortex is required for the integration of acoustic evidence. *Current Biology : CB, 30*(17), 3293–3303.e4. https://doi.org/10.1016/j.cub.2020.06.017

Yovel, G., Tambini, A., & Brandman, T. (2008). The asymmetry of the fusiform face area is a stable individual characteristic that underlies the left-visual-field superiority for faces. *Neuropsychologia, 46*(13), 3061–3068. https://doi.org/10.1016/j.neuropsychologia.2008.06.017

Yucel, K., Taylor, V. H., McKinnon, M. C., MacDonald, K., Alda, M., Young, L. T., & MacQueen, G. M. (2007). Bilateral hippocampal volume increase in patients with bipolar disorder and short-term lithium treatment. *Neuropsychopharmacology, 33*(2), 361–367. https://doi.org/10.1038/sj.npp.1301405

Zhou, H.-X., Chen, X., Shen, Y.-Q., Li, L., Chen, N.-X., Zhu, Z.-C., Castellanos, F. X., & Yan, C.-G. (2020). Rumination and the default mode network: Meta-analysis of brain imaging studies and implications for depression. *NeuroImage, 206*, 116287. https://doi.org/10.1016/j.neuroimage.2019.116287

Zimmerman, E. M., & Konopka, L. M. (2013). Preliminary findings of single- and multifocused epileptiform discharges in nonepileptic psychiatric patients. *Clinical EEG and Neuroscience, 45*(4), 285–292. https://doi.org/10.1177/1550059413506001

Zimmerman, E. M., Golla, M. A., Paciora, R. A., Epstein, P. S., & Konopka, L. M. (2011). Use of multi-modality imaging and neuropsychological measures for the assessment and treatment of auditory verbal hallucinations: A brain to behavior approach. *Activitas Nervosa Superior, 53*(3–4), 150–158. https://doi.org/10.1007/bf03379939

USING THE EXPRESSIVE THERAPIES CONTINUUM AS A FRAMEWORK IN THE TREATMENT OF TRAUMA

Influence of Creativity on Resilience

Lisa D. Hinz and Vija B. Lusebrink

Author note: It is with great sadness that I write that my friend and mentor, Vija Lusebrink passed away in June 2022. As was her nature as a lifelong scholar, Vija was reading, writing, and editing until the very end of her life. She was an inspiration in determination in the face of adversity and most importantly a true creative genius. Her creative spirit will be greatly missed.

Psychological trauma has been defined as the occurrence of an event or series of events that overwhelm an individual's ability to cope (American Psychiatric Association, 2013). Trauma survivors often have difficulty expressing themselves verbally, especially if they have experienced early trauma which may have interfered with haptic perception and the development of elemental language skills (Hauser, 2021). Childhood maltreatment or neglect contributes to understimulation or overstimulation of the developing brain, thus disrupting the development of the ability to regulate emotion, process pain, and maintain attention (Hauser, 2021). Although art therapy has been used to treat the effects of trauma and post-traumatic stress disorder (PTSD), Baker and colleague's recent review of the efficacy of all creative art therapies and PTSD indicated that the quality of studies was low and therefore the results difficult to interpret and generalize (Baker et al., 2018). The authors of the review advised that more systematically planned investigations and scientific rigor in general are needed. The Expressive Therapies Continuum could be used to structure art therapy intervention strategies and research to address these concerns. This chapter addresses the art therapy treatment of trauma in the context of two systems-based concepts: Expressive Therapies Continuum (ETC) and large-scale brain networks (LSBN) (Lusebrink & Hinz, 2020). We illustrate how understanding the ETC theory can refine and individualize the art therapy treatment of trauma using various art media and methods. It is further proposed that, in the context of a supportive therapeutic relationship, art therapy can uniquely enhance resilience through engaging clients in creative activities that lead to Flow experiences (Csikszentmihalyi, 2008) and provide opportunities for post-traumatic growth.

3.1   THE ETC AND BRAIN FUNCTIONS

The Expressive Therapies Continuum (ETC) (Kagin & Lusebrink, 1978; Lusebrink, 1990, 2016), with its conceptual approach to the multi-leveled nature of visual expression, facilitates the individualization of art therapy treatment strategies with trauma patients. The three developmentally progressive levels of the ETC,

DOI: 10.4324/9781003348207-3

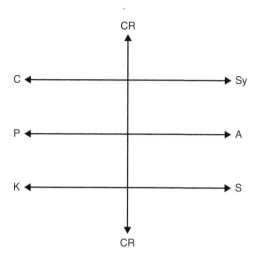

FIGURE 3.1 The Expressive Therapies Continuum. K refers to kinesthetic component, S – sensory, P – perceptual, A – affective, C – cognitive, Sy – symbolic, CR – creative

namely kinesthetic/sensory, perceptual/affective, and cognitive/symbolic, reflect the increasing complexity of visual expression and information processing through imagery formation (see Figure 3.1).

Lusebrink (2004, 2010) proposed that the different levels of the ETC dovetail, in a "bottom-up" manner, the sequence of brain areas and functions involved in the creation and processing of visual expressions. The processing of sensory information proceeds from the analysis of elementary sensory features in the primary sensory cortices, to that of associated features in a given modality in respective unimodal association cortices (visual, somatosensory, motor, and audio). Processing across several sensory and non-sensory modalities occurs in the transmodal or multimodal association cortex in the parietal lobe and subsequently is forwarded to the frontal cortex (Fuster, 2005). Based on data from visual information processing and imagery formation, the regions and functions of the brain presumed to be associated with each level of the ETC are addressed in their general, schematically predominant manner. This approach presumes the fact that the brain operates in a holistic manner with many reciprocal interactions between the different parts. Each ETC level is described as a continuum between two polarities representing gradations and variations in visual expression (see Figure 3.1).

3.2   KINESTHETIC/SENSORY (K/S) LEVEL

The K/S level represents simple motor expressions with art media and their corresponding visual manifestations of energy and sensory involvement. Because of the bipolar nature of ETC levels, an emphasis on the kinesthetic (K) component of the K/S level decreases awareness of sensory functioning. On the other hand, an emphasis on the sensory (S) component of this level decreases and slows down kinesthetic action because the focus of attention is directed to the experience of sensations. Lusebrink

(2010) hypothesized that the K component reflects the predominant involvement of the basal ganglia and the primary motor cortex. The sensory component of visual expression focuses attention on the sensory exploration of materials, surfaces and textures, and appears to involve the primary sensory-motor cortex. Brain activity on the K/S level appears to be fundamental to imagery formation in the brain. Damasio (Damasio, 2012; Meyer & Damasio, 2009) proposed that imagery formation involves basic visual, sensory, motor, and audio components, thus supporting the importance of kinesthetic and sensory involvement with art media in art therapy (Hinz, 2019; Lusebrink, 2014). In trauma treatment, K/S work can aid in the release of tension, awaken the senses, elicit preverbal bodily memories, and establish healing rhythms (Malchiodi, 2020).

3.3   PERCEPTUAL/AFFECTIVE LEVEL (P/A)

The perceptual (P) component of the P/A level is characterized by figure/ground differentiation with a focus on feature analysis and the differentiation of forms, whereby forms are defined by lines and/or color as boundaries. This information is combined and analyzed in the primary and secondary visual cortices, and then divided into two streams of analysis. The lower or ventral stream goes to the visual association cortex in the inferior temporal lobe that responds to features and shapes and integrates their forms and colors. The upper or dorsal stream responds to spatial locations and goes to the visual association cortex in the parietal lobe and the multimodal association cortex (Christian, 2008; Fuster 2005; Lusebrink, 2004, 2010). This distinction is important in understanding visual expressions in art therapy because it separates form or "what is it?" and spatial location or "where is it?" Both streams have direct reciprocal connections with the prefrontal cortex (PFC).

The affective (A) component of the P/A level is characterized by increasing involvement with emotion and its expression, and the affective modification of forms. The presence, differentiation, and transformation of affect are indicated by increases and/or variations in the use of hues and their values. The affective component appears to primarily reflect the processing of emotions in the amygdala, located in the subcortical limbic system, and its influence on the visual stream (Christian, 2008; Lusebrink, 2004). Input from the amygdala is modified by the hippocampus and two cortical structures, namely, the cingulate cortex and the orbitofrontal cortex. The amygdala has direct connections to the prefrontal cortex (PFC) and indirect connections to the right orbitofrontal cortex (OFC) through the thalamus (Fuster, 2005). The interplay between the P and A components in visual expression involves the transition from feature-based information processing at the P polarity on the left side of the ETC schema, to the amygdala-based information processing at the A polarity on the right side. The interchange between these two ETC components is critical in trauma work as exposure to trauma elicits affect and structured P work organizes and contains it.

3.4   COGNITIVE/SYMBOLIC LEVEL (C/SY)

The cognitive component (C) of the C/Sy level emphasizes cognitive operations and is characterized by concept formation, categorization, problem solving, and the differentiation of meaning of objective images and abstractions (Lusebrink,

2004, 2010). The C component of the ETC presumably reflects the activity of the PFC and the OFC. The PFC performs the integrative functions of working memory. In addition, the PFC is responsible for maintaining attention and inhibition, including integrating information from the posterior cortex, namely the multimodal parietal cortex, and the different sensory information stored in the temporal cortex and occipital cortex (Dietrich, 2004). The C component of the ETC also appears to reflect the regulatory "top-down" influences of the dorsolateral prefrontal cortex (dlPFC) and possibly the anterior part of the cingulate cortex (ACC) (Christian, 2008; Lusebrink, 2010). The OFC receives direct input from part of the ventral stream whereas another part of the ventral stream goes to the thalamus and the cingulate cortex before it reaches the OFC area (Christian, 2008; Fuster 2005). The OFC is likely involved in emotional regulation, whereas areas of the PFC have been conceptualized as dealing with affective working memory and anticipating the consequences of positive and negative emotions (Herringa, 2017).

The symbolic (Sy) component of the C/Sy level emphasizes intuitive processing of experiences and visual information by involving input from sensory and affective sources, autobiographical processing, and symbolic expressions. It is characterized by symbolic affective images, symbolic use of color, symbolic abstractions and intuitive, integrative concept formation (Lusebrink, 2004, 2010). The Sy component appears to reflect predominantly the processes of the OFC and possibly the posterior part of the cingulate cortex and the ventromedial part of the PFC. The integrative function of the OFC includes the retrieval of autobiographical consciousness. Both the Sy and C aspects of the C/Sy level are necessary for processing memories in therapy, and both aspects rely on information stored in the multimodal cortex in the parietal lobe (Fuster, 2005). C/Sy work in trauma can aid in constructing a meaningful and coherent trauma narrative (Howie, 2016; Rubinstein & Lahal, 2022), cognitive restructuring (Steele & Kuban, 2012) and in teaching appropriate coping skills (Rosal, 2016).

3.5   CREATIVE DIMENSION (CR)

The creative (CR) dimension of the ETC is conceptualized as a perpendicular intersection of all three levels. The CR dimension can be present on each of the levels at the intersection between the two polarities; at the same time, it can involve information processing from all of the ETC levels. Artistically, creative visual expression can encompass the characteristics along the whole continuum spanning any level or component of the ETC, whereby the preference for a particular component is reflected in the artistic style (Hinz, 2019; Lusebrink, 1990). Critical reviews of the cognitive neuroscience of creativity (Dietrich, 2004; Perryman et al., 2019; Vartanian et al., 2020) assert that the creative process consists of many interactive cognitive processes and emotions, and that the right and left hemispheres of the brain are equally active in most creative tasks. The thoughtful application of art therapy interventions can result in increased creative self-confidence which may have a mediating role in the development of post-traumatic growth (Orkibi & Ram-Vlasov, 2019).

3.6   LARGE-SCALE BRAIN NETWORKS

Over the past decade, research in neuroscience has demonstrated that early conceptualizations of single brain structures corresponding to specific functions are no longer adequate to explain complex brain activities. Current knowledge emphasizes the conjoint functioning of multiple brain areas working together as *large-scale brain networks* (Bressler & Menon, 2010; Menon, 2011, 2015) or intrinsic connectivity networks (Lanius et al., 2020). Large-scale brain networks (LSBN) have been defined as "a collection of interconnected brain areas that interact to perform circumscribed functions" (Bressler & Menon, 2010, p. 281). The discovery of these coordinated neurological networks helped to explain how functionally connected *systems* both activate and constrain cognitive functions (Koziol et al., 2014; Menon, 2011).

According to Menon's (2011) *triple network model*, the main core neurocognitive networks are the central-executive network (CEN), salience network (SN), and default mode network (DMN), which differ in brain structural involvement, as well as functional significance. The DMN has main anchors in the medial prefrontal cortex (mPFC) and the posterior cingulate cortex (PCC), and prominent nodes in the medial temporal lobe and angular gyrus. The DMN is viewed as an unified neurological system supporting emotional processing, autobiographical memory, and self-referential thought leading to a coherent sense of self. It is the DMN that allows people to consider and gain insight from their own behavior as well as mentalize the thoughts and behaviors of others (Lanius et al., 2020). DMN activity is likened to daydreaming and has been associated with mind wandering, divergent thinking, and creativity (Beaty et al., 2016; Sun et al., 2022). The DMN is operational at rest and during tasks that involve passive sensory processes and internally directed processes (Lanius et al., 2020). Further, the DMN shows reduced activity when tasks require high CEN involvement (Hass-Cohen & Findlay, 2015; Lanius et al., 2020). In fact, the DMN and CEN have been described as having an antagonistic relationship such that when one is operational the other is deactivated (Bressler & Menon, 2010; Koziol et al., 2014; Menon, 2015). However, cooperation between the networks has been noted in some creative tasks (Beaty et al., 2016; Vartanian et al., 2020).

The CEN is centered around the dorsolateral prefrontal cortex (dlPFC) and is involved in a wide range of externally oriented cognitive tasks. The CEN is important for higher order executive functioning such as cognitive control of thought/rumination, emotion regulation, and working memory. It is active in rule-based problem solving and decision making in the context of goal-directed behavior.

The SN contains areas partially overlapping with the CEN, but also shows a distinct pattern of connectivity across different cortical and subcortical areas. The two principal nodes of the SN are the anterior insula (AI) and the dorsal-anterior cingulate cortex (dACC). The AI has been described as a multimodal convergence area for diverse sensory information and it is integral in attention/arousal, interoceptive awareness and autobiographical memory. The dACC is a fundamental part of the limbic system involved with reward-based decision making (Menon, 2015; Vartanian et al., 2020). The SN is involved in detecting, integrating, and prioritizing relevant interoceptive information and directing other networks, including the CEN, to engage in goal-directed behavior. It is especially important for the detection of personally relevant stimuli. The SN contributes to communication, self-awareness, and social behavior through its ability to assimilate cognitive, emotional, and sensory input (Koziol et al., 2014; Menon, 2011).

In summary, the CEN and DMN have an inverse relationship with one another such that when one is activated, the other is deactivated. Typically, the DMN is operational when the brain is "task negative" or not involved with external activities or involved only with the processing of internal stimuli. The CEN is viewed as "task positive," activated with the processing of external stimuli. The SN is seen as acting as a dynamic switching mechanism between these two LSBNs because input to the AI from subcortical areas provides stimuli-relevant information about the saliency of information to the self and prompts appropriate action.

Lusebrink and Hinz (2020) proposed similarities between the LSBNs involved in cognition and the C/Sy level of the ETC. Both are systems-based theories and as such, a change in one aspect of the system has implications for other parts of the system. Specific similarities include first that the symbolic component of the ETC appears to parallel the DMN. The DMN deals with episodic memory related to self and self-directed thoughts involving affective input from the insula and the amygdala. The symbolic component diverts attention from external reality to internal thoughts. Work with the symbolic component of the ETC involves the formation of symbols and metaphors related to inner experiences, the creation of self-symbols, and engagement with personal, intuitive, or universal symbols, similar to the self-referential mental activity of the DMN.

The cognitive component, which deals with the cognitive aspects of visual expression without affective input (Lusebrink, 2010, 2016), demonstrates similarities with the CEN. Art therapy with the C component utilizes problem solving, decision making, and planning activities much like the CEN. Similar to the inverse relationship between the CEN and DMN, functioning with the C component inhibits symbol formation with the Sy component (Hinz, 2019; Lusebrink, 2016).

Due to its involvement with saliency cues, the SN could be particularly important in art therapy because it integrates interoceptive information with cognition and facilitates the selection of emotionally charged images significant to the self. The process of transitioning between the perception of internal images and their externalization through art could reinforce the function of the SN, in that it emphasizes the dynamic switching from the internally oriented DMN to the externally oriented CEN. The role of the SN is not specifically discussed in the ETC model (Lusebrink & Hinz, 2020). Nevertheless, the self-salience activity of SN could occur in the creative transition area of the ETC, where both C and Sy processing contribute to creative and therapeutic experiences (Lusebrink, 2016). The ETC model suggests that disrupted connections between components are associated with deficits in psychological functioning (Hinz, 2019; Lusebrink, 2016). Similarly, disrupted functional connectivity within and between the three core neurocognitive networks (DMN, SN, CEN) significantly contributes to many psychiatric disorders (Menon, 2011).

3.7   LSBN AND TRAUMA

The experience of trauma causes neuroendocrine responses that can result in structural and functional changes in the developing brain (Hauser, 2021; Herringa, 2017; Weems et al., 2019). Studies of the effects of childhood trauma on brain structures and functions demonstrate disrupted connections within LSBNs and among the three intrinsic brain networks important in cognition (Herringa, 2017; Lanius et al., 2015; Nicholson et al., 2020; Sheynin et al., 2020; Weems et al., 2019; Zhao et al., 2021). Moreover, the presence of PTSD symptoms has been correlated with disrupted within-DMN connectivity and greater DMN–SN connectivity (Sheynin et al., 2020). Functional disruptions in the DMN can be related to negative self-referential thought, as well as changes in autobiographical memory and social cognition (Nicholson et al., 2020; Sheynin et al., 2020). SN disturbances have been associated with hypervigilance and hyperarousal, as well as with overmodulation of affect and emotional detachment. According to Nicholson et al. (2020), *increased* connection with the mPFC has been associated with greater emotion regulation and dissociative symptoms, while *decreased* connection with the mPFC has been associated with emotional reactivity. It appears that the experience of childhood trauma may impair the ability of the prefrontal cortex to exert control over limbic system responses through the prefrontal cortex (PFC)–amygdala-hippocampal network. Consequently, unregulated signals from the amygdala may lead to excessive anxiety due to insufficient cognitive discrimination, resulting in emotional deregulation (Weems et al., 2019). In addition, trauma is associated with alterations within the CEN and the connections between the CEN and other LSBN. These disruptions are associated with reduced cognitive functioning across multiple domains and resulting under regulation of emotion (Nicholson et al., 2020). Alternatively, overmodulation of affect in PTSD has been associated with over recruitment of CEN areas related to emotion regulation (Nicholson et al., 2020).

In summary, in the aftermath of trauma, intrinsic network functioning is characterized by decreased intra-network and inter-network functional connectivity with the most outstanding interference seen in connections involving the SN (Zhao et al., 2021). Hallmark features also include a weakened DMN and CEN, and inefficient modulation between DMN and CEN. SN disruptions could account for hypervigilance due to increased stimulus saliency. CEN disruptions may contribute to the presence of intrusive thoughts and other cognitive processing difficulties (Zhao et al., 2021). Decreased emotion regulation is likely related to inefficient modulation between DMN and CEN, and is reflected in hyperarousal and attending to task irrelevant features during cognitive processing (Herringa, 2017; Weems, 2019; Zhao et al., 2021). At the same time, overmodulation of affect in PTSD has been associated with over recruitment of CEN areas related to emotion regulation (Nicholson et al., 2020). Interestingly, resilience following childhood trauma has been associated with increased integrity of the SN, especially with a strong connection between the left dACC and the bilateral lingual gyrus, brain areas related to declarative memory and the processing of emotional stimuli (van der Werff et al., 2013).

Aside from reducing problematic symptoms of PTSD, the ability to engage creatively and to achieve Flow, resilience, and eventually post traumatic growth requires coordinated activity among all three LSBN involved in cognition (van der Linden et al., 2021). Thus, the DMN would be enlisted to encourage idea generation, autobiographical memory, and self-referential meaning making. Appropriate SN functioning would help integrate internal or interoceptive/emotional cues, discern individual emotional salience, and add personal relevance. The CEN would aid in convergence on a combination of internal/external input that would provide information for further exploration and self-discovery. This coordinated creative activity can lead to Flow, resilience, and ultimately post traumatic growth (Hinz et al., 2022; van der Linden et al., 2021).

3.8   THE USE OF THE ETC IN THE TREATMENT OF TRAUMA

Understanding the cognitive neuroscience underlying brain functioning and more specifically, the neurobiological effects of trauma, can increase the effectiveness of art therapy for PTSD as clients can better understand and accept symptoms and decrease self-judgment (Perryman et al., 2019). The ETC has been used to structure group art therapy treatment for traumatized children (Feen-Calligan et al., 2020) and art therapy was demonstrated to have a small effect on therapeutic outcome. The individualized use of the ETC may better ensure the effectiveness of art therapy for PTSD. The three-tiered structure of the ETC, which may partially reflect LSBN organization, is based on the idea that several component functions may be involved in visual expression, but one component or level is usually predominant. In using the ETC as a framework for creative arts therapies, it is important to distinguish which of the components of client expression reflect strengths in artistic expression and which reflect respective deficits. It is believed that personal resources or shortcomings demonstrated in ETC component processing mirror preferences in the reception, processing, integration, and expression of information, emotion, and action in other aspects of life (Hinz, 2019).

This overview indicates that the strengths or challenges seen with ETC components also could reflect optimal functioning or disruptions in intrinsic brain network connectivity or functioning. The focus of art therapy in the context of the ETC is to enhance and work with client strengths on different levels, while at the same time expanding or reinforcing areas of weakness (Hinz, 2019; Lusebrink, 2004, 2010). Typically art therapy begins with the component process where clients demonstrate strengths, moving in a stepwise fashion to enhance less well developed areas of functioning (Hinz, 2019; Lusebrink, 1990, 2016). The use of the ETC model allows for the customization of therapeutic interventions and goals in the treatment of trauma. The ETC encourages individualized choices of media, art interventions, and treatment goals. Effective trauma treatment allows for the controlled exposure to trauma triggers and associated affect, alternated with opportunities for conscious withdrawal and containment (Homer, 2015; Howie; 2016; Lanius et al., 2015). The ETC model proposes that information processing on the right side of the ETC permits exposure through A and/or Sy channels; processing on the left provides containment and restructuring through P and C functions.

The three levels of the ETC also can be considered for their "top-down" and "bottom-up" methods of action. The bottom-up manner of information integration proceeds from the K/S level of sensory-motor responses to feature analysis and affective input on the P/A level in the unimodal cortices to their multimodal integration in the parietal cortex, followed by cognitive integration in the PFC on the C/Sy level. The top-down sequence of information processing starts on the C/Sy level with activity in the PFC and is followed by a gradual differentiation of form, affect, and sensory-motor-based information in the parietal, temporal, and occipital cortices on the P/A and K/S levels respectively. The top-down treatment approach gradually allows clients to become comfortable with their emotions and physical bodies, and to achieve a degree of control or emotion regulation. In contrast, the bottom-up direction aids in emotion regulation through increased cognitive processing (Hinz, 2019). Therapeutic gains in the treatment of trauma also can be made through horizontal shifts among the ETC components.

3.9   CREATIVITY, FLOW AND POST-TRAUMATIC GROWTH

Ultimately, integration of information processing using all of the different levels of the ETC can contribute to healing and post-traumatic psychological growth. It is hypothesized that the fluid transition between the two sides and the different levels of the ETC could reflect the experience of "Flow" (Csikszentmihalyi, 2008; Hinz et al., 2022; Lee, 2015). Flow is an optimal state of functioning in which clients are challenged by a task, engage in problem-solving behavior to adjust skills and goals, and are able to achieve mastery (Lee, 2015). While in Flow clients experience highly focused behavior, an altered sense of time, and moments of peak joy. The occurrence of Flow is intrinsically rewarding and is followed by long-lasting periods of increased well-being (Csikszentmihalyi, 2008). Increased well-being is exemplified by more satisfying interpersonal relationships, an enhanced view of the self, and changes in life philosophy which are three cardinal features of post-traumatic growth (Kilmer, 2014). The following case studies demonstrate the processes by which two brothers emerged from childhood trauma and demonstrated greater resiliency via creativity and Flow experiences in art therapy.

3.10   CASE STUDIES DEMONSTRATING THE USE OF THE ETC

Introduction to Two Brothers: Art Therapy Approaches to Trauma

Two brothers, ages 7 (Steven, a pseudonym) and 8 years (Ed, also a pseudonym), were referred for art therapy by their social services case worker. The boys had been removed from their mother's custody following disclosure by Ed that they were being sexually abused by the mother's live-in boyfriend. The children first were placed with their biological father and his girlfriend, but Ed ran away from that living situation because the girlfriend was physically and emotionally abusive. The brothers were placed in separate foster homes and referred for therapy exhibiting symptoms of PTSD. After introductory sessions to establish safety and a therapeutic rapport and to familiarize the boys with the art materials and art therapy, Figures 3.2 and 3.3 were the first free drawings completed by the brothers. Both boys drew houses and their drawings demonstrate that although the brothers underwent similar traumatic experiences, their depictions and their preferred ways of processing information were diametrically opposed.

Ed described his house (Figure 3.2) as being surrounded by a tornado. Alternating energy and control can be seen in his precise coloring of the house and his expansive creation of the swirling storm. Prominent features of the drawing also include the use of many colors, the pointed black roof, and a gutter drawn on the

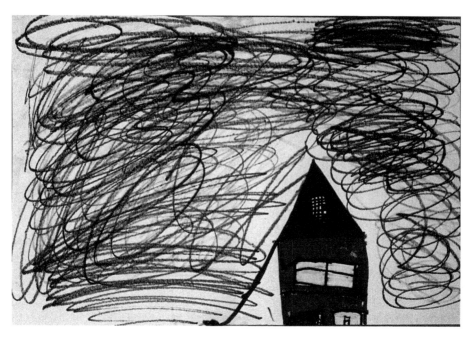

FIGURE 3.2 Ed's first free drawing, "House"

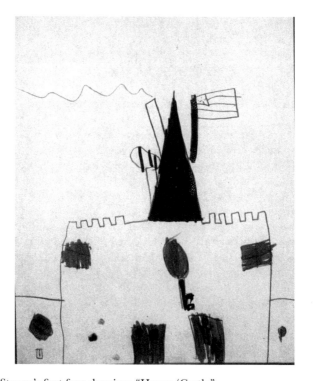

FIGURE 3.3 Steven's first free drawing, "House/Castle"

side of the house to allow "dirty water to escape." Based on this drawing, Ed was characterized as energetic, assertive, expansive, action-oriented, an externalizer of emotion, and as experiencing unpleasant thoughts and emotions needing expression. Using the framework of the ETC, one could say that although the house drawing was on the C/Sy level, kinesthetic action was Ed's predominant mode of processing emotionally threatening information. It is suggested that Ed might have been experiencing difficulties switching between DMN and CEN and that these neurocognitive disruptions were reflected in hyperarousal, attending to task irrelevant features during cognitive processing, and reduced emotion regulation.

In contrast, 7-year-old Steven characterized his house as a castle and added that it had many windows and doors, including the key-shaped window in the center. Additionally, he pointed out an intruder on a ladder trying to gain access to the house. Prominent features of this drawing include geometric shapes, two chimneys, and a dearth of color. The drawing indicated that this boy was tentative, thought or fantasy oriented, an internalizer of emotion, possibly experiencing guilt, self-blame, and depression. Steven preferred working on the C/Sy level of the ETC and it is possible that the overmodulation of affect seen in this drawing was associated neurocognitively with over recruitment of CEN areas related to emotion overregulation.

These two different client presentations naturally required different therapeutic approaches, but with the same ultimate goals for weekly art therapy: the expression of trauma-related thoughts and feelings, including expression and integration of the nonverbal traumatic memories encoded as sensations, the organization of a trauma narrative, and psychological growth allowing the freedom to choose appropriate coping skills based on a positive sense of self-esteem. One brother presented with tremendous energy and kinesthetic involvement. He had to discharge a great deal of energy before he could learn to express emotion appropriately and later coherently relate his trauma narrative. The second brother was comfortable using cognitive strategies to keep emotions under control. It was important to meet him at the C/Sy level where his strategies could be respected and reinforced before eliciting emotional and K/S learning.

A "Bottom-up" Approach to Trauma Therapy: Art Therapy with Ed

Ed began art therapy being guided to work with clay as an appropriate artistic outlet for energy release. In the first sessions he merely pounded, pushed, pinched, rolled, and tossed the clay. Resistive media, those that require energetic manipulation, can help manage the sensory excitation of traumatic memories and allow for a sense of personal control. In addition, Ed achieved a release of energy that was evident in his calm facial expression as he left the sessions. Although these meetings were dominated by action, Ed drew pictures as well. Figure 3.4 demonstrates pent up energy awaiting discharge in one of the early art therapy sessions. As work continued and he was able to release energy in a controlled and acceptable fashion, Ed's drawings indicated decreased energy and increased sensory involvement as seen in the rhythmic horizontal strokes of yellow color shown in Figure 3.5.

In the next phase of art therapy, Ed was educated about the natural presence and purposes of emotions. Psychoeducation combined with art expression allowed Ed to understand that emotions are signals that require accurate reception and

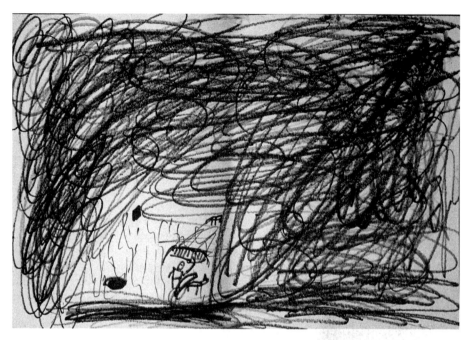

FIGURE 3.4 Ed's drawing showing pent up energy awaiting release

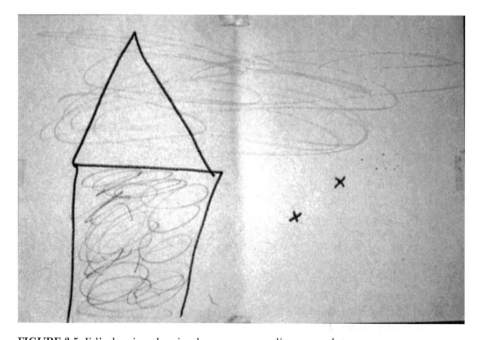

FIGURE 3.5 Ed's drawing showing less energy needing an outlet

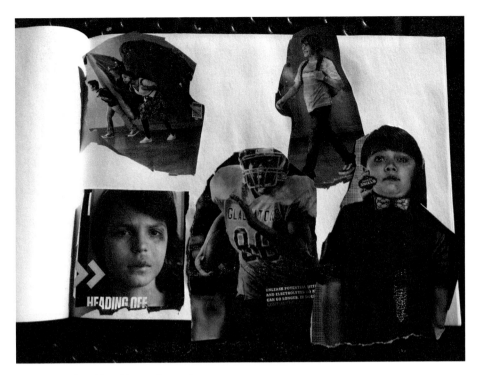

FIGURE 3.6 Ed's collage of emotions

appropriate expression. Ed created collages of facial expressions such as the one depicted in Figure 3.6 in order to learn about the range of emotions that persons might feel. Each emotion was examined individually with respect to the event(s) that might have caused it, and what appropriate action might be taken in response to the emotion. Ed also created paintings of emotions that he personally experienced and began to separate and discriminate what he previously felt as the undifferentiated, swirling storm. In addition, the P/A work involved teaching the use of art as a method for recognizing bodily sensations of emotion through the use of body feelings maps and continued psychoeducation regarding appropriate responses to various emotional signals followed.

In a subsequent stage of therapy, Ed created clay animal figures and told stories about their lives, some of which he also illustrated with drawings (see Figure 3.7). These stories formed the basis of Ed's trauma narrative; the metaphoric telling allowed enough reflective distance for him to safely tell his trauma story. The stories also allowed for purposeful cognitive restructuring as the art therapist witnessed the original stories, helped Ed to recognize themes and emotions, and asked Ed to create new chapters or endings that emphasized his strengths and inner resources. For example, the story that accompanied the drawing in Figure 7 was this: *Two dogs are traveling and they get lost. They end up on two sides of this big river. The little dog cries to the big dog, I don't know how to swim! The big dog tells him to shut up and he (the little dog) gets caught by the dog catcher. The big dog tries to find his way home, but there are too many signs pointing in different directions. He doesn't know the way.*

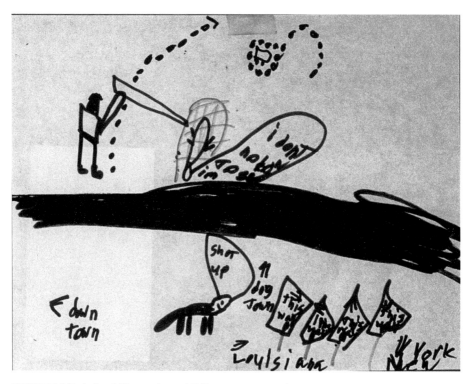

FIGURE 3.7 Animal illustration of Ed's trauma narrative

Clearly Ed was expressing guilt about leaving his brother Steven behind when he ran away from their father's abusive girlfriend and perhaps other instances where he was not able to help his younger brother. Steven suffered more abuse and eventually the boys were placed in separate foster homes. The art therapist commented on how guilt is often manifested as anger at the victim and helped Ed identify positive resources and skills that might be employed if the situation were encountered in the future. Subsequent sessions involved further exploring adaptive coping strategies and using cognitive restructuring techniques. Ed created a subsequent chapter that allowed the big dog to help the small dog and an additional chapter in which the two dogs together found their way home. The new images were reminders of positive and more rewarding approaches to difficult situations and reinforced personal resilience.

Following the animal stories, Ed used clay to create human figures that he arranged in teams to play basketball or soccer. He engaged the art therapist on the opposing team and the games provided opportunities for teaching appropriate coping skills (e.g., cooperation alongside competition; compassion; creation instead of destruction). These sessions in particular offered experiences of Flow. Human figures were more challenging than animals to create and manipulate. Therefore, Ed was engaged in decidedly focused behavior, problem solving, and mastery. His stories featured boys who were proud and positive role models. Ed demonstrated intense enjoyment of his abilities and further, his precise artistic behavior was very different from the unfocused, action-oriented behavior characteristic of the first art therapy sessions.

The course of Ed's treatment vis-à-vis the ETC is graphically depicted in Figure 3.8. Ed began art therapy manipulating clay at the K/S level. In the first sessions his work was utterly kinesthetic: he pounded, pushed, pinched, rolled, and tossed clay. The bipolar nature of the K/S level necessitates that as participation with kinesthetic activity increases, sensory involvement naturally will decrease. Therefore, if the sensory nature of clay evoked trauma memories as has been hypothesized, kinesthetic action with the clay provided a necessary release of tension. Pictures drawn during these early meetings demonstrated that after the kinesthetic work and the additional release of energy, Ed was able to focus on form and art therapy work naturally moved to the P/A level in order to identify, discriminate, appropriately express, and soothe emotions.

At first Ed was encouraged to identify and discriminate among other people's emotions through the use of collage images. The appropriate selection of both task and media encouraged the reflective distance that allowed the experiences to remain more perceptual (contained) than affective (expansive). When Ed demonstrated some familiarity with emotions in general, he was encouraged to express his personal emotions through painting and the experiences became more affectively charged. Again, the art therapist's choices of tasks and media helped move the experience in the desired direction.

Although in the final stages of this "bottom-up" approach to trauma mastery Ed again used clay, his work with the material was more refined than previously in terms of the figures created and the stories imagined (see Figure 3.7). Previously his work was action-oriented and haphazard; the creation of form was not integral to the experiences. In the later phase of art therapy, Ed created figures of animals, and created detail pictures and stories to accompany them. He invested time and energy in the creative process and was rewarded by experiences incorporating the CR dimension

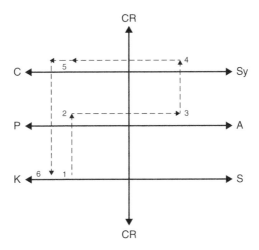

FIGURE 3.8 Representation of Ed's sequence of visual representations on the ETC schema

(Hinz et al., 2022). The investment can be seen graphically by comparing Figures 3.4 and 3.5 with Figure 3.7. The better developed and positively elaborated figures and stories demonstrated Ed's increasing ability to master his trauma experience through symbolic and creative expression. In addition, through cognitive restructuring, the art therapist encouraged prefrontal cortex control over limbic system processing, thus over time establishing increased conscious control over emotional responding.

The creative dimension was accessed and Flow experiences were achieved throughout these final experiences as Ed used clay on the C/Sy level, and were further encouraged during his active and constructive engagement with the art therapist in team play. Ed showed greater problem solving skills and mastery of challenges encountered with the art materials and processes; he demonstrated important aspects of resiliency gained through his interactions in art therapy. In dramatic contrast to the trauma narrative related above in which the big dog tells the crying little dog to "shut up," Ed showed growth in his ability to demonstrate cooperation and compassion in his interactions with the art therapist.

A "Top-down" Approach to Trauma Therapy: Art Therapy with Steven

Steven's first images in art therapy mimicked the style seen in Figure 3.3: line drawings with scattered random colors used mainly to outline forms. After a few sessions, Steven began experiencing nightmares. Therefore, he was asked to draw his nightmares and create response drawings to them in an attempt to cognitively restructure these highly emotional experiences. In the response drawings, Steven was instructed to change negative images into ones that were more manageable or ones in which he was in control of the outcome. For example, in one dream his father's girlfriend was a giant who aggressively pursued Steven. Steven drew a picture of the giant shown in Figure 3.9, then he "cut her down to size" (Figure 3.10). In a ensuing series of drawings (not pictured), the perpetrator became smaller and smaller until she was merely a dot that disappeared into the white expanse of paper. Nightmares are common among trauma survivors; they are one way in which the body re-experiences trauma and the drawing technique helped Steven manage the anxiety that he felt as he recounted his dreams in therapy. Consequently, he was coached to use the technique at home so that his sleep gradually was less disrupted.

Because the nightmares included many trauma-related incidents, Steven was encouraged to create a trauma narrative with the goals of organizing the story, increasing understanding, expressing affect, and restructuring self-image from victim to survivor. Unlike his brother who created emotional distance by telling his story symbolically, Steven told his trauma story in factual pictures as he remembered it over the course of several weeks, each week adding new details and incidents until he felt that the story was complete. It was apparent from his images that Steven was encountering his story with very little emotion. He typically used one marker to create a line drawing, focusing on the details of the scene but not using color realistically. After illustrating his story, Steven was engaged in cognitive restructuring as the art therapist asked him to create different views of abusive incidents or create alternative responses. Thus, Steven began to develop and incorporate different views of situations, people, himself, and his coping skills. These activities afforded exposure to the trauma but safe retreat into the structure and details of the drawings or the

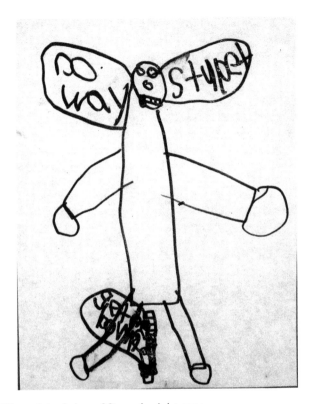

FIGURE 3.9 The original view of Steven's nightmare

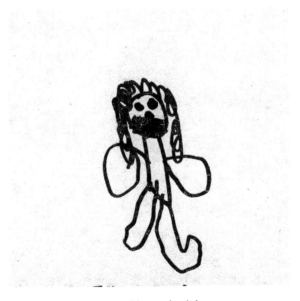

FIGURE 3.10 Cognitive restructuring of Steven's nightmare

cognitive restructuring activities. His growing mastery of the emotion associated with trauma experiences can be seen in the improved line quality and increased developmental level of the drawings in his early, compared to his later drawings.

Steven was encouraged to elaborate his drawings with the addition of color which was a first step in moving him from the C/Sy to the P/A level. One example can be seen in Figure 3.11. This picture, of Steven imagining his mother's boyfriend going to jail following Steven's court testimony, was originally made with only a blue marker that was neither color-appropriate nor particularly emotionally expressive. At the therapist's suggestion, Steven added more color to the image; he subsequently indicated greater satisfaction with his expression and willingly added color to subsequent drawings. He next created a collage of faces portraying feelings as described above in work with Ed. Collage was chosen as a nonthreatening introduction to the identification and discrimination of emotions on the P side of the P/A level. Subsequently, Steven identified his own feelings through the use of 'mazin' collage images and later paired feeling pictures with his own experience of emotions. The next step was a depiction of four primary emotions in marker which is shown in Figure 3.12. Markers were chosen because they are somewhat fluid and capable of evoking emotion, while at the same time they are familiar and manageable enough to allow for the containment of affect. The emotions depicted by Steven were from top left, in clockwise order: fear, sadness, anger, and happiness. He then drew and colored body

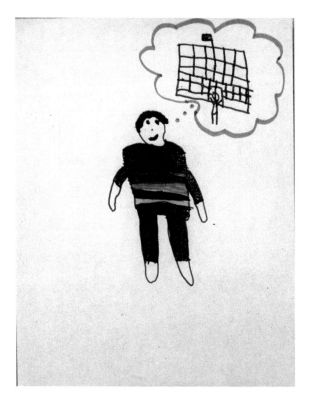

FIGURE 3.11 Adding color to enhance emotional responding

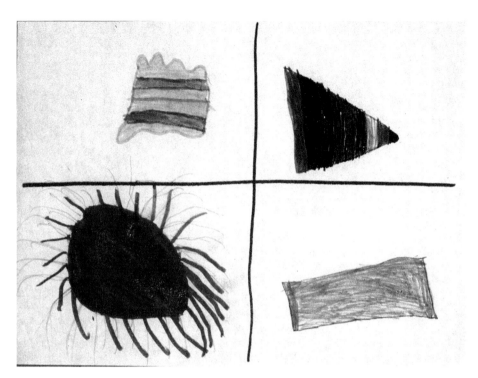

FIGURE 3.12 Steven's four primary feelings picture. From top left, in clockwise order: fear, sadness, anger, and happiness

maps of feelings indicating where and how he experienced his own emotions. The intention of these sessions was to help awaken and restore interoceptive awareness and personal saliency detection. Several sessions followed in which feelings were further discriminated through paintings. The use of a more fluid media, low complexity, and low structure tasks (e.g., paint what you are feeling) encouraged more direct access to and expression of emotion.

Following three missed visitations by his mother, Steven created the drawing shown in Figure 3.13 that he named, "Alien." His description of the drawing was: *This guy is an alien; you see, his blood is blue and not red. His heart is upside down. No one loves him. He has super powers to kill. His knife is bloody; he is going to kill.* Depersonalization experiences, or feeling like an alien, can be seen when disconnections within the DMN lead to difficulties in somatic self-referential processing (Launius et al., 2020). Further exploration of the alien figure led to the discovery that Steven was suicidal. He was hospitalized to ensure his safety and treatment continued on an in-patient basis where Steven was able to express a combination of emotion and energy in various activities. Creating handmade paper and papier-mâché were two activities that helped lead to Flow experiences. Steven was challenged by the activities and yet masterful as he worked with the art therapist to create meaningful and beautiful products. He developed a sense of power and control, enjoyed the experience and wanted to continue it in subsequent sessions. Like his brother, Steven demonstrated a level of focused activity that was not present at the beginning of treatment and

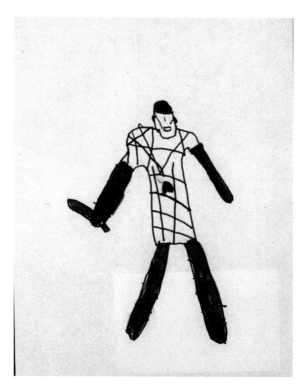

FIGURE 3.13 Steven's drawing of the "Alien"

which seemed to indicate that he was in Flow. After approximately one year Steven left art therapy with a greater sense of self-esteem, a greater understanding of his experiences, and a more complete arsenal of coping skills contributing to increased resilience.

The sequence of visual representations in Steven's art therapy treatment is shown in Figure 13.14. A "top-down" approach to the art therapy treatment of trauma can be helpful when clients present in a cognitively controlled fashion with little access to emotion, possibly indicating over-recruitment of CEN areas related to emotion regulation. The goal of such an approach is to begin with high CEN involvement (C component of the ETC) and gradually expose clients to affect in ways that at first emphasize control and mastery. Art therapy with Steven began with with symbolic material presented both in free drawings such as the Castle/House in Figure 3.2, and in dreams. However, image formation and information processing quickly moved to the C component where he seemed most comfortable creating. Responding to nightmares presented the first opportunity to employ cognitive restructuring (Rosal, 2016; Lanius et al., 2015; Steele and Kuban, 2012). Steven was able to draw scenes from his nightmares such as the one in Figure 3.9 and then use drawing materials to make the images manageable. With time the nightmares were eliminated indicating a degree of emotional regulation and resilience.

Steven was then engaged in the creation of a pictorial trauma narrative with factual drawings that helped him develop a sense of order to and increased

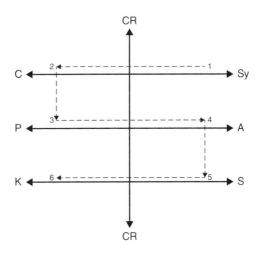

FIGURE 3.14 Representation of Steven's sequence of visual expressions on the ETC schema

understanding of life events (Howie, 2016; Neimeyer, 2014). The minimal use of color and increased attention to detail and attention to irrelevant details could indicate SN dysfunction and probably functioned to regulate affect. The next step in art therapy was to help Steven transition to functioning on the right-hand side of the ETC (P/A level) in order to integrate the experience of emotion and therefore he was asked to integrate color into his trauma narrative drawings. Interestingly, color was added in a very structured fashion (see Figure 3.11), and this controlled use of color pervaded his four primary emotions drawing as can be seen in Figure 3.12. Increased affect was further encouraged through the use of watercolor. New trauma of three failed visits by his mother caused Steven to experience overwhelming feelings of rejection and suicidal depression reflected in regression to his original Sy style shown in Figure 3.13 of the alien. Art therapy continued on an in-patient basis progressing to sensory and kinesthetic processing allowing for the release of tension, and the integration of sensation and emotion. Thus, as is demonstrated in Figure 3.14, Steven started treatment on the right side of the ETC, then slowly integrated information processing and functions from both sides, ending up at the K/S level.

3.11 COMPARISON OF TWO BROTHERS: ART THERAPY APPROACHES TO TRAUMA

These two descriptions demonstrate that not all trauma survivors can be treated in the same fashion to achieve equivalent therapeutic results. Two brothers who experienced similar abusive situations presented with very different images in their first art therapy sessions. These differences in artistic production indicated differences in underlying brain functioning and preferred information processing strategies. Ed's traumatic memories were apparently encored predominantly as sensory-motor memories on the K/S level indicating predominant encoding in the posterior cortex. Alternatively, Steven's memories of the trauma were presented as predominantly affective symbolic images on the Sy pole of the C/Sy level as confirmed by his nightmare drawings, indicating the predominant involvement of the limbic system and amygdala. Although therapeutic goals were similar, the approaches to art therapy with the two boys were different.

A "bottom-up" strategy was used with Ed which began on K/S level, allowing for the release of energy and tension. Therapy then moved up to the P/A level to aid in the recognition of interoceptive cues to emotion, the containment and appropriate expression of emotion, and to the C/Sy level to support the integration of new information and skills. Interestingly, in the final stages of therapy, creative integration occurred on the C/Sy level and included significant K/S involvement through the use of clay. Steven was treated with a "top-down" approach that began on at the C/Sy level, worked down to the P/A level to awaken and restore interoceptive awareness and saliency detection, and to invite contained expression of affect, and finally approached the K/S level to allow release of energy and the thoughtful integration of sensation through creative work involving sensory-motor activity. Again, the creative integration in this case of trauma recovery and resilience was characterized by significant K/S involvement which some have argued is an essential element in effective trauma treatment (e.g., Hass-Cohen & Findlay, 2015; Ogden, 2018).

Art therapy helped both boys experience Flow as an important healing component of art therapy. Over the course of a year in treatment, the brothers were able to incorporate a more positive sense of self and improved interpersonal relationships, possibly indicating strengthening of the DMN. Demonstrated increases in focused behavior, mastery, and self-esteem, as well as lengthening periods of attention and concentration could signify strengthened within-network CEN connections. Both boys were better able to attend to relevant internal and external stimuli as it applied to art therapy which could have resulted in the enhanced interoceptive awareness, saliency detection, and emotional regulation skills demonstrated over the course of art therapy and possibly reflected greater SN connectivity (Lanius et al., 2015). Optimal connections between the three LSBN can set the stage for Flow (van der Linden et al., 2020). It is certain that the boys were more resilient as a result of their creative experiences and it is possible that they experienced post-traumatic growth as they underwent positive changes that seemed to surpass adjustment to a new life, and to indicate the learning of effective coping skills in the face of adversity (e.g., Kilmer, 2014).

3.12   CONCLUSIONS

Art therapy as a sensory-motor and visually based expressive modality addresses two important aspects of therapy with trauma survivors: the integration of the non-verbal sensory-motor-based traumatic memories and the temporal organization of segmented verbal memories. The ETC with its three hierarchical levels, provides a structure for the gradual organization and integration of trauma memories in a bottom up or top down manner. The three levels of the ETC could reflect parallel brain activity in the posterior cortex, specifically, the occipital, temporal, and parietal cortices, and the prefrontal cortex. This chapter also considered similarities with three core intrinsic brain networks involved in a wide range of cognitive tasks: DMN, CEN, and SN. DMN is "task negative" in that it is active during mind-wandering and daydreaming. The CEN is a "task positive" network active during tasks involving working memory, executive functioning, and goal-directed behavior. The SN functions as a switching mechanism between the other two networks. The experience of childhood trauma causes disruptions in these networks and resulting cognitive and emotional dysregulation, as stimulus saliency cues are not appropriately attended causing hyper- or hypoarousal. As was demonstrated in the case studies, art therapy can possibly provide experiences to help re-regulate these neurocognitive systems and provide relief from PTSD symptoms. It appears that in the two cases described, creative integration occurred on the basic level of the ETC, namely on the K/S level, thus involving the basic components of sensory encoding. Due to the fact that early trauma experiences can be stored in the body without conscious verbal associations, sensory involvement has been hypothesized to be a significant component of effective trauma treatment (e.g., Ogden, 2018). Future studies can use the ETC to systematically explore possible advantages that art therapy has over verbal therapies because of its kinesthetic and sensory qualities.

REFERENCES

American Psychiatric Association. (2013). *Diagnostic and statistical manual of mental disorders* (5th ed.). Author.

Baker, F. A., Metcalf, O., Varker, T., & O'Donnell, M. (2018). A systematic review of the efficacy of creative arts therapies in the treatment of adults with PTSD. *Psychological Trauma: Theory, Research, Practice, and Policy, 10*(6), 643–651.

Beaty, R. E., Benedek, M., Silvia, P. J., & Schacter, D. L. (2016). Creative cognition and brain network dynamics. *Trends in Cognitive Sciences, 20*(2), 87–95.

Bressler, S. L., & Menon, V. (2010). Large scale brain networks in cognition: Emerging methods and principles. *Trends in Cognitive Sciences, 14*, 277–290.

Christian, D. (2008). The cortex: Regulation of sensory and emotional experience. In N. Hass-Cohen & R. Carr (Eds.), *Art therapy and clinical neuroscience* (pp. 62–75). Jessica Kingsley.

Csikszentmihalyi, M. (2008). *Flow: The psychology of optimal experience*. Harper.

Damasio, A. (2012). Neuroscience and psychoanalysis: A natural alliance. *Psychoanalytic Review, 99*(4), 591–594.

Dietrich, A. (2004). The cognitive neuroscience of creativity. *Psychonomic Bulletin & Review, 11*(6), 1011–1026.

Feen-Calligan, H., Ruvolo Grasser, L., Debryn, J., Nasser, S., Jackson, C., Seguin, D., & Javanbakht, A. (2020). Art therapy with Syrian refugee youth in the United States: An intervention study. *The Arts in Psychotherapy, 69*, 1–16.

Fuster, J. M. (2005). *Cortex and mind: Unifying cognition*. Oxford University Press.

Hass-Cohen, N., & Findlay, J. (2015). *Art therapy and the neuroscience of relationships, creativity, and resiliency: Skills and practices*. Norton.

Hauser, M. D. (2021). How early life adversity transforms the learning brain. *Mind, Brain & Education, 15*(1), 35–47.

Herringa, R. J. (2017). Trauma, PTSD, and the developing brain. *Current Psychiatry Reports, 19*(10), 1–9.

Hinz, L. D. (2019). *Expressive Therapies Continuum: A framework for using art in therapy* (2nd ed.). Routledge.

Hinz, L. D., Rim, S., & Lusebrink, V. B. (2022). Clarifying the creative level of the Expressive Therapies Continuum: A different dimension. *Arts in Psychotherapy, 78*, 101896.

Homer, E. S. (2015). Piece work: Fabric collage as a neurodevelopmental approach to trauma treatment. *Art Therapy: Journal of the American Art Therapy Association, 32*(1), 20–26.

Howie, P. (2016). Art therapy with trauma. In D. E. Gussak and M. L. Rosal (Eds.), *The Wiley handbook of art therapy* (pp. 375–386). Wiley Blackwell.

Kagin, S. L., & Lusebrink, V. B. (1978). The Expressive Therapies Continuum. *Art Psychotherapy, 5*(4), 171–180.

Kilmer, R. P. (2014). Resilience and posttraumatic growth in children. In *Handbook of posttraumatic growth* (pp. 264–288). Routledge.

Koziol, L. F., Barker, L. A., Joyce, A. W., & Hrin, S. (2014). Structure and function of large scale brain systems. *Applied Neuropsychology: Child, 3*(4), 236–244.

Lanius, R. A., Frewen, P. A., Tursich, M., Jetly, R., & McKinnon, M. C. (2015). Restoring large-scale brain networks in PTSD and related disorders: A proposal for neuroscientifically-informed treatment interventions. *European Journal of Psychotraumatology, 6*(1), 27313.

Lanius, R. A., Terpou, B. A., & McKinnon, M. C. (2020). The sense of self in the aftermath of trauma: Lessons from the default mode network in posttraumatic stress disorder. *European Journal of Psychotraumatology, 11*(1), 1807703.

Lee, S. Y. (2015). Flow indicators in art therapy: Artistic engagement of immigrant children with acculturation gaps. *Art Therapy: Journal of the American Art Therapy Association, 32*(3), 120–129.

Lusebrink, V. B. (1990). *Imagery and visual expression in therapy.* Plenum Press.

Lusebrink, V. B. (2004). Art therapy and the brain: An attempt to understand the underlying processes of art expression in therapy. *Art Therapy: Journal of the American Art Therapy Association, 21*(3), 125–135.

Lusebrink, V. B. (2010). Assessment and therapeutic application of the Expressive Therapies Continuum: Implications for brain structures and functions. *Art Therapy: Journal of the American Art Therapy Association, 27*(4), 168–177.

Lusebrink, V. B. (2014). Art therapy and neural basis of imagery: Another possible view. *Art Therapy: Journal of the American Art Therapy Association, 31*(2), 87–90.

Lusebrink, V. B. (2016). Expressive Therapies Continuum. In D. E. Gussak and M. L. Rosal (Eds.), *The Wiley handbook of art therapy* (pp. 57–67). Wiley Blackwell.

Lusebrink, V. B., & Hinz, L. D. (2020). Cognitive and symbolic aspects of art therapy and similarities with large scale brain networks. *Art Therapy: Journal of the American Art Therapy Association, 37,* 3, 113–122.

Malchiodi, C. A. (2020). *Trauma and expressive arts therapy: Brain, body, and imagination in the healing process.* Guilford.

Menon, V. (2011). Large scale brain networks and psychopathology: A unifying triple network model. *Trends in Cognitive Sciences, 15*(10), 483–506.

Menon, V. (2015). Large scale functional brain organization. In A. W. Toga (Ed.), *Brain mapping: An encyclopedic reference*, Vol. 2 (pp. 449–459). Amsterdam: Elsevier.

Meyer, K., & Damasio, A. (2009). Convergence and divergence in a neural architecture for recognition and memory. *Trends in Neurosciences, 32*(7), 376–382.

Nicholson, A. A., Harricharan, S., Densmore, M., Neufeld, R. W., Ros, T., McKinnon, M. C., Frewen, P. A., Theberge, J., Rakeshletly, D. P., & Lanius, R. A. (2020). Classifying heterogeneous presentations of PTSD via the default mode, central executive, and salience networks with machine learning. *NeuroImage: Clinical, 27,* 102262.

Neimeyer, R. A. (2014). Re-storying loss: Fostering growth in the posttraumatic narrative. In *Handbook of posttraumatic growth* (pp. 68–80). Routledge.

Ogden, P. (2018). Play, creativity, and movement vocabulary. In T. Marks-Tarlow, M. Solomon, & D. J. Siegel (Eds.), *Play and creativity in psychotherapy* (pp. 92–109). Norton.

Orkibi, H., & Ram-Vlasov, N. (2019). Linking trauma to posttraumatic growth and mental health through emotional and cognitive creativity. *Psychology of Aesthetics, Creativity, and the Arts, 13*(4), 416.

Perryman, K., Blisard, P., & Moss, R. (2019). Using creative arts in trauma therapy: The neuroscience of healing. *Journal of Mental Health Counseling*, 4(1), 80–94.

Rosal, M. (2016). Cognitive behavioral art therapy revisited. In D. E. Gussak and M. L. Rosal (Eds.), *The Wiley handbook of art therapy* (pp. 68–76). Wiley Blackwell.

Rubinstein, D., & Lahad, M. (2022). Fantastic reality: The role of imagination, playfulness, and creativity in healing trauma. *Traumatology*. https://doi.org/10.1037/trm0000376

Sheynin, J., Duval, E. R., Lokshina, Y., Scott, J. C., Angstadt, M., Kessler, D., … & Liberzon, I. (2020). Altered resting-state functional connectivity in adolescents is associated with PTSD symptoms and trauma exposure. *NeuroImage: Clinical*, 26, 102215.

Steele, W., & Kuban, C. (2012). Using drawing in short-term trauma resolution. In C. A. Malchiodi (Ed.), *Handbook of art therapy* (2nd ed) (pp. 162–174). Guilford.

Sun, J., He, L., Chen, Q., Yang, W., Wei, D., & Qiu, J. (2022). The bright side and dark side of daydreaming predict creativity together through brain functional connectivity. *Human Brain Mapping*, 43(3), 902–914.

van der Linden, D., Tops, M., & Bakker, A. B. (2021). Go with the Flow: A neuroscientific view on being fully engaged. *European Journal of Neuroscience*, 53(4), 947–963

van der Werff, S. J. A., Pannekoek, J. N., Veer, I. M., van Tol, M.-J., Aleman, A., Veltman, D. J., Zitman, F. G., Rombouts, S. A. R. B., Elzinga, B. M., & van der Wee, N. J. A. (2013). Resilience to childhood maltreatment is associated with increased resting-state functional connectivity of the salience network with the lingual gyrus. *Child Abuse & Neglect*, 37(11). https://doi.org/10.1016/j.chiabu.2013.07.008

Vartanian, O., Saint, S. A., Herz, N., & Suedfeld, P. (2020). The creative brain under stress: Considerations for performance in extreme environments. *Frontiers in Psychology*, 11, 2861.

Weems, C. F., Russell, J. D., Neill, E. L., & McCurdy, B. H. (2019). Annual research review: Pediatric posttraumatic stress disorder from a neurodevelopmental network perspective. *Journal of Child Psychology and Psychiatry*, 60(4), 395–408.

Zhao, H., Dong, D., Sun, X., Cheng, C., Xiong, G., Wang, X., & Yao, S. (2021). Intrinsic brain network alterations in non-clinical adults with a history of childhood trauma. *European Journal of Psychotraumatology*, 12(1), 1975951.

CHAPTER 4

THE IMAGE COMES FIRST

Treating Preverbal Trauma with Art Therapy

Linda Gantt and Tally Tripp

Editor's Note: *Louis W. Tinnin, MD, originally the lead author, died February 21, 2014. Tally Trip LCSW, ATR-BC, the second author, died Dec 6, 2023. We dedicate this chapter to their memories. The writers thank Jennifer Sweeton, PsyD, for her help and comments on aspects of this chapter.*

Our chapter describes how art therapy is essential to the treatment of preverbal traumas, illustrated with a case example. We discuss the importance of first processing foundation traumas (those occurring prior to three years of age) before tackling other traumatic events. Recent neurobiology research supports the idea that a nonverbal approach, such as art therapy, is ideally suited for working with early developmental trauma (Chapman, 2014). Our case study demonstrates how a foundation trauma (in this case, a birth trauma) can be quickly and effectively processed in a short time by using a trauma treatment approach based on the Instinctual Trauma Response® (ITR) pioneered by Linda Gantt and Louis Tinnin in their outpatient clinic in Morgantown, West Virginia.

4.1 BRIEF HISTORY OF THE TREATMENT OF EARLY TRAUMA

Trauma treatment has made tremendous strides in the last 40 years. As recently as the 1980s it was assumed that talking about the trauma was optimal for producing a cathartic experience, which was the only avenue for healing. We now realize that talking about trauma can, at best, be a difficult experience, and at worst, be re-traumatizing (Center for Substance Abuse Treatment, 2014). Early, severe trauma often results in highly dissociative states that leave the individual with myriad debilitating symptoms, including the inability to connect to feelings. Since the 1990s, coined the "Decade of the Brain," there has been increased accessibility to neuroimaging studies, and the resulting neuroscience research has greatly impacted our understanding and treatment of psychological trauma. Important to our work as art therapists, it is now a widely accepted view that traumatic memory is encoded in visual imagery and bodily sensations, rather than through language or cognition, and that unresolved traumatic memory can severely compromise cognitive functioning (Ogden et al., 2006; van der Kolk, 2006, 2014). Neuroscience studies provide compelling evidence supporting the utility of a "bottom-up" (nonverbal) rather than "top-down" (cognitive) approach for working with traumatic memory (Ogden & Fisher, 2015). This aligns with our long-standing assumption that art therapy is an ideal treatment for trauma resolution and, as an approach that does not rely on verbalization, we feel it is particularly beneficial for working with early, preverbal traumas.

DOI: 10.4324/9781003348207-4

Many contemporary writers have described the enduring effects of the earliest childhood traumas (Gaensbauer, 1995; Karr-Morse & Wiley, 1997; Lipsitt, 2012; Perry & Szalavitz, 2007; Perry, 2009; Terr, 1988, 1990). In *The Trauma Spectrum*, neurologist Robert Scaer (2005) offers an entire chapter on preverbal trauma in which he describes the traumatizing effects of modern medical treatment, starting with hospital delivery. Delima and Vimpani (2011) describe childhood maltreatment in terms of "acts of omission" and "acts of commission" that, especially when prolonged and begun early in life, can adversely affect brain development and result in a significant increase in mental health disorders across the lifespan. Preverbal traumas can include being neglected by drug-addicted parents (Burton, 1992), witnessing domestic violence (Bogat et al., 2006; Fantuzzo et al., 1997; Miller-Graff et al., 2016), or being sexually or physically abused (Gale et al., 1988). These early experiences of maltreatment, particularly when chronic or sustained, can negatively impact all brain-mediated activity including speech and motor functioning, as well as social, emotional, and behavioral regulation (De Bellis & Zisk, 2014; Perry, 2009).

As recently as the end of the 20th century, the erroneous assumption that the infant brain was not mature enough to recognize pain dictated our understanding about early trauma related to birth, circumcision, and surgery (Anand & Hickey, 1987; Chamberlain, 1989; Williams & Lascelles, 2020). It was a widely held misconception by doctors and psychologists that infants and young children did not experience physical pain and, even if they did, they would not remember traumatic events (Philo, 2015). To this day, many therapists do not routinely assess for early traumas, much less treat them systematically. However, we concur with LeDoux who suggests that traumatic memory is long-lasting and "an indelible form of learning" (1996, p. 204). The very structure of the human brain is such that traumas are especially enduring if they occur before age three (Cozolino, 2014). Such foundation experiences are termed "preverbal traumas" as they occur within the earliest time of life while the brain is undergoing major developmental changes, before verbal skills and cognitive processes are fully on-line. The impact of early traumatic childhood experiences has been well documented through the landmark Adverse Childhood Experiences (ACE) study, which demonstrates a strong correlation between adverse events in childhood (such as sexual and physical abuse, addiction, or mental illness in either parent, various forms of neglect, or witnessing domestic violence) and negative health outcomes in middle age (Felitti et al., 1998). Furthermore, research suggests there is a robust and cumulative correlation between exposure to ACEs in childhood and the current expression of trauma-related symptomatology associated with post-traumatic stress disorder (PTSD) (Messina & Schepps, 2021) and with post-traumatic stress syndrome (PTSS) occurring within 30 days of a traumatic event (Sparks, 2018). Another consideration is the contribution of racism and other cultural issues to the cumulative load (Bernard et al, 2021). These foundation traumas are essentially preverbal attachment wounds that are held in the body via implicit memory and may not be accessible or readily resolved through traditional verbal therapies. Understanding the impact of early trauma and how implicit memories affect the mind and body throughout the lifespan should motivate us to refine our methods of trauma treatment (Barnett et al., 2020).

4.2   BASIC TENETS OF THE ITR APPROACH

Rather than using art therapy as an ancillary therapy, as often occurs with other approaches, in Instinctual Trauma Response® we consider art therapy to be a primary means of treatment. Furthermore, we boldly assert that trauma symptoms can be eliminated, not just diminished, when the source for those symptoms is identified as coming from the ITR® (see section below). Creating imagery that puts the fragments of a trauma back into the context of a specific event causes these bits that we call *mental shrapnel* to lose the power to create intrusive symptoms. This art therapy tool is designed to access, reconsolidate, and resolve trauma through the creation of a Graphic Narrative® that externalizes the trauma and transforms it into a coherent, visual form. Although our case example focuses on a birth trauma, the procedures and concepts we describe here can be used for treating any trauma.

Our basic tenets for working with preverbal trauma can be stated as follows:

1   **Preverbal traumatic memories are stored in the nonverbal brain.**

These nonverbal memories consist primarily of body experiences of the animal survival instincts that we call the Instinctual Trauma Response®. (See the section on the ITR below.) These evolutionarily acquired survival behaviors are shared with reptiles and mammals (Gazzaniga & Volpe, 1981; MacLean, 1990; Tinnin & Gantt, 2014). During trauma, the structure and functioning of the brain under stress favors firing of subcortical neural networks focused on survival tasks, making explicit narrative and executive functioning choices unavailable or outside conscious awareness.

2   **Preverbal memories are blocked from awareness and are inaccessible to verbal probes.**

Through creative activities such as artmaking and expression through an Externalized Dialogue® with parts of self, people can access traumatic memories without reliving them. Through this process, we can recover the preverbal traumatic experience and embed it in a coherent narrative that will provide closure and subsequent storage in long-term verbal memory. The reconsolidated trauma memory is retired when converted to past tense, and the emotional arousal connected to the memory becomes neutralized. The mental shrapnel is no longer able to provoke flashbacks or other intrusive symptoms because it is put into context.

3   **In the nonverbal (emotional) brain, imprints of trauma memory lack linear sequence and narrative structure and, therefore, lack narrative closure.**

Preverbal traumatic memory may last a lifetime if not treated. When activated, imprints of trauma or implicit memories may be experienced as occurring in the present (a flashback). People may be "triggered" by overwhelming feelings with dissociative responses such as emotional numbing, amnesia, depersonalization, derealization, and even identity alteration. Art therapy can enable a creative response to traumatic memory that offers both a sense of control and distance from the past, thus transforming the overwhelming experience into something manageable (Hass-Cohen et al., 2018; Tripp et al., 2019). As an active and mindful approach, art therapy can help to bring the client's attention back into the present. Furthermore, it provides the means to retrieve preverbal traumatic memory and to integrate it in a verbal auto-biography which can be externalized and made tangible in an art form. In helping a client construct the Graphic Narrative® (GN), the therapist provides the necessary structure and linear sequence of the traumatic event. The functional connectivity of the emotional, memory, and cognitive systems is changed during trauma (Daniels et al., 2010; Hermans et al., 2014). Even the structure of the hippocampus and the amygdala can be altered (Ben-Zion et al., 2023). When the GN is re-presented the client can *hear and see* that the event is truly history; it is no longer felt to be present tense. Not only is the vertical connection of the right hemisphere's cortical and sub-cortical limbic systems functionally restored, but intrahemispheric communication can be enhanced. We hypothesize that the verbal brain has an obligatory rejection of the nonverbal brain's implicit memories (especially with infants and young children when the corpus callosum has not been fully myelinated) that can be overcome. This process can be explained by considering the neurobiological construct of "memory reconsolidation" as a means of revising the subjective experience of traumatic mem-ory (J. Sweeton, personal communication, April 7, 2023). Through the creation and repetition of new neural connections, new circuits begin to override the old ones, thus new learning changes the brain by reconsolidating the memory (Ecker et al., 2012). One might think about dealing with files on a computer, whereby the unman-ageable emotional learning is revised or updated before it can be saved.

4.3   BRAIN STRUCTURE AND HEMISPHERIC ASYMMETRIES

The structure of the modern human brain shows its evolutionary history from its bottom to top and its specialization for language through its left/right asymme-tries. In a model originally formulated in the 1960s, MacLean (1990) described the theory of the "triune brain." This theory has been criticized as being overly simplistic, although we acknowledge it can be useful as a general description for therapists when providing psychoeducation to their clients. More recent findings in neuroscience have spurred theorists and researchers to propose that the term "triune brain" be discarded and replaced with the "adaptive brain" (Steffen et al., 2022). In this new formulation, the adaptive brain consists of interdependent net-works that evolved together rather than as three mostly separate structures. These various networks are dynamic in that certain networks can work together or shut down others.

Understanding the interconnections between these various regions of the brain and the role of these structures in response to trauma has been extremely valuable for trauma therapists. Also of great significance are the neuroscience studies of the 1980s that produced important work on hemispheric asymmetry in the brain (Gazzaniga & Volpe, 1981; Geschwind & Galaburda, 1986; Sperry, 1985). Such work confirmed a supposition extant as early as the 4th century BC – that the two sides of the human brain have different functions (Ornstein, 1997). According to Siegel (1999), the right hemisphere, for example, is the more holistic of the two, includ-ing expression of emotion and the nonverbal and bodily processes, whereas the left hemisphere is more concerned with linguistic processing and narrative information. While it is useful to consider the different roles of the two hemispheres when looking at the emotional versus cognitive responses to trauma, for example, overgeneralizing about the left/right brain differences can be overly simplistic (Ornstein, 1997; Siegel, 1999; Springer & Deutsch, 1993). A more nuanced way to understand the role of the two hemispheres is that, in adults, both hemispheres contribute to complex activities such as language production and comprehension (Hertrich et al., 2020) and that both hemispheres receive and process bodily information (Power et al., 2011). And, thanks to the brain's neuroplasticity, a person can recover from certain physical and emotional injuries through creating new neural connections in the brain (Voss et al., 2017).

Two contemporary theorists especially important to our discussion are Daniel Siegel (a child psychiatrist: 1995, 1996, 1999, 2001) and Allan Schore (a neuropsychoanalyst: 1994, 1997, 2000, 2001, 2002, 2003, 2009, 2019). Siegel was instrumental in developing *interpersonal neurobiology*, a multidisciplinary field that combines concepts from mindfulness, attachment, and brain structure/function to give the neurobiological underpinnings of interpersonal experience. Schore has written extensively about affect regulation, brain development, and attachment. Of particular interest is that both authors stress the contributions of the right hemisphere in early childhood development. Since the right hemisphere is more active before age 3 (Schore, 2000, 2019), this has implications for the genesis and treatment of early traumas that we call *foundation* traumas in this chapter.

As Schore explains (2009), before the left hemisphere becomes more active, the right hemisphere performs the crucial role of developing the emotional self and of forming a secure attachment with a caregiver. If an infant experiences trauma(s) in early life, traumatic residue may press for expression through body sensations such as anxiety that has no root in the present day. While the corpus callosum begins myelination at 4 months of age, it does not finish the process until 25 or 30 years of age (Young et al., 2019). Therefore, its efficiency in transmission is compromised. This underscores the necessity of treating preverbal trauma. The insula plays a crucial role in interoception as it transmits nonverbal material such as the basic emotions of happiness, joy, and anger to other parts of the brain. Some of the other contributions of the insula (which is found in both hemispheres) are: providing context to social cues, generating a sense of self, perceiving pain, and achieving motor control (www.spinalcord.com). Interoceptive awareness (being able to sense bodily states) may point to fundamental mechanisms in art making and art therapy.

Siegel (1999) emphasizes that normal brain functions are integrated: "In neurologically intact individuals, the activity of both sides … contributes to the functioning … as a whole with greater or lesser degrees of interdependent activity" (p. 185). Siegel also points out the problems of disconnection or inhibition as contributing to certain psychological conditions, including PTSD.

The rapidly developing neurosciences now take us far beyond simple right/left descriptions of brain structure. Now, general right/left distinctions have limited utility. What matters more in terms of theory are the emotional/rational and verbal/nonverbal divisions and the functional neural networks that are generated from them.

When we offer an abbreviated description of the architecture of the brain and the general neuroscience of trauma, we find people are grateful for the basic message that their responses to trauma are universal survival strategies and their brain and body responded instinctively. This, of course, minimizes the likelihood of experiencing shame and stigmatization around a trauma response. Many clients find it quite a relief to know they are not crazy!

4.4   THE INSTINCTUAL TRAUMA RESPONSE®

We postulate that the Instinctual Trauma Response® (ITR) is a universal response to overwhelming, life-threatening events (Tinnin et al., 2002; Tinnin & Gantt, 2014). The fundamental components of the ITR are the following: the startle, the thwarted intention to fight or flee, the freeze, an altered state of consciousness, automatic obedience (animal submission), and attempts at self-repair. A person may face a potentially traumatizing situation, but if he/she is successful in fighting off an attacker or escaping, the freeze will not occur and the body is able to respond to the fight/flight response resulting from the activation of the sympathetic nervous system. However, at times the person (or animal) is not able to fight or is unsuccessful with flight, and in such situations, the freeze response is the last hope for survival (Roelofs, 2017). Sometimes a predator loses interest in the frozen prey, but there is a cost to pay. Even if the person survives the attack, there may be traumatic memory and fear in the system that is not adequately discharged or processed. In these situations, when the person is rendered helpless over the fearful situation, he or she falls into an altered state of consciousness. Those who experience such peritraumatic dissociation are more likely to develop PTSD (Breh & Seidler, 2007; Thompson-Hollands et al., 2017). In the ITR, the explicit and implicit memories of the event become dissociated, and symptoms including affect dysregulation, depersonalization, derealization, numbness, and amnesia are common responses.

We stress that the ITR is not a strategy that involves an active choice but is an evolutionarily acquired survival mechanism. For example, if an individual could use thinking to avert a trauma, such as successfully hiding from an attacker or swerving to avoid an oncoming car, then the person might be temporarily shaken. However, this would not likely result in a post-traumatic state. If, on the other hand, the person were trapped and/or unable to mount a behavioral response to the activation of sympathetic nervous system by that traumatic stressor, the body would naturally go into a parasympathetic state of freeze (Roelofs, 2017) and the cascade of the rest of the ITR would occur. Dissociation, a response to overwhelming trauma, has generally been characterized as a defense mechanism and a final survival response to life-threatening events. We see dissociation as a brain process that ensues when the verbal brain goes offline, agreeing with Meares who states, "dissociation, at its first occurrence, is a consequence of a 'psychological shock' or high arousal" (1999, p. 1853). According to LeDoux (1996) this process favors the "low road" from the sensory input of the thalamus to the amygdala because it is much faster than the "high road" to the amygdala through the sensory cortex. Similarly, Schore sees dissociation as "the loss of the integrative capacity of the vertically organized emotional right brain" (2009, p. 126).

The rather recent capacity for language (that is, recent in terms of human evolution), is housed for most people in Broca's area in the left frontal lobe and Wernecki's area in the left temporal lobe. These language areas of the brain "include(s) verbal consciousness as the uppermost and most recently acquired part" (Tinnin

& Gantt, 2014, p. 22). It is important to note that analogous structures in the right hemisphere can also develop language (Olulade et al., 2020).

During trauma, the language centers and other areas of the brain fail in reverse order of their evolution. This is what the famed neurologist Hughlings Jackson termed "dissolution" (Meares, 1999). If one cannot think one's way out of a potential trauma, then animal instincts take over. The parasympathetic division of the autonomic nervous system links the major organs of the body via the large vagal nerve. According to the polyvagal theory of Porges (2011), the ventral vagal complex of this nerve controls the social-engagement processes that are higher order functions. However, life-threatening situations interfere with these functions and disable the verbal brain. The organization of the right hemisphere is such that it responds to any stimuli more quickly than the left (Buklina, 2005; Cozolino, 2014), calling upon the fight/flight instincts. This is mediated by the sympathetic nervous system. However, when fight/flight does not work, the parasympathetic vagal system (the dorsal vagal complex) is evoked (Porges, 1995, 2011) resulting in a state of freeze or collapse.

As clinicians, we offer clients an understanding of the impact of trauma on the nervous system that can help de-stigmatize and normalize responses to trauma triggers. This can reduce self-judgment and internal messages that a heightened or shutdown response means that "something is wrong with me."

4.5   TRAUMA PROCESSING ACCORDING TO THE ITR THEORY

We contend that a complete trauma resolution must use an approach to restore the integration of up/down and whole brain networks by making a visual and verbal narrative to be stored in the frontal cortices. When using ITR, the trauma processing is complete when the perceptual, emotional, memory, and language elements of the trauma are wholly integrated. The person can see that a specific trauma is undisputedly over. In the terms of our processes as described below, by using a series of specified drawings (the Graphic Narrative® and its re-presentation), the story is finished at last. Through those drawings the GN allows us to access the traumatic memories that were not stored as episodic verbal memories. This allows the person to perceive the event in linear order, with a time orientation for the first time, thus creating new neural pathways. Finally, the experience is integrated in the brain with the Externalized Dialogue® by repeatedly exercising those new pathways, making them strong and resilient. This is an example of the brain's neuroplasticity.

Treating Foundation Traumas First

A *foundation trauma* is not simply a trauma that occurs during the preverbal period but one that sets the stage for later life. Like a house made of bricks, the cracks that originate in the walls are akin to the problems (e.g., symptoms) that therapy routinely addresses. Such damage may be clearly observable and seem relatively easy to repair. However, those that actually begin in the foundation are "below grade" and may be invisible. So it is with early trauma. Such damage cannot be completely repaired if the actual source of the damage has not been found. Also, once foundation traumas are processed it is then easier to address subsequent ones.

How does one know one might be dealing with foundation traumas? In general, the symptoms are those that have been associated with what had been termed neuroses, or diagnoses such as borderline personality disorder or avoidant personality disorder in previous editions of the DSM. Life-long features such as having chronic anxiety, emotional outbursts, depression, indecisiveness, unstable moods, difficulty in relationships, impulsiveness, problems regulating affect, toggling between intense love and intense hate for another person, feelings of emptiness or boredom, extreme responses to actual or perceived abandonment, or lack of self-worth point to the possibility of foundation traumas. Early trauma can also be linked with dissociation with up to 80% of individuals diagnosed with borderline personality disorder experiencing transient dissociative symptoms including depersonalization, derealization, psychological numbing, and analgesia (American Psychiatric Association, 2013; Krause-Utz, 2022). Factors contributing to more severe dissociative symptomatology include earlier age of onset and longer duration of abuse (Krause-Utz, 2022). Here are some examples of people who struggled with the persistent effects of foundation traumas:

- A young woman processed her birth trauma when she recognized that she was already "a burden" to her parents even before she was born. She gave her first GN the title "What Am I Here For?";
- A middle-aged man experienced extreme anxiety for routine medical check-ups that were determined to be remnants of an unfinished story as the result of a surgery in infancy. ITR helped him gain perspective and self-compassion for his wounded part who suffered the impact of preverbal trauma;
- A young man unpredictably fled uncomfortable situations, first running away as a teenager, then as a college student, and finally, as a postulant, leaving his religious community without permission. ITR helped him visualize the drive to escape, as it mirrored a history of multiple surgeries within the first days of life from which he never felt safe or protected; and
- A woman who had surgery within days of her birth for pyloric stenosis, a life-threatening stricture that blocks food from entering the small intestine and that can result in death. As this procedure was performed in the early 1950s when infants were not anesthetized (Chamberlain, 1989), we worked with the lifelong problems that she had as a result: feeling she was "born broken"; being preoccupied with her breathing and the inside of her body (Was she "dead or alive?"); feelings of being helpless and hopeless at different times of her life; and dealing with the effects of several suicide attempts.

Early preverbal trauma is not unusual but requires specialized tools for treatment. These individuals mentioned above all carried unresolved trauma-based symptoms into adulthood that manifested in shame, extreme anxiety, attachment difficulties, dissociation, and feelings of "not being safe" or "not being good enough." These issues cannot easily be explored with traditional verbal or insight focused therapies as they relate to memories that may not be readily accessible through talk therapy. In such cases, ITR helps individuals take a closer look at the experience of early trauma without being re-traumatized and facilitates a completion of the story that brings closure to the traumatic stress.

Many individuals know of specific preverbal traumas because family member verify events (such as a difficult birth, surgery, neglect, severe illness on the part of a caretaker, or abuse). Other people desire to do ITR because their years of talk therapies have not addressed the intrusive, arousal, and avoidant symptoms of PTSD. Still others are referred by therapists who feel inadequately trained in handling this type of treatment. Those who are unlikely to benefit from ITR are people with an active substance use disorder, an eating disorder requiring weight management, or an underlying psychotic disorder. These acute conditions have to be addressed first. When they are under control and a person is stable (and without dissociative regression), ITR can be commenced.

4.6   DESCRIPTION OF THE ITR APPROACH

The essential components of our treatment are the Graphic Narrative® (GN), the re-presentation of the GN, and the Externalized Dialogue® (ED). Each trauma is processed using the same techniques in the same order. Generally, we deal with the traumas in chronological order, starting with the foundation traumas.

The Graphic Narrative® and Its Re-presentation

The Graphic Narrative® is a structured series of drawings based on the Instinctual Trauma Response® (ITR). The ITR encompasses what we hypothesize to be a universal response to overwhelming trauma. The minimum drawings should be: a *Before* and an *After* scene, plus one for each ITR component (the startle, the thwarted intention of fight or flee, the altered state of consciousness, the automatic obedience, and the attempts at self-repair). It is helpful to put the body sensations in each picture, but a client can also make a separate drawing just focusing on those sensations. Other pictures can be included in the GN, such as a transition drawing showing a change of location, a map picture showing the environment of the event, and a close-up drawing depicting important details.

We cannot emphasize enough the importance of doing the drawings first, before any extensive verbal details about the trauma are given. Otherwise, the verbal brain will dominate the process and stifle important emotional material. Work with split-brain patients shows that the so-called "silent" hemisphere can communicate by drawing as well as by pointing to cue cards or making hand gestures (Schiffer, 2022). This suggests the potential for individuals with intact interhemispheric function to bypass using language. Many highly verbal people often say, "I don't know," when they really mean, "I don't have words for my experience." Symptoms such as having difficulty identifying and naming emotional states (alexithymia), and experiences of depersonalization and fragmentation of experience (dissociation) are often seen in clients with chronic, interpersonal trauma histories (Minshew & D'Andrea, 2015). Our approach recognizes that, while explicit memory may not be available, we can invite the individual to access implicit or unconscious processes simply by "letting the hand draw what your mind forgot."

By using the ITR as the outline for processing a trauma story, a person can likely capture those implicit memories that are the raw material of flashbacks and other intrusive experiences. We have found that these interruptions (or triggers) are fragments of specific events. When they are put into context in a GN and thoroughly processed with the re-presentation, such triggers cease to generate overpowering intrusive responses.

The GN not only provides structure but also affords an opportunity for psycho-education since it is based on the ITR. Although there are variations, all traumatic events meeting the DSM-5 TR and ICD-11 criteria will have the basic ITR components. Fundamentally, all the components are nonverbal and based on the body's responses to a life-threatening event (whether experienced first-hand or observed in another person).

The re-presentation part of the process truly brings the trauma to a close. Unlike with most art therapy processing sessions during which the artist tells about a picture, or in verbal therapy where the client is expected to talk about their story, in our method it is the therapist who witnesses and listens to the story as told through art and then repeats the narrative back to the client in a "re-presentation." It is important that the series of pictures are displayed in temporal sequence on the wall, and the therapist tells the story in the client's words without adding any interpretation or commentary. Some dramatic elements can be used, such as prosody, pitch of voice, pacing, and repetition which resonate with the right hemisphere (Schiffer, 2022). It is important to keep the re-presentation narrative true to the linear sequence of the ITR, and that the story is told from a third-person point of view keeping it "in the past," confirming that the traumatic event is indeed over. Cheftez describes the process of creating coherence in psychotherapy and his words apply doubly so to the re-presentation: "Left- and right-brain elements of experience are knitted into a coherent narrative by the left brain's ability to interpret what the right brain's emotionality generates but can't name" (2015, p. 46).

The re-presentation provides an opportunity to use memory reconsolidation (mentioned briefly above). According to van der Kolk, there are two brain-based systems that deal with self-awareness but are in two different brain regions – one that "keeps track of the self across time and one that registers the self in the present moment" (2014, p. 236). We hypothesize that, in addition to these two networks, others such as the visual network, the frontoparietal control network, and the dorsal attention network can be engaged by the re-presentation, resulting in a new understanding of the story as it is put into working memory.

The Externalized Dialogue®

After a GN is completed and re-presented, it is time for an *Externalized Dialogue*® (ED). The ED is similar to the Gestalt therapy process of the empty chair (Perls, 1969) in that the focus is an exchange between a person and an imagined entity. In contrast, in the ED the participants in the exchange are the parts of the client. As van der Kolk says, "A part is considered not just a passing emotional state or customary thought pattern but a distinct mental system with its own history, abilities, needs, and worldview" (2014, p. 281). The concept of internal parts can be traced back to Jung and Freud. Contemporary practitioners of this are Richard Schwartz (1995) who developed Internal Family Systems and van der Hart, Nijenhuis, and Steele (2006) who describe a theory of Structural Dissociation.

Setting up the ED is quite simple, and there are several useful variations depending on the age and preferences of the client. Originally, we used a video dialogue in which the client spoke into a video camera to record one part and then watched the replay, before responding for another part. Changing the view from a wide-angle to telephoto focus made the replay a dramatic conversation between older and younger parts of the person. Puppets, drawn portraits of the parts, and sculptures can be used instead of actual video footage of the client. The entire videotaped dialogue can be viewed so that it flows, as would a conversation between two people.

The written version of the ED is quite portable and easy to teach. Using writing paper and pens or markers in at least two different colors of ink, the client alternates hands to explore the different parts of self (Schwartz, 1995). The guidelines are also simple: Take turns, do not interrupt, and be civil. The first two of these can be quite difficult for those who are highly dissociative and have multiple streams of consciousness that compete for attention. The client is asked to use the dominant hand in making a written invitation to that part with which he/she wishes to talk. Then the person switches hands and the color of ink or marker to reply on behalf of the part. It is common for a person to be uncomfortable with the writing task and possibly find using the non-dominant hand difficult. A negative response at the beginning of the process ("Hell, no, I don't want to talk!") should not be a deterrent. In fact, a strong response is usually a good prognosis since some heretofore unexpressed thoughts and emotions have quickly surfaced. Often, people are intrigued when they are told about the connection of the hands to the opposite side of the body from the two hemispheres. (Of course, it is not as simple as having only one half of the brain control the other side of the body because there is some innervation to the same side as well.) However, many people have been surprised to experience the non-dominant hand-writing responses that are totally unexpected but are revelatory, wise, supportive, or challenging.

Here's a simplified version of what we tell clients about how ITR works. The GN allows for the emotional brain to deal with bits and pieces of trauma memory that have previously gone round and round in a repetitive "limbic loop" (the amygdala, hippocampus, and cingulate gyrus). The GN stops the looping and *shows* the logical brain what happened. These pieces get rearranged in a linear sequence, and are time-stamped, thus logically stored in explicit memory as past history. The re-presentation tells what happened during the trauma and includes thoughts, feelings, and body sensations. This gives the whole brain a new and much more integrated way to understand the full story with a beginning, middle, and end. Finally, accessing parts in the ED, the whole brain can communicate about past experiences and create healthy new patterns of reactions and responses to use for situations in the future.

We describe our approach as an empowerment model that lasts far beyond the formal therapy sessions. Once a person has done several GNs and EDs, they can do others on their own. We stress that these ITR processes are "tools for life" that can be accessed whenever needed.

4.7   A CASE STUDY

We present here a case of a woman who was able to use intensive trauma therapy to access and integrate preverbal traumatic experiences using a structured, trauma-sensitive art therapy approach. Prior to beginning this treatment, the client had largely avoided dealing with her traumatic past, a behavior consistent with her PTSD diagnosis. We contend that ITR facilitated a means to approach, actively uncover, and finally face the feared traumatic material. Ultimately the client was able to uncover new insight to her early trauma and find successful resolution.

Kim (a pseudonym), an attractive, well-educated, professional woman, was 37 years old when she was referred to Tally (second author) for trauma-focused art therapy following many years of conventional verbal psychotherapy. The referral was made because Kim and her previous therapist felt that their work had reached an impasse; furthermore, it was apparent that the focus needed to be redirected to deal with the pre-verbal trauma that had not been sufficiently addressed in earlier treatment.

Like many clients with early relational trauma, Kim was quite guarded in the initial months of therapy and it took time to develop any safety or sense of trust in the therapeutic alliance. Although she had intentionally sought out working with Tally and using art therapy with the goal of working on traumas that may have been difficult to verbalize, her behavior indicated a more ambivalent stance. She most often avoided using art as an expressive vehicle, instead focusing on keeping safe, managing her fluctuating feelings, and attempting to stay emotionally grounded. For Kim, distancing and intellectualization were ready defenses; she avoided the potential vulnerability that could accompany the unknown realm of connection through nonverbal expression.

As treatment progressed, however, a much younger ego state began to emerge that held and expressed significant unmet childhood longings and vulnerabilities. In this "child" state, Kim demonstrated a strong dependence upon Tally. In so many words, she continually looked for cues and asked for proof that Tally truly cared about her.

The younger "dependent" self-state and the older "self-reliant" one were in dramatic opposition to one another. Sessions were marked by intense vacillation where Kim would, on the one hand, express an overwhelming yearning for Tally's care and attention (for example, begging Tally to take her home) followed by periods of distance, immense rage, and feelings of disappointment (such as when Tally did not give in to her pleas, or when Tally set boundaries or otherwise disappointed her with some perceived lack of attunement).

Therapeutic boundaries were extremely challenging to maintain in this therapy, and limits were often perceived by Kim as "cold hearted, uncaring" even when offered with compassion. The therapeutic relationship became stressful for both client and therapist and themes of transference and countertransference had to be consistently addressed. Kim's attempts to forge some kind of special relationship with Tally (and her disappointment when these wishes were not met) seemed to be directly based on her childhood experiences with her parents where a cold/aloof mother or a demanding/inappropriate father were her most significant role models.

Kim was quite certain that she had experienced some preverbal trauma in her life, but her earliest memories were diffuse, consisting mainly of vague, unsettling somatic body sensations and intrusive imagery. She reported having frequent and disturbing flashbacks, experiencing feelings of depersonalization and derealization, and seeing unsettling, frightening, and often sexual images in everyday things. One disturbing memory came from a dramatic, all-black image she drew called "Mother's

Crotch." In the center of the paper is a "Y" shape with the three points of the "Y" touching the edges of the paper, done in heavy strokes of black charcoal. On either side of the "Y" are somewhat lighter applications of color, giving the suggestion of looking at a close-up of a woman's genitals and the tops of her legs. This powerful image emerged spontaneously and seemed to represent a traumatic birth story, triggering further feelings and associations about the early neglect and abuse.

Kim did have some explicit recall of sexual play that occurred between the ages of 3 and 5 with her brother and other children, as well as at least one incident of sexual abuse by a teenage male babysitter when she was 8. This incident with the babysitter was later reported to her mother who minimized its impact, stating, "Well, it was not your fault," and then walking away, thereby urging Kim to move on and not dwell on her feelings. Further sexual trauma occurred in an early adult relationship when Kim was victimized in a relationship with a controlling boyfriend.

Kim's parents were fundamentalist Christian ministers; her upbringing was strict and without demonstrated affection. She felt particularly pushed away by her narcissistic, self-involved mother and thus perceived herself as a burden. Her father, on the other hand, spent more time with Kim, making her feel *special* but inappropriately so, as he would take her out to show her off or buy her clothes and behave in a sexualized way that was confusing. Growing up in a family where neither parent was appropriate or available, where boundaries were either too rigid or too loose, Kim spent most of her childhood trying to manage, attempting to blend in without disrupting the balance. In describing her experience with her family, she once said: "I evaporate and meld into what they expect me to be, so I can blend in. I become tall, thin, and intelligent, whatever they need me to be so that I can match up with what they expect. Camouflage—that is my first language. It is what I do best."

Themes of not being seen, heard, validated, or comforted permeated Kim's early history and these themes persisted into her adult life. For example, she recalled a traumatic memory from age 4 when she choked on a piece of spinach and believed she was going to die. The terror she felt from her father's lifting her upside down by the heels and shaking her vigorously until she threw up, and of her mother's backing away from the scene, without comforting her or even explaining what had happened, resulted in conflicts for many years around eating, throwing up, and feeling unsafe and out of control.

Kim coped with stress by building a wall between herself and others. In an attempt to create a healthy boundary, Kim severed relationships with her parents and brother, based on unresolved feelings about her early childhood trauma and neglect. Her emotional life was quite constricted; she was inflexible and rigid. Avoiding expressing needs and feelings, she was extremely uncomfortable in social settings and had no real friends. At the start of treatment, Kim had been married for about five years to a kind but passive man with whom she was unable to have any kind of sexual relationship. Interestingly, this lack of sexual intimacy did not bother either of them.

While her external appearance was neat and polished, Kim's internal state was highly anxious and agitated. She could get to her high-pressure job on Capitol Hill most days because there was a clear expectation and structure about it, but coming to therapy proved to be more challenging, probably because it was less structured and required introspection. In her therapy sessions, Kim preferred sitting on the floor to sitting in a chair, and so spent many sessions seated on the floor in this child state leaning up against Tally's chair, where she seemed most comfortable. Interestingly, in this position she was not able to have eye contact with Tally. Also, Kim was not forthcoming with her own feelings or ideas. Instead, she would defer to Tally, often asking Tally to discuss what she was noticing about Kim or what theory she was using in treatment. Kim believed that anything that Tally could offer would be helpful because she, Kim, was so diffuse in her identity. The work of finding a self truly began when Tally did not fully gratify Kim's wish to have the theoretical base explained or to be told who Tally thought Kim was. Instead, Tally encouraged Kim to be patient and curious about her own experience and to believe that she would eventually find the answers within. This belief came from the assumption that a more adult self-state would eventually find a way to be present and offer some answers to move the process forward.

Early Artwork: Smearing, Primitive, and Unformed

Kim's early art therapy consisted of experimenting with the materials and dealing with the process of not knowing. Like a child's art works, many of Kim's early expressive pieces were blended, smudged non-representational pictures with layers of color and no distinguishable form. The smearing was done in a regressive state, and Kim often seemed to dissociate while layering her preferred medium, chalk pastel, on the page. She rarely had words to describe these scenes. The process of creating seemed to give her some pleasure and often resulted in messy hands, fingerprints, and chalk dust everywhere.

Preparing for an ITR Intensive

Kim saw Tally once or twice per week in art psychotherapy for about two years, during which time she ultimately moved from the regressive child state toward an increasingly adolescent or adult one, although there continued to be variability in her dependency and feelings toward Tally.

Judith Herman's groundbreaking book *Trauma and Recovery* outlines a three-phase model of "safety, remembrance and mourning [trauma processing], and reconnection" (1992, p. 156) that has become a model for sequencing trauma treatment. Together Tally and Kim accomplished some of Herman's important Phase 1 treatment goals, working on the extremely difficult task of developing a trusting therapeutic relationship in which there were simultaneously firm boundaries and consistency. Tally navigated a sensitive transference line of being perceived at times as the cold, distant mother and, at other times, as the inappropriate, demanding father. It was clear that working with years of developmental trauma would require a solid base, especially since so many of Kim's memories were implicit ones that had no explicit verbal recall. Gradually, Tally was able to help Kim find a more curious, adult stance and look inward to gain some access to her hidden emotional life.

Experientially based art therapy facilitated this process, and for Kim, the art making became increasingly expressive and took on meaning where she discovered freedom and joy in the process. Kim also began making moves towards independence, taking community-based art classes, and joining a Survivors of Incest support group. The biggest change in her life, however, came just months before Tally recommended more focused trauma work. Kim had become increasingly stressed with the expectations of her full-time lobbying position, finding the work extremely draining and the involvement with clients exhausting. She notified Tally that she planned to leave her job and find work as a dog walker so she would not have to deal with "difficult" people. This meant a substantial salary loss and significant changes in her lifestyle. Despite Tally's initial reservations about the decision, this proved to be the right move for Kim. The relationship Kim was able to develop with animals was overwhelmingly positive in contrast to her difficulties with human interactions. The dogs were unconditional in their loyalty and love. Furthermore, Kim's engagement with them created an experience of "limbic regulation," a term coined by Lewis et al. (2000, p. 98) to describe the life-sustaining way that pets and their owners can read each other's emotional cues, be comforted and soothed by one another, and even regulate one another's physiology. The therapeutic work deepened when Kim brought in video clips of the animals, showing Tally vignettes of her happy and uncomplicated interactions with pets, and demonstrating her ability to experience an emotional connection with them. Sharing these videos provided a nice vehicle through which Kim could be attuned to, appreciated, and seen.

At this point, Tally felt Kim was ready to do some of the trauma processing work and begin to address the early issues that were at the core of her interpersonal struggles. Linda and Lou happened to be lecturing at the university art therapy clinic that was a training clinic for Tally's trauma classes, and they agreed to see Kim as a teaching case. The team felt the ITR approach was ideal in that it typically starts with a graphic narrative of the earliest, most foundational trauma – a preverbal memory of the earliest moments of experience. Because Kim had sketched out the image of "Mother's Crotch" during her art therapy with Tally, the birth trauma story offered a good place to start. For others, they can be told that we will begin with a practice story and we will prompt them to "Imagine yourself as a baby in diapers in distress." Then, they are helped to do a story using the ITR as its structure.

Although we are not claiming that Kim or any client can recall the explicit events of a birth, we do recognize that birth is a first traumatic experience for everyone, and particularly for individuals where secure attachment is lacking. Thus, in the graphic narrative process, being invited to *imagine* the experience of birth or other preverbal experiences through the instinctual trauma lens, using what is known about parents, their circumstances, early history, and the setting into which they were born, can provide us with much insight into the foundational experiences, beliefs, and circumstances for any client.

Kim's Graphic Narrative

We began the session showing Kim a handout describing the essential components of ITR where each "stage" of the process has a precise function: the startle (the moment when there is a recognition that something potentially traumatic is happening), the thwarted intention (the attempt to fight or flee), the freeze (a sudden shutdown state), the altered state of consciousness (with feelings of being detached from the body), automatic obedience (where actions are moving in robot-like submissive response), body sensations (somatic cues throughout), self-repair (when the person gets back to feeling "self"). With this template, Kim modified the drawings in her GN to fit the circumstances of her own birth – the imagined experiences of her mother in labor, a picture of her birth, and the first moments of human consciousness.

Kim's drawings showed each of the components of the trauma response on separate sheets of 12" x 18" paper. The series began with a *Before* picture to set the stage and an *After* picture to show, once and for all, that the event is over. Putting body sensations and thoughts and feelings on each page completes the GN. Kim added her drawing of "mother's crotch" as an integral part of the series. Kim described this as a "horrifying, terrifying image" that she believed to mirror herself in her newborn state, undifferentiated from her mother. Kim's drawings were abstract but extremely effective in depicting her subjective experience of feeling the pressures of her mother's labor. The structure of the ITR approach seemed to offer Kim a way to map the events in some sort of order, which was different from the diffused stories, so overwhelming and confusing, that she had been unable to address previously.

Kim's Response to the Re-presentation: "I'm Pink, Not Black"

After Kim finished her GN we taped the drawings to the wall in sequential order to prepare for the re-presentation. As Linda, who was standing, explained the process to be used, Kim stopped her, saying, "You just became my mother!" Kim identified that Linda's standing up and "teaching" sparked her negative response (maternal transference). This was interesting to observe, as Tally was sitting by Kim (in a supportive role) and Linda (in the therapist role, re-presenting the work) became a fearful object (her unresponsive, cold mother). Fortunately, Linda quickly attuned to Kim's concerns and sat down, thus assuring Kim that the team was listening to her and was respectful of her needs. Kim was comfortable with this dynamic and allowed Linda to continue in her role as therapist and continue to re-present the artworks.

Linda told the story of "About-To-Be-Born Kim," using as many of Kim's own words about her drawings as possible. A typical ITR processing of any trauma story provides several passes over the content: the client's general description of the event in preparation for processing, the drawing of the GN, and the therapist's review of the GN (with the client) in preparation for the re-presentation. The task for the therapist is to stay as close to the client's material as possible but also to weave into the story the elements of the ITR, especially the nonverbal aspects of the body sensations that accompany it. In the middle of the re-presentation, Kim pointed to one of the darkest drawings and emphatically said: "That's me! That's what I see to be me – instead of looking into my mother's eyes and seeing *her*, I see *me*. That's the me!" She then had an extraordinarily important insight that the black drawing was not, in fact, a reflection of her, but of her mother. In what seemed to be an instant, Kim's fundamental assumptions about herself began to shift. For the first time, she saw how she had entered the world as a pure, "pink" baby untainted and born with fresh potential. She recognized that she was not the ugly black smudge that she had seen in her mother. This marked a nascent experience of individuation and allowed us to work with new parts in the continued work of the session.

The Externalized Dialogue®

Following the GN and re-presentation, Kim was instructed to create a written version of the ED. The following is her ED between the dominant hand (DH) and non-dominant hand (N-DH):

DH: Hi Newborn Kim. I heard your story today and saw what you saw. Is there anything else you want me to know today?

N-DH: *I like pink.*

DH: Was there more of you inside before you came out?

N-DH: *I was pink and everywhere.*

DH: There were lots more fingerprints behind where you were born. Was that all you too?

N-DH: *Yes, I had our fingers.*

[After some coaching and getting some reassurance that she was doing the ED "right," Kim resumed it.]

DH: Hello again Newborn Kim. I will keep trying to write with you – so we can see each other better.

N-DH: *OK.*

Kim's positive (and seemingly immediate) response to the ITR processes boded well. She could see for herself that the idea she was evil and damaged came, not from her own sense of self, but from her mother's projections onto Kim at birth. In the ITR program it is not uncommon for the first story to provide a theme that encapsulates a person's trauma history and sets the stage for the work to come.

Intensive Therapy at the ITR Clinic

About six months later, Kim agreed to participate in two weeks of intensive trauma therapy at the ITR clinic in Morgantown, West Virginia. The goal was for Kim to work on the issues she had begun to address in outpatient therapy with Tally and to gain more information about her preverbal trauma experiences. The treatment team consisted of Linda and Lou as well as others of the Morgantown staff who participated in a few of the sessions. As part of her training in ITR methods, Tally supported Kim's work by attending all sessions for the first week of the intensive, observing the process and assisting with the overall treatment.

Externalized Dialogues with "Warthog"

We invited Kim to select several stuffed animals or puppets from ITR's well-stocked playroom to use in the Externalized Dialogue process. Kim had used her own stuffed animals for a resource in the earlier session at the university clinic, so we felt puppets would be helpful as a projection of parts of self. Kim immediately eyed the warthog puppet that was "so ugly she was cute." Although she also used other animals, Warthog was clearly her favorite. We came to understand that Warthog was the tangible representation of Kim's preverbal self.

In her EDs Kim showed exquisite concentration and emotional intensity. She would position a pad of paper in front of her on the table and place Warthog in her lap so she could peer into Warthog's eyes. Aside from the initial instruction about the ED and some occasional coaching when she got stuck, the therapists said little in the sessions, instead playing the role of "enlightened witness" (Miller, 1990).

Figure 4.1 shows the beginning of the first ED. It is a meet-and-greet that is reminiscent of a young child showing him/herself to a new adult. Kim's statement ("I felt what you were feeling yesterday and I know that it was all encompassing and bad") refers to a preverbal trauma processed the day before. Figures 4.2 through 4.11 are presented as they occurred in the dialogue process.

It is tempting to try to determine more of the specific content of Warthog's responses. However, we contend that what is most important is the communication *between the verbal and nonverbal parts of the brain*, which allows the preverbal experience to be expressed and responded to by internal parts within the session. In our approach, while there is less emphasis on interactions between the therapist and the client, we highlight the significance of the implicit right interhemispheric processing that seems to promote healing. This is the kind of support that Kim needed – to be witnessed by adults who viewed her seriously and to simultaneously discover the adult self-state who could also fill that role.

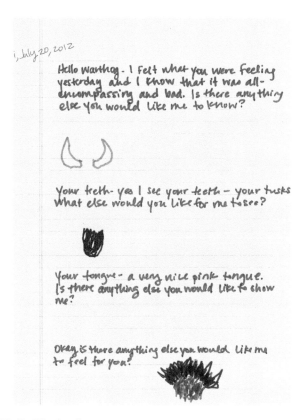

FIGURE 4.1 "Hello Warthog"

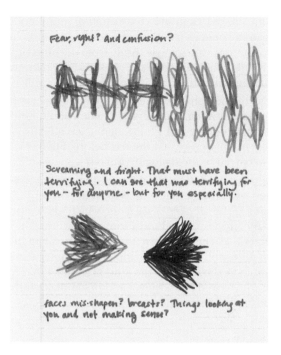

FIGURE 4.2 "Fear and Confusion"

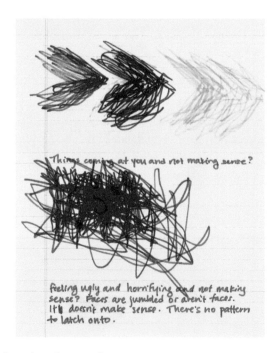

FIGURE 4.3 "It doesn't make sense"

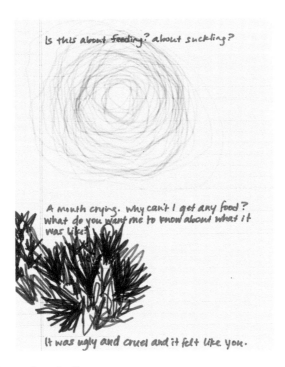

FIGURE 4.4 "A mouth crying"

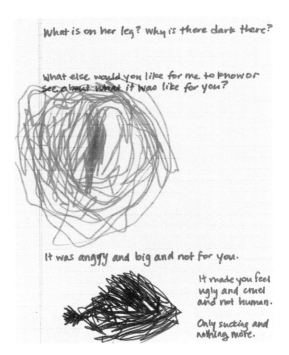

FIGURE 4.5 "What was it like for you?"

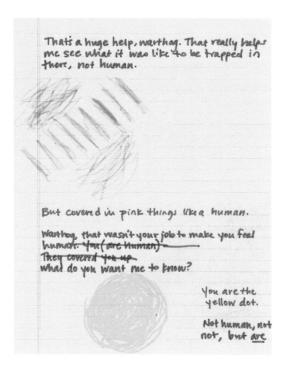

FIGURE 4.6 "That's a huge help, Warthog"

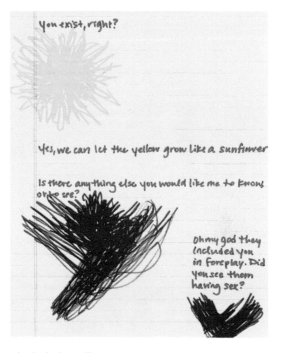

FIGURE 4.7 "They included you!"

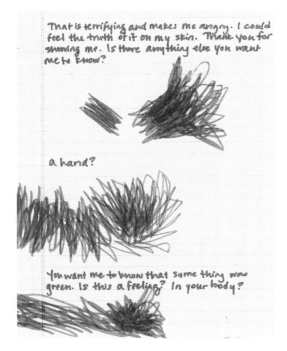

FIGURE 4.8 "Thank you for showing me"

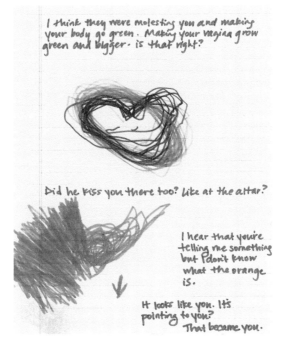

FIGURE 4.9 "I hear that you are telling me something"

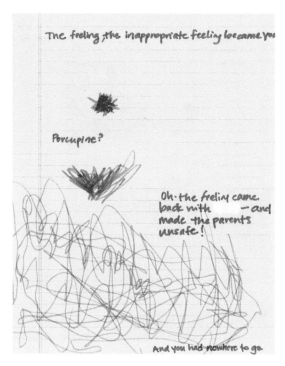

FIGURE 4.10 "The inappropriate feeling became you, and you had nowhere to go"

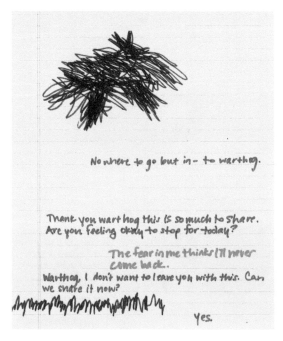

FIGURE 4.11 "Thank you Warthog, this is so much to share!"

Kim's Response to the ITR Experience

Using the GN process, Kim addressed several early traumas, but most of the work in the two-week intensive program involved EDs. The experience in West Virginia facilitated a vast shift in the way Kim saw herself and the way she trusted her internal processes and nonverbal experience. In describing the GN in a post-treatment interview, Kim remarked: "The Graphic Narrative made it [the trauma] something you could look at … Before, it was just a feeling of chaos and confusion that didn't know it had a place or a source. It [the GN] calmed a fault line at the very base of me." She added that before the intensive therapy, she would "fall through" such a fault line. This was a beautiful description of repairing a foundation trauma.

Kim continued to progress greatly in her outpatient therapy with Tally. After ITR, she left her dependent relationship with her husband because, upon her return, she found he would not listen to her and stated he was not able to believe her story about the early trauma. Kim decided she needed to be with people who understood her and believed her story. Kim discovered a new strength of self-awareness that probably would not have happened, and certainly not as quickly, had she not done the intensive work on the foundation trauma.

The puppet Warthog gave Kim critical information to help her heal and to deal with that information without becoming destabilized. Even without the day-to-day relationship with her husband, Kim was noticeably stronger, more independent, and less easily triggered. Eventually she established some friendships and sought out a new community through church and other activities. Although feelings of anxiety continued to come and go, she felt "prepared" and believed that living on her own was "not as scary" as she thought it might be.

In describing the art therapy process and her experience at ITR, Kim stated:

> It [the experience] is coming from inside the client. Art is creating a language on paper and making it make sense. As I do it, it becomes something that makes sense. I can tell a story. So the process of doing it accesses information that is projected into the picture, and then it becomes real. Warthog – she expressed a bunch of scribbles that meant something – [my] left hand and Warthog had no words.

Follow-up on the Case

After the ITR experience, Kim continued to work for several years with Tally in outpatient therapy. Warthog made the transition with Kim back to her apartment and came to therapy sessions for a few months until Kim felt her beloved puppet was no longer needed. She continued her work as a dog walker and was promoted to a staff position at the dog day care center. She began to expand her social spheres making several meaningful friendships and finding great satisfaction working with the animals and their owners. Most significantly, the rigid, anxious, and shut-down version of Kim gave way to a self that was notably more flexible, open, and resilient and that was able to negotiate life in a much more adult state.

When reflecting on her experiences in treatment, Kim remained curious about the early traumas and was willing to address these issues directly. She admitted that she was not sure if she would ever know the explicit truth behind these preverbal

experiences, but that she felt much more able to live life as a complete person knowing that her story had been expressed and witnessed. As she attended to the previously fragmented images and memories, she found the experience to be not as
threatening or destabilizing as it had been in the past.

4.8   DISCUSSION

Memories are stored in several places in the brain. It is theorized that explicit memories are stored in the hippocampus, prefrontal cortex, and amygdala (Eichenbaum,
2017). The amygdala and cerebellum are involved in emotionally salient and implicit
memory (Kandel et al., 2021, Fastenrath et al., 2022). Researchers are now finding
that traumatic memories apparently change the structure as well as the function
of the brain particularly with respect to neural networks (Baron, 2021; Power et al,
2011). Investigators are linking an understanding of these effects to clinical applications (Postel et al., 2021).

We assert that the expressive therapies, because they can access these implicit
memories and do not rely on thinking and verbalization, are a treatment of choice
for trauma-related disorders (Gantt & Tinnin, 2009; Tripp, 2007). Art therapy can
bypass some of the difficulties inherent in traditional verbal psychodynamic psychotherapy because the emphasis on the art-making process allows the therapy to
attend to the images and metaphors produced, rather than focusing primarily on
the therapeutic relationship. Survivors of trauma often resist engaging in trauma
work because they fear becoming dysregulated by the intense range of feelings
that may be unearthed, and because they distrust any intimate relationship. Art
therapy can provide a holding space to reduce anxiety and can safely help manage and contain overwhelming and dysregulating feelings (Tripp et al., 2019). It
can be a pleasurable process that can build self-confidence in the artist who ultimately, through the action of art making, takes control of the expression and any
subsequent interpretation of the material. The intensive trauma approach further
assists the client by providing a structured template through which feelings can be
expressed (the GN and ED), thus facilitating the process of telling the trauma story
without becoming overwhelmed.

Kim's experience with the ITR methods shows the importance of treating foundation traumas. It also shows how rapidly changes can be accomplished when the
focus is on communication between the verbal and nonverbal parts of the brain.

4.9   CONCLUSION

The specific methods we have outlined for drawing and writing are straightforward
and simple. Once a person has had some practice during art therapy sessions, he or
she can easily do the same techniques outside the sessions. The ED is flexible and
highly adaptable to a client's situation. We recommend that the EDs be used preemp-
tively as well (for example, checking in with identified self states when a big event is
coming up, such as a family reunion or an evaluation at work, or when the person
needs to make a major decision).

Kim's case illustrates the gains that are possible when preverbal (foundation) traumas are processed using the GN and ED. Knowledge of brain structure and function permits the development of approaches that take advantage of this understanding. However, as Siegel points out, "What we are concerned with is the subjective experience of minds, not merely the functional anatomy of the brain" (1999, p. 199). The job of an attuned therapist working with complex trauma is to assist a client in finding a way to confront, express and rework the traumatic material. The goal is not to engage in a treasure hunt to find specific, hidden information, but rather to collaborate with the client in an experiential and creative process. Ultimately, we find our methods help the clients co-create a story that provides a beginning, middle, and ending for the trauma, and make it clear, once and for all, that the past is past.

4.10   TRAINING AND ASSESSMENTS FOR ITR

While the steps of the ITR protocol are fairly simple, one does need specific training to use this approach. For more information about ITR training and assessments, go to www.ITRtraining.com. For people seeking to be treated with ITR, we require getting a thorough trauma history and filling out trauma assessments, along with an initial screening and an intake interview. The assessments used by ITR are self-report questionnaires.

At the time of Kim's treatment, the ITR clinic used the following assessments:

Toronto Alexithymia Scale (TAS)

Symptom Checklist-45 (SCL)

Dissociative Regression Scale (DRS)

Trauma Recovery Scale (TRS)

Dissociative Experiences Scale (DES II)

Impact of Events Scale-R (IES-R)

REFERENCES

American Psychiatric Association (2013). *Diagnostic and statistical manual* (5th edition). Author.

Anand, K., & Hickey, P. (1987). Pain and its effects in the human neonate and fetus. *New England Journal of Medicine, 317*, 1321–1329. https://doi.org/10.1056/NEJM198711193172105

Barnett, M. L., Kia-Keating, M., Ruth, A., & Garcia, M. (2020). Promoting equity and resilience: Wellness navigators' role in addressing adverse childhood experiences. *Clinical Practice in Pediatric Psychology, 8*(2), 176.

Barron, H. (2021). Neural inhibition for continual learning and memory. *Current Opinion in Neurobiology, 67*, 85–94. https://doi.org/10.1016/j.conb.2020.09.007

Ben-Zion, Z., Korem, N., Spiller, T., Duek, O., Keynan, J., Admon, R., Harpaz-Rotem, I., ... Hendler, T. (2023). Longitudinal volumetric evaluation of hippocampus and amygdala subregions in recent trauma survivors. *Molecular Psychiatry, 28*(2), 657–667. https://doi.org/10.1038/s41380-022-01842-x

Bernard, D. L., Calhoun, C. D., Banks, D. E., Halliday, C. A., Hughes-Halbert, C., & Danielson, C. K. (2021). Making the "C-ACE" for a culturally-informed adverse childhood experiences framework to understand the pervasive mental health impact of racism on Black youth. *Journal of Child & Adolescent Trauma, 14*, 233–247.

Bogat, G., DeJonghe, E., Levendosky, A., Davidson, W., & von Eye, A. (2006). Trauma symptoms among infants exposed to intimate partner violence. *Child Abuse & Neglect, 30*(2), 109–125.

Breh, D., & Seidler, G. (2007). Is peritraumatic dissociation a risk factor for PTSD? *Journal of Trauma & Dissociation, 8*(1), 53–69. https://doi.org/10.1300/J229v08n01_04

Buklina, S. (2005). The corpus callosum, interhemispheric interactions, and the function of the right hemisphere of the brain. *Neuroscience & Behavioral Physiology, 35*, 473–480.

Burton, L. (1992). Black grandparents rearing children of drug-addicted parents: Stressors, outcomes, and social service needs. *The Gerontologist, 32*(6), 744–751.

Center for Substance Abuse Treatment (2014). *Trauma-informed care in behavioral health services*. Substance Abuse and Mental Health Services Administration. [Treatment Improvement Protocol (TIP) Series, No. 57.] Chapter 5, Clinical Issues Across Services. Available from: www.ncbi.nlm.nih.gov/books/NBK207185/

Chamberlain, D. (1989). Babies remember pain. *Pre- & Perinatal Psychology, 3*(4), 297–310.

Chapman, L. (2014). *Neurobiologically informed trauma therapy with children and adolescents: Understanding mechanisms of change.* W.W. Norton.

Chefetz, R. (2015). *Intensive psychotherapy for persistent dissociative processes: The fear of feeling real.* W.W. Norton.

Cozolino, L. (2014). *The neuroscience of human relationships: Attachment and the developing social brain* (2nd ed.). W.W. Norton.

Daniels, J., McFarlane, A., Bluhm, R., Moores, K., Clark, C., Shaw, M. … Lanius, R. (2010). Switching between executive and default mode networks in posttraumatic stress disorder: Alterations in functional connectivity. *Journal of Psychiatry & Neuroscience, 35*(4), 258–266. https://doi.org/10.1503/jpn.090175

De Bellis, M., & Zisk, A. (2014). The biological effects of childhood trauma. *Child & Adolescent Psychiatric Clinics of North America, 23*(2), 185–222. https://doi.org/10.1016/j.chc.2014.01.002

Delima, J. F., & Vimpani, G. V. (2011). The neurobiological effects of childhood maltreatment. *Family Matters*, Issue No. 89.

Ecker, B., Ticic, R., & Hulley, L. (2012) *Unlocking the emotional brain: Eliminating symptoms at their roots using memory reconsolidation.* Routledge.

Eichenbaum, H. (2017) Memory: Organization and control. *Annual Review of Psychology, 68*, 19–45. https://doi.org/10.1146/annurev-psych-010416-044131

Fantuzzo, J., Boruch, R., Beriama, A., Atkins, M., & Marcus, S. (1997). Domestic violence and children: Prevalence and risk in five major U.S. cities. *Journal of the American Academy of Child & Adolescent Psychiatry, 36*(1), 116–122.

Fastenrath, M., Spalek, K., Coynel, D., Loos, E., Milnik, A., Egli, T., Schicktanz, N., Geissmann, L., Roozendaal, B., Papassotiropoulos, A., & de Quervain, D. J.-F. (2022). Human cerebellum and corticocerebellar connections involved in emotional memory enhancement. *Proceedings of the National Academy of Sciences, 119*(41), e2204900119.

Felitti, V., Anda, R., Nordenberg, D., Williamson, D., Spitz, A., Edwards, V., … Marks, J. (1998). The relationship of adult health status to childhood abuse and household dysfunction. *American Journal of Preventive Medicine, 14*, 245–258.

Gaensbauer, T. (1995). Trauma in the preverbal period: Symptoms, memories and developmental impact. *Psychoanalytic Study of the Child, 50*, 122–149.

Gale, J., Thompson, R., Moran, T., & Sack, W. (1988). Sexual abuse in young children: Its clinical presentation and characteristic patterns. *Child Abuse & Neglect, 12*, 163–170.

Gantt, L., & Tinnin, L. (2009). Support for a neurobiological view of trauma with implications for art therapy. *The Arts in Psychotherapy, 36*, 148–153.

Gazzaniga, M., & Volpe, B. (1981). Split brain studies: Implications for psychiatry. In S. Arieti (Ed.), *American Handbook of Psychiatry* (2nd ed., Vol. 7). Basic Books.

Geschwind, N., & Galaburda, A. (1986). *Cerebral lateralization: Biological mechanisms, associations, and pathology*. MIT Press.

Hass-Cohen, N., Bokoch, R., Clyde Findlay, J., & Banford, A. (2018). A four-drawing art therapy trauma and resiliency protocol study. *The Arts in Psychotherapy, 61*, 44–56.

Herman, J. (1992). *Trauma and recovery*. Basic Books.

Hermans, E., Battaglia, F., Atsak, P., de Voogd, L., Fernandez, G., & Roozendaal, B. (2014). How the amygdala affects emotional memory by altering brain network properties. *Neurobiology of Learning & Memory, 112*, 2–16.

Hertrich, I., Dietrich, S., & Ackermann, H. (2020). The margins of the language network in the brain. *Frontiers in Communication, 5*, Sec. Language Sciences.

Kandel, E. R., Koester, J. D., Mack, S. H., & Siegelbaum, S. A. (2021). *Principles of neural science* (6th ed.). McGraw Hill.

Karr-Morse, R., & Wiley, M. (1997). *Ghosts from the nursery: Tracing the roots of violence*. Atlantic Monthly Press.

Krause-Utz, A. (2022). Dissociation, trauma, and borderline personality disorder. *Borderline Personality Disorder and Emotional Dysregulation, 9*(1), 14).

LeDoux, J. (1996). *The emotional brain: The mysterious underpinnings of emotional life*. Simon & Schuster.

Lewis, T., Amini, F., & Lannon, R. (2000). *A general theory of love*. Random House.

Lipsitt, L. (2012). Long-term consequences of perinatal trauma (pp. 422–426). *Encyclopedia of trauma*. SAGE Publications.

MacLean, P. (1990). *The triune brain in evolution: Role in paleocerebral functions*. Plenum Press.

Meares, R. (1999). The contribution of Hughlings Jackson to an understanding of dissociation. *American Journal of Psychiatry, 156*, 1850–1855.

Messina, N. P., & Schepps, M. (2021). Opening the proverbial "can of worms" on trauma-specific treatment in prison: The association of adverse childhood experiences to treatment outcomes. *Clinical Psychology & Psychotherapy, 28*, 1210–1221.

Miller-Graff, L., Galano, M., & Graham-Bermann, S. (2016). Expression of re-experiencing symptoms in the therapeutic context: A mixed-method analysis of young children exposed to intimate partner violence. *Child Care in Practice, 22*, (1), 64–77.

Miller, A. (1990). *Banished knowledge: Facing childhood injuries* (L. Vennewitz, Trans.). Anchor/Doubleday. (Originally published in 1988)

Minshew, R., & D'Andrea, W. (2015). Implicit and explicit memory in survivors of chronic interpersonal violence. *Psychological Trauma: Theory, Research, Practice and Policy, 7*(1), 67–75.

Ogden, P. & Fisher, J. (2015). *Sensorimotor psychotherapy: Interventions for trauma and attachment*. W.W. Norton & Co.

Ogden, P., Minton, K., & Pain, C., (2006) *Trauma and the body: A sensorimotor approach to psychotherapy*. W. W. Norton.

Olulade, O., Seydell-Greenwald, A., Chambers, C., Turkeltaub, P., Dromerick, A., Berl, M. … Newport, E. (2020). The neural basis of language development: Changes in lateralization over age. *PNAS, 11*(38), 23477–23483.

Ornstein, R. (1997). *The right mind: Making sense of the hemispheres*. Harcourt Brace.

Perls, F. (1969). *Gestalt therapy verbatim*. Real People Press.

Perry, B. (2009). Examining child maltreatment through a neurodevelopmental lens: Clinical applications of the neurosequential model of therapeutics. *Journal of Loss & Trauma, 14* (4), 240–255.

Perry, B., & Szalavitz, M. (2007). *The boy who was raised as a dog*. Basic Books.

Philo, J. (2015). *Does my child have PTSD?* www.familius.com

Porges, S. (1995). Orienting in a defensive world: Mammalian modification of our evolutionary heritage. A polyvagal theory. *Psychophysiology, 32*, 301–318.

Porges, S. (2011). *The polyvagal theory: Neurophysiological foundations of emotions, attachment, communication and self- regulation.* W.W. Norton.

Postel, C., Mary, A., Dayan, J., Fraisse, F., Vallée, T., Guillery-Girard, B., Viader, F., … Gagnepain, P. (2021). Variations in response to trauma and hippocampal subfield changes. *Neurobiology of Stress, 15,* 100346.

Power, J., Cohen, A., Nelson, S., Wig, G., Barnes, K., Church, J., … Petersen, S. (2011). Functional network organization of the human brain. *Neuron, 72*(4), 665–678.

Roelofs, K. (2017). Freeze for action: Neurobiological mechanisms in animal and human freezing. *Philosophical Transactions of the Royal Society B Biological Sciences, 372,* 20160206.

Scaer, R. (2005). *The trauma spectrum: Hidden wounds and human resiliency.* W.W. Norton.

Schiffer, F. (2022). Dual brain psychology: A novel theory and treatment based on cerebral laterality and psychopathology. *Frontiers of Psychology, 13,* 986374.

Schore, A. (1994). *Affect regulation and the origin of the self: The neurobiology of emotional development.* Erlbaum.

Schore, A. (1997). Early organization of the nonlinear right brain and development of a predisposition to psychiatric disorders. *Development & Psychopathology, 9,* 595–631.

Schore, A. (2000). The self-organization of the right brain and the neurobiology of emotional development. In M. D. Lewis & I. Granic (Eds.), *Emotion, development, and self-organization: Dynamic systems approaches to emotional development* (pp. 155–185). Cambridge University Press.

Schore, A. (2001). The effects of early relational trauma on right brain development, affect regulation, and infant mental health. *Infant Mental Health Journal, 22*(1–2), 201–269.

Schore, A. (2002). Dysregulation of the right brain: A fundamental mechanism of traumatic attachment and the psychopathogenesis of posttraumatic stress disorder. *Australian & New Zealand Journal of Psychiatry, 36,* 9–30.

Schore, A. (2003). *Affect dysregulation and disorders of the self.* W.W. Norton.

Schore, A. (2009). Attachment trauma and the developing right brain: Origins of pathological dissociation. In P. Dell & J. O'Neil (Eds.), *Dissociation and the dissociative disorders: DSM-V and beyond.* Routledge.

Schore, A. (2019). *Right brain psychotherapy.* W.W. Norton.

Schwartz, R. (1995). *Internal family systems therapy.* Guilford.

Siegel, D. (1995). Memory, trauma, and psychotherapy: A cognitive science view. *Journal of Psychotherapy Practice & Research, 4,* 93–122.

Siegel, D. (1996). Dissociation, psychotherapy and the cognitive sciences. In J. Spira (Ed.), *The treatment of dissociative identity disorder* (pp. 39–80). Jossey-Bass.

Siegel, D. (1999). *The developing mind: Toward a neurobiology of interpersonal experience.* Guilford.

Siegel, D. (2001). Toward an interpersonal neurobiology of the developing mind: Attachment relationships, "mindsight," and neural integration. *Infant Mental Health Journal, 22*(1–2), 67–94.

Sparks, S. (2018). Posttraumatic stress syndrome: What is it? *Journal of Trauma Nursing, 25*(1), 60–65.

Sperry, R. (1985). Consciousness, personal identity, and the divided brain. In D. Benson & E. Zaidel (Eds.), *The dual brain: Hemispheric specialization in humans.* Guilford.

Springer, S., & Deutsch, G. (1993). *Left brain, right brain* (4th ed.). Freeman.

Steffen, P. R., Hedges, D., & Matheson, R. (2022). The brain is adaptive not triune: How the brain responds to threat, challenge, and change. *Frontiers of Psychiatry, 13,* 802606.

Terr, L. (1988). What happens to the memories of early trauma? A study of twenty children under age five at the time of documented traumatic events. *Journal of the American Academy of Child and Adolescent Psychiatry, 27,* 96–104.

Terr, L. (1990). *Too scared to cry.* Harper & Row.

Thompson-Hollands, J., Jun, J., & Sloan, D. (2017). The association between peritraumatic dissociation and PTSD symptoms: The mediating role of negative beliefs about the self. *Journal of Traumatic Stress, 30*(2), 190–194.

Tinnin, L., & Gantt, L. (2014). *The instinctual trauma response and dual brain dynamics: A guide for trauma therapy.* Available through Create Space on Amazon Books.

Tinnin, L., Bills, L., & Gantt, L. (2002). Short-term treatment of simple and complex PTSD. In M. B. Williams & J. G. Sommer (Eds.), *Simple and complex post-traumatic stress disorder: Strategies for comprehensive treatment in clinical practice* (pp. 99–118). Haworth Press.

Tripp, T. (2007). A short-term therapy approach to processing trauma: Art therapy and bilateral stimulation. *Art Therapy: Journal of the American Art Therapy Association, 24*(4), 176–183.

Tripp, T., Potash, J., & Brancheau, D. (2019). Safe place collage protocol: Art making for managing traumatic stress. *Journal of Trauma & Dissociation, 20*(5), 511–525.

van der Hart, O., Nijenhuis, E., & Steele, K. (2006). *The haunted self: Structural dissociation and the treatment of chronic traumatization.* W.W. Norton.

van der Kolk, B. A. (2006). Posttraumatic stress disorder and the nature of trauma. In M. Solomon & D. Siegel (Eds.), *Healing trauma: Attachment, mind, body and brain* (pp. 168–195). W.W. Norton.

van der Kolk, B. A. (2014). *The body keeps the score: Brain, mind, and body in the healing of trauma.* Viking.

Voss, P., Thomas, M., Cisneros-Franco, J., & De Villers-Sidani, E. (2017). Dynamic brains and the changing rules of neuroplasticity: Implications for learning and recovery. *Frontiers in Psychology* (Sec. Auditory Cognitive Neuroscience), Volume 8.

Williams, M., & Lascelles, B. (2020). Early neonatal pain: A review of clinical and experimental implications on painful conditions later in life. *Frontiers in Pediatrics* (February 6).

Young, D., Neylan, T., Chao, L., O'Donovan, A., Metzler, T., & Inslicht, S. (2019). Child abuse interacts with hippocampal and corpus callosum volume on psychophysiological response to startling auditory stimuli in a sample of veterans. *Journal of Psychiatric Research, 111,* 16–23.

CHAPTER 5

PRINCIPLES OF MEMORY RECONSOLIDATION

Advanced Art Therapy Relational Neuroscience Perspectives

Noah Hass-Cohen

5.1 INTRODUCTION

Trauma-conditioned and altered neurobiological functions may frequently retraumatize as they rekindle fear and invasive memories (Hass-Cohen & Clyde Findlay, 2015; Lanius et al., 2011). In this way traumatic memories may create a vicious cycle of intrusive and disturbing negative emotions and cognitions (Ehlers & Clark, 2000). This cycle reconsolidates old fears, fragments autobiographical memories, prevents contextualizing the trauma as a past event, and constrains interpersonal functions (Lane et al., 2015).

Memory recall and processing destabilizes established memories, temporarily making them susceptible to change, and supporting reconsolidation (Schwabe et al., 2014). During memory recall, proteins in the fear and memory synapses of the brain (the lateral amygdala and the hippocampus) become labile for several hours and can therefore be modulated by protein synthesis in the hippocampus (Nader et al., 2000; LeDoux, 2003). Consequently, as traumatic memories are processed visually or verbally, they may fade away or contextually update and integrate with other autobiographical memories (Lee et al., 2017) allowing for continuous reorganization and recovery (Moscovitch & Gilboa, 2022). This kind of reconsolidation is not a one-time event but rather is repeated with subsequent activation of memories (Nader et al., 2000; Tronson & Taylor, 2007). The theory has been partially supported by pharmacological and psychedelics research (Astil et al., 2021; Kindt et al., 2009; Lonergan et al., 2013).

Research has suggested that the application of specific treatment principles has the potential of updating recalled memories so that they become non-threatening (de Oliveira Alvares & Do-Monte, 2021; Herry et al., 2010; Lanius et al., 2010; Lane et al., 2015; Schiller et al., 2010; Schwabe et al., 2014). In general, achieving and maintaining actual and perceived safety and affect regulation while engaging in contextualized traumatic memory processing has been shown to be critical for trauma informed care (Herman, 1997; Lanius et al., 2010). It is the balance between contextualized representations and non-contextualized sensory-based representations that contributes to the integrity or fragmentation of episodic and semantic memory recall (Brewin et al., 2010). Thus, memory reconsolidation treatment guidelines for safe and positive memory reconsolidation include (a) avoiding further activation of traumatic memories by pairing them with new non-threatening information, (b) developing close supportive relationships, (c) balancing and regulating of out-of-control responses by increasing the capacity for positive emoting, and (d) compassionate relapse prevention. To counteract the persistent nature of fears, mindfulness softening, curiosity, and positive acceptance of traumatic memories are needed

DOI: 10.4324/9781003348207-5

throughout (Briere & Scott, 2015; Hass-Cohen & Clyde Findlay, 2015; Hass-Cohen, Bokoch, & McAnuff, 2022; King et al., 2013).

5.2 ART THERAPY RELATIONAL NEUROSCIENCE MODEL FOR MEMORY RECONSOLIDATION

Art therapy relational neuroscience (ATR-N) based theoretical principles are designed to provide a good foundation for traumatology-based memory reconsolidation goals (Hass-Cohen & Clyde Findlay, 2015). ATR-N interventions can be designed to take advantage of the neural linkages between ruptured functions of traumatic memories and creativity (Hass-Cohen et al., 2018).

This chapter describes constraining and supportive ATR-N principles for memory reconsolidation which are grounded in pertinent neuroscience (Hass-Cohen & Clyde Findlay, 2015). The ATR-N approach includes six CREATE theoretical principles: (1) creative embodiment, (2) relational responding, (3) expressive communicating, (4) adaptive responding, (5) transformative integration, and (6) empathizing and compassion (Hass-Cohen, 2008).

The principle of adaptive responding incorporates the secure remembrance model (SR-5), which has five expressive arts goals/tasks: (1) safety, (2) relationships, (3) remembrance, (4) reconnection, and (5) resiliency and relapse prevention (Hass-Cohen & Clyde Findlay, 2015; Hass-Cohen et al., 2014) (Figure 5.1). In therapy, the SR-5 goals are not necessarily set or achieved consecutively. Although establishing safety is the first task in traumatology work, developing and maintaining safety and the therapeutic relationship are reiterative tasks. In the same vein, remembrance, which focuses on trauma memory processing, may not be possible for some

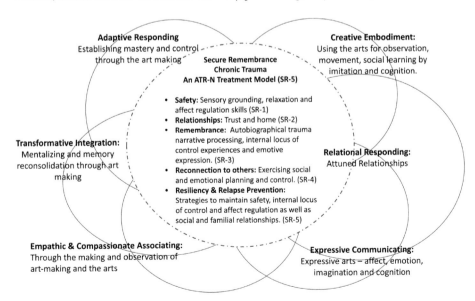

FIGURE 5.1 Summary of the ATR-N principles and secure remembrance (Noah Hass-Cohen)

traumatized people; for others, remembrance may start the first day of treatment (King-West & Hass-Cohen, 2008).

5.3   RELATIONAL RESONATING

Security

Survivors of trauma and abuse often express ongoing painful relational experiences with others, including a lack of support and outright disbelief, devaluation, and betrayal (Perry et al., 1995). The recall of these traumatic memories constrains memory reconsolidation as during the necessary recall adrenal and cortisol discharge may recondition and strengthen fear and trauma-based memories. Throughout therapy, rekindled symptoms threaten the therapist–client relationship contributing to a sense of mistrust, resignation, defeat, guilt, and shame. Trauma survivors have most likely have never had positive relational mirroring, and likely interpret body gestures as threats to security rather than empathic ones (Lane et al., 2015; Markowitz et al., 2009).

Lacking these empathizing and mentalizing skills likely affects the way that survivors interact with the world. The individual may develop negative relational generalizations that leave her feeling overwhelmed even in a therapeutic setting. Hence establishing a strong relationship that can mediate the implicit emotional turmoil that explicit narrative trauma processing may entail is critical (Missirlian et al., 2005).

Social and instrumental imitation involves prefrontal motor mirror neuron (MN) activation (Mukamel et al., 2010). MN fire in recognition and anticipation of one's own and others' purposeful and successful movements involving the hands and mouth. Early research had suggested that mirror neurons are also activated in the development of empathy (Rizzolatti et al., 2001). Others have suggested that the function of MN is only linked to observation and imitation of motor tasks (Heyes & Catmur, 2022). However, this research has not explored the context in which gestures, actions, and use of implements occur. Moreover, people with a history of trauma and neuropsychiatric disorders may experience dysfunctions in mirror neuron systems (MNS) (Ferrari et al., 2017; Walsh et al., 2021). In art therapy, client–therapist gestures provide a unique therapeutic opportunity to mend such relational ruptures. Recognizable movements, media, and tools associated with active art making also likely activate MNS, presenting an opportunity for social embodiment (Hass-Cohen & Clyde Findlay, 2015; Singer, 2004). So, for example when therapists engaged in reflections grounded in mimicking, their empathic resonance increased (Agarwal, 2021). MNS activation is particularly sensitive to significant others, gestures, actions, and situations (Duschek et al., 2019; Coan et al., 2006). This broader mirroring function is an intersubjective function by which clients can then start to utilize therapy as a way of stabilizing and feeling interpersonally secure (Ammaniti & Gallese, 2014). The trusted therapist becomes an auxiliary-self that reduces heightened fear activation and habituation and shapes new self-memories (Knol et al., 2020). Directives from the therapist can also progressively promote an exploration of safe relationships such as "draw a safe place, including growing and changing places such as gardens" and "represent a soothing and trusting living relationship." That is, the therapist self becomes a reparative mirror for the client (Ellingsen et al., 2020; Hass-Cohen, 2007).

Interpersonal and intersubjective mirroring is supported by connectivity and familiarity (Feng et al., 2022). Familiarity and respect can be developed slowly through instrumental and task-oriented accidental or deliberate mutual touching, for example, of the same piece of paper used for art (Hass-Cohen et al., 2015). Symbolic and physical art-mediated-interpersonal-touch and-space (AMITS) is one of art therapy's advantages (Hass-Cohen et al., 2014). For example, positive and safe AMITS include sharing materials and touching one's own artwork or a client's artwork, as well as expressing a positive interest in the tactile aspects of artwork (Hass-Cohen et al., 2014). Several opportunities exist to express closeness, interest, curiosity, and support in this way. Early in a therapeutic relationship, the art therapist may suggest that the client touch a smudged pastel area on the therapist's own page. Alternatively, he or she might ask to touch a client's page to stabilize it as the client's scribbling moves it or ask to hold a ball of clay made by a client to sense its weight and power. While the first line of relational support lies in this implicit therapeutic relationship, support can evolve and become symbolized and explicit through dual and dyadic drawing techniques (Bat-Or, 2010; Fish, 2012; Franklin, 2010; Gavron, 2013; Kaiser & Deaver, 2009).

In therapy, fingertips brushing against another person's fingertips is another example of how the art therapist's "third hand" (Kramer, 1990), in assisting the client, can provide mirroring reassurance, comfort, and security. In dual drawings, therapists and clients also touch the same page as they gesture to each other to co-create. MN assist in establishing a sense of familiarity with the art therapist's activities; these include provision, structuring, and handling of the art materials and the invitation to engage in simple art-making tasks, such as coloring pre-made shapes. Under therapy conditions, the client's reactions to these movements build connectivity. MN, which typically function to recognize purposeful actions, can boost clients' recognition, anticipation, and creative imagination of what will happen next. In therapy, this intersubjective function carries a supportive, non-threatening role and may present as the following internal dialogue: "I do what you do; I can do what you do; and I can recognize and anticipate what you will do." Once this relational familiarity is established, the therapist can initiate specific safety-oriented directives. Interventions such as "make an anchor from clay," "depict a safe place, space, thing, or pet," or "use visual arts [dance, moment, theater, or music] to show how you might feel under safe circumstances" are also appropriate (Hass-Cohen & Clyde Findlay, 2015). These arts-based requests are used to trigger the imagination of diverse representations of safeness. Choosing to "make, show, and tell" one of these representations most likely engages creative- and task-based neurocircuitry that also contributes to reducing rumination and depression.

5.4   ENGAGING IN INTERPERSONAL SOCIAL RELATIONSHIPS

Some treatment approaches suggest that outreach to others may be best attempted after successful narrative trauma processing (Herman, 1997), which in this case would be following memory reconsolidation. However, information from the neuroscience of post traumatic growth suggests that social interaction can directly contribute to the onset of adaptive allostasis, responding by regulating cortisol and catecholamine levels and supporting updating of memories (Schelling et al., 2006; Tsai et al., 2014). As described later in this chapter, hormonal levels of cortisol and catecholamine increase in response to acute stress, and can become dysregulated in response to chronic stress. While positive and supportive social environments regulate the feedback loops associated with these hormones, negative social interactions continue to dysregulate (Duax et al., 2014; McGaugh & Roozendaal, 2002; Sapolsky, 2004). Thus, it is incumbent that therapists use the art to interact relationally with clients, invite symbolic representations of relationships, and encourage reaching out to social networks. Guidelines for such interactions may be for clients to slowly familiarize themselves with a social milieu and perhaps start with dyadic interactions as well as develop skills to escape or leave uncomfortable situations (Schulkin, 2011). Schulkin's research suggested that engaging in unfamiliar or unclear situations can increase cortisol secretion, whereas avoidance of potentially threatening events will decrease cortisol. Other research found that having three or more regular social contacts has been linked with lower allostatic load scores (Seeman et al., 2002).

5.5 ADAPTIVE RESPONDING

Immobilization and Engagement

The freeze response is an immobilized response which is characterized by a collapse of mobility (Kozlowska et al., 2015). From a sympathetic nervous system perspective, the person is not able to engage in a stress flight or fight response, is mostly aware of the situation and continues to be scared. Executive, fear, memory, and modulatory centers of the brain (medial prefrontal cortex, amygdala, hippocampus and hypothalamus) contribute to freezing and deactivation of motor areas. In this conceptualization the freeze response comes after an initiation of a stress response and is part of the sympathetic and neuroendocrine nervous system. The response may become habituated and traumatizing (Kozlowska et al., 2015).

There is another freezing, more primitive, response which is mediated by the parasympathetic nervous system and described as a freeze-or-faint (Porges, 2001, 2009). These responses may relate to branches of the vagus nerve which directly innervate the heart. Freeze responses triggered by the unmyelinated dorsal vagal complex (DVC)-based reactions are automatic and non-conscious, as are all ANS functions. These down regulated heart rhythms can be dangerous. The polyvagal system, which acts though the parasympathetic nervous system, has two branches. An activated dorsal vagal complex (DVC) brings on a primal immobilizing response. This face–heart connection is impacted by social interactions, which then serve visceral bodily states (Porges, 2022). The DVC function contrasts to the myelinated ventral vagal complex (VVC) relaxation response, associated with interpersonal and social connectivity (Figure 5.2).

Threat-based responses can be observed in non-expressive facial expressions such as a permanently downward facing mouth, lack of prosody and vocal intonation, hypersensitivity to low frequency background noises and sensory cues, and difficulty attuning to the human voice. Other clues include consistent negative or aroused appraisals of day-to-day situations (Porges, 2001; 2009).

Clinically it may or may not be possible to ascertain the neuroscientific type of freeze which may also shift from a sympathetic to a parasympathetic response. First and foremost, it is critical to convey a positive non-threatening interaction. To do so the

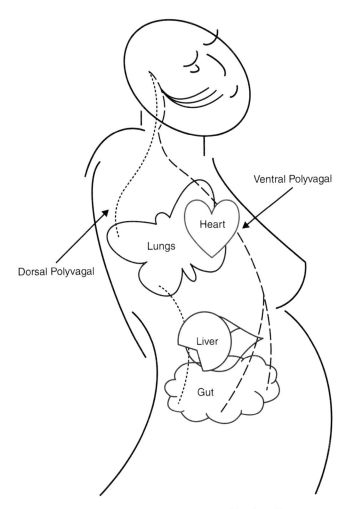

FIGURE 5.2 Schematic polyvagal system. Front, ventral broken line represents the social ventral vagal complex (VVC). To the back of the figure, dorsal dotted line represents the immobilizing dorsal vagal complex (DVC). The polyvagal, the longest cranial nerve, innervates the heart as well as the lungs (represented as a butterfly form), the liver (represented by tear shapes), and the gut (represented by a cloud form). Together with other cranial nerves the polyvagal innervates the face and influences facial expressions (Noah Hass-Cohen)

therapist should use a consistent, sincere, and soft voice as well as caring facial expressions, such as genuine smiling that naturally activates the eye muscles (Ekman, 1992). These kinds of social interactions facilitated by gaze, facial expressions, and other socially based sensory cues can mediate dysregulated autonomic states (Porges, 2013).

Overall structuring the art therapy environment to support safety and relational resonating is also needed. The therapist needs to provide clients with information on the protective utility of the freeze response, reminding them that in the past an immobilized response may have saved them from abuse and danger (Porges, 2013). Within the art therapy studio, reduced glare and low frequency noises can calm the DVC reaction and open opportunities for VVC social engagement. Background music with vocals can help the client attune to human interaction (Porges, 2013). Soft materials can further soothe and calm (Hass-Cohen et al., 2022a; Hass-Cohen et al., 2022b).

Stress Reduction

Clients' felt and perceived sense of security has been directly associated with positive versus negative outcomes (Meekums, 1999). Short-term as well long-term stress responses contribute to this threat. Experiencing fear, trauma related stress or non-specific stress both before or after memory reactivation may impact reconsolidation as stress-associated neurochemicals may either enhance or impair memory functions (Schwabe et al., 2014; Sutherland & Bryant, 2005). A negative reconsolidation of memory rekindles traumatic responding in multiple neuropathways and needs to be avoided.

The fight or flight short term stress response involves activation of the sympathetic-adreno-medullar (SAM) axis (Sapolsky, 2004; Sorrells & Sapolsky, 2007) (Figure 5.3). Other areas in the sympathetic autonomic nervous system are the amygdala as well as adrenaline and noradrenalin release. SAM is an aroused activation coping response. Relevant to memory reconsolidation, adrenaline and noradrenalin dampen the prefrontal responses. This reduced cognitive response constrains memory reconstruction. The hypothalamic-pituitary-adrenal (HPA) axis is part of the neuroendocrine system and involves the release and circulation of glucocorticoids, meaning cortisol (Figure 5.3).

Pertinent to memory reconsolidation, high and continuous levels of cortisol impair memory retrieval and consolidation. This may again constrain updating of memories (Sapolsky 2004; Sorrells, S. F., & Sapolsky, 2007). Furthermore, the HPA axis is sensitive to early trauma impacts and may have an altered function in survivors (Godoy et al., 2018). While the long-term stress response has clearly been associated with loss and depression, the two responses are not mutually exclusive.

The resolution of short- and long-term stress responses has been associated with proactive social responses whereas an altered chronic long-term stress function has been associated with chronic social avoidance and defeat (Stephen et al., 2021; Wood et al., 2010). Reducing allostatic load requires learning a range of strategies (Schulkin, 2003; Sterling & Eyer, 1988). Addressing these goals for the client who operates from the more evolved stress response, whether short- or long-term, is somewhat of a different task than for the polyvagal oriented client. This is because stress responses occur on an axis of mastery and control that can be mediated by cognitive functions. Therefore, alternative learned responses, such as reduced reactivity to external sensory inputs and internal bodily sensations, may contribute to reduced sympathetic and neuroendocrine arousal. Such adaptive responding and resiliency are associated with rapid resolution of short- and long term-stress responses. The skills necessary for this resolution include these: (1) learning and engaging in relaxation and grounding, i.e. affect regulation techniques, (2) practicing mastery and control in the therapy environment, and (3) repeated actual and perceived

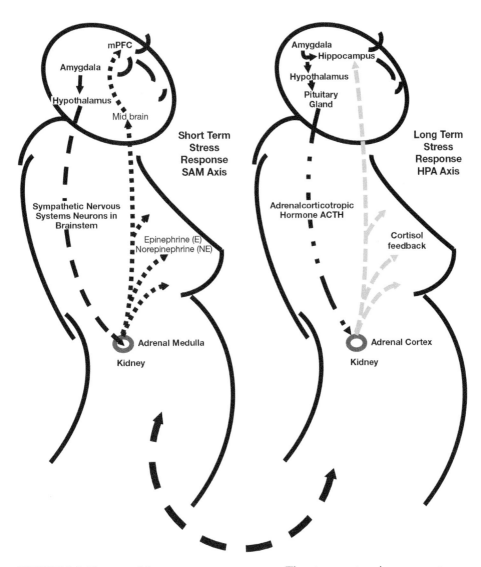

FIGURE 5.3 Short- and long-term stress response. The stress system is an neurotransmitter and endocrine system that involves the short-term sympathetic adrenomedullary (SAM) axis stress response (left) as well as the long-term hypothalamic-pituitary-adrenal (HPA) axis response (right). Activation of SAM releases norepinephirne (NE) whereas that of the HPA releases cortisol. As shown by the lower dotted semi curve, the two systems work in tandem (Noah Hass-Cohen)

behavioral mastery and cognitive perception of control outside of the therapy context (de Kloet et al., 2005). The acquisition of these three skills supports renewed social interactions, narrative trauma processing, secure remembrance, and relapse prevention (Strouse et al., 2021). In addition, creative art making can be used as a self-care practice that contributes to allostatic adjustment.

Relaxation, Safeness, and Comfort

While safety is associated with hypervigilance which is intended to avoid stress and danger triggers, safeness represents as an emotional self and other warm interpersonal and loving connection. Starting and ending art therapy meetings with brain-based relaxation techniques such as a mindfulness self-compassion break, mindfulness interventions, mindful movement can support self-regulation and a sense of safeness (Emerson, 2015; Hass-Cohen et al., 2022). Soothing materials and the creation of soft products such as cloth attachment albums may bring on a sense of quietness and calm (Hass-Cohen, 2008; Lucre & Clapton, 2021). The art making can also provide a time of rest which would include drawing images from nature and/or any other studio art-based work not directly related to the trauma history (Petersen et al., 2007). For some, the prompt to imagine and create safe and stable experiences has a similar effect (Hass-Cohen & Clyde Findlay, 2009).

Safeness can also be established by meeting distress in session with soft materials and compassion (Hass-Cohen et al., 2022c). The idea is to partner soft, ephemeral materials that may trigger feeling unsafe, with a compassionate reaction. For example, a ten-week group curriculum which offered non-structured materials, specifically, water, clay, and paint before engaging with structured media and prompts showed continuing significant improvement in self-compassion and cognitive and affective mindfulness with no reported aversive reactions. These results suggested that the traditional structured media approach to safeness may be inverted. Potentially disturbing psychophysiological reactions to media are viewed as an opportunity to practice self-compassion (Hass-Cohen et al., 2022c).

Control

Counterbalancing negative short-term stress responses, positive excitation such as therapeutic art making could potentially have positive effects on memory reconsolidation as the art expression offers vivid interfering material, which can be accompanied by positive excitation, which contributes to a balanced stress response. Experiences and or perceptions of escapable stress involve active coping, which regulates the stress response, whereas inescapable stress involves passive coping and behavioral inhibition. Repeatedly asking clients if they wish to proceed with processing and gently reminding them that they can stop or proceed as quickly or as slowly as they would like to, may increase clients' sense of control, and reduce the likelihood of re-traumatization. It is also critical to work with the client to make sure that he or she does not feel trapped. This is because connections from the dorsal raphe nucleus and mPFC to the amygdala modulate fear expression of escapable or inescapable situations (Hartley et al., 2014; Phelps & Ledoux, 2005). Reminding clients that traumatic memory reconsolidation and processing are upsetting now can help clients differentiate between past and current threat and regulate affect. Another way the therapist can reduce the risk of current threat reconsolidation is to avoid any pressures or demands on the client to ascertain the truth or provide a complete picture of what has happened.

Neurobiologically, excitation, such as that which might be experienced with heightened sense of control as well as a short-term stress response, is expressed as a low-level cortisol and NE release (McEwen, 2007, 2012). It is associated with allostasis and eustress. In addition to providing energy, excitation is also associated with heightened attention and focus and the forgetting of traumatic memories. In other words, under the right conditions, the stress response, manifested as excitation, can be beneficial (McEwen, 2007, 2012). Extrapolating from information about the stress response, the therapist may want to introduce novelty and excitation by helping the client maintain a slower pace (Hass-Cohen & Clyde Findlay, 2015). As appropriate, it is important to explore on paper or through other media, escape, and avoidance routes; these are correlated with lower levels of internalized symptoms (Shahar et al., 2012).

Increased sense of control has been demonstratively associated with post traumatic growth (Dekel et al., 2011). As the active coping area of the amygdala receives visual and auditory information (Hass-Cohen & Clyde Findlay, 2015; Pessoa & Adolphs, 2010), it is likely that art therapy practices can play a strong role in deconditioning the amygdala. Indeed, empirically proven trauma-focused cognitive behavioral therapy (TF-CBT) often includes art and play therapy (Deblinger et al., 2006). All these types of interventions must be repeated (Perry, 2006) to support affirmative memory reconsolidation.

Mastery

Interventions can provide a sense of safety and pleasure and generate experiences of coping, mastery, and control supporting cognitive and emotional flexibility (Chapman et al., 2001; Chapman, 2014; Gil, 2010; Gray, 2011; Klorer, 2005; Moon, 2001; Hass-Cohen, 2008; Hass-Cohen & Clyde Findlay, 2015; Kashdan et al., 2004; King-West & Hass-Cohen, 2008; Malchiodi & Crenshaw, 2017; Meekums, 1999). Recovery may also be mediated by the appreciation of beauty (Peterson et al., 2007).

Scaffolded according to the clients' interests and ability, an art therapy approach, which includes the development of artistic mastery, is appropriate (Kramer, 1990). The verbal discussion of artistic mastery in addition to a psychological exploration of the content may help cement these competencies. In therapy, the art making assists in transforming avoidant or negative responses into positive or assertive striving for control responses (Henry & Wang, 1998). For example, clients' refusals to draw or making quick marks on the page may indicate adaptive efforts and should not be interpreted negatively. Another example is large gesture drawings. Those gestures may embody fight or flight fantasy and yet represent coping as the exploration of this imagery may increase a sense of mastery. Furthermore, because resiliency is associated with the ability to successfully anticipate the need for coping, it is possible for clients to identify pertinent scenarios and imagine how they might utilize coping strategies (Lahad, 1993). Highlights of contextual processing include transforming implicit imagery, supporting reflexive mentalizing, and making the implicit explicit. The goals are to make the most painful memories speakable, to maintain self-regulation, and to coherently narrate current experiences. This kind of controlled exposure to traumatic memory is considered a necessary ingredient of art-based trauma processing. Within the studio, such exposure, through excitation, can be safe and therapeutic as the client controls it. Guided by the principle of expressive communicating, the art therapist relies on multimodal expressive means, including dance, music, drama, and crafts to stimulate divergent creative expressions and engage in positive emotions. For example, movement and positive mental states trigger dopamine in the reward system as described earlier (Jung et al., 2013).

In the reward system, the raphe nucleus, the locus coeruleus, and the ventral tegmental area connect to the cerebellum, an area responsible for movement. These connections are crucial to affect processing and positive emotions (Konarski et al., 2005; Villanueva et al., 2021). From a reward system perspective, tactile pleasant experiences, sensory vividness, and mastery contribute to pleasurable feelings. Movements and extroversive expression are triggered by expressive arts interventions; possibly they stimulate dopamine (DA) release and limbic activity that are linked to positive emotions and reinforcement. A generalization effect may occur as the generation of positive emotions may prompt the emergence of additional positive emotions. In addition, pride in the art product likely stimulates the brain's natural reward systems, which can then continue to generate positive responses. A part of instinctual, survival-based reactions, emotions contribute to physiological equilibrium and homeostasis (Panksepp & Burgdorf, 2006).

Therefore, for the client who repeatedly perceives threat in session, the recommendation is to focus on the art making and initially, avoid processing the content and meaning of the art. This intervention may support increase in positive rewards and decrease in negativity.

5.6 EXPRESSIVE COMMUNICATION

Novelty and Creativity

If memory reactivation is not immediately followed by learning of interfering material, episodic memories may be strengthened. Creativity plays a major role in successful positive memory reconsolidation. In fact, brain structures that are involved in the three functions of autobiographical memory also involve regions of the default mode network (DMN), which is associated with creativity (Jung et al., 2013). DMN activation involves the medial prefrontal cortex (mPFC), midline frontal and lateral parietal structures, and medial and lateral temporal-limbic regions (Spreng & Grady, 2010) (Figure 5.4). Autobiographical self-referential processing also occurs in cortical midline structures, particularly in the mPFC (St. Jacques, 2012).

According to developing research, it is likely that in tandem with alterations in the mPFC, alterations in the DMN are predictive and/or a result of PTSD (Lanius et al., 2010; Qin et al., 2012); in trauma-impaired mPFC, the capacity for fear extinction is compromised (Yehuda & LeDoux, 2007). Contextual processing and expressive communication that focuses on how the narrative is actively processed, rather than on the content of the narrative, also more likely allows memories to be put aside or placed in the past (Gold, 2008; Hass Cohen & Clyde Findlay, 2015). Art-based contextual memory processing seeks coherent and contextual narration of the memory rather than a focus on the content of the memory. Therefore, it behooves the therapist to work with the client to access only the necessary upsetting memories and not the full picture of what had happened, who was involved and who was responsible. Furthermore, for chronic trauma survivors who may have for many years sought to find the truth or the reason for what had happened continuing in this vein is likely not recommended.

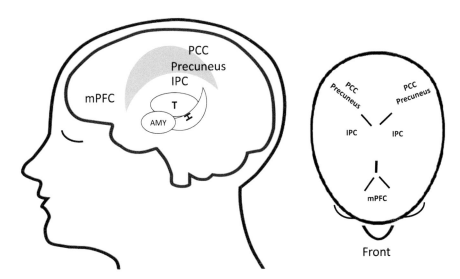

FIGURE 5.4 Midline neurocircuitry of autobiographical memories, mentalizing, and creativity. Shown on the left side view is the shared midline pathway from the medial prefrontal cortex (mPFC, self-center), through midline frontal and lateral parietal structures, and medial and lateral temporal-limbic regions – crescent shape – which include the inferior parietal cortex (IPC), the posterior cingulate cortex (PCC) and the precuneus, which borders on the visual cortex. Top view on the right demonstrates same areas. Lines within images represent the ventricles, which are provided for orientation purposes. Also shown are the amygdala (AMY), fear center; hippocampus (H), memory center; and the thalamus (T), gateway of sensory processing (Noah Hass-Cohen)

Positivity

Expressive communication and positive emoting will likely produce positive outcomes as well as to negate negative outcomes (Fredrickson et al., 2000). Experiencing positive emotions supports psychological and physical well-being (Lyubomirksy et al., 2005; Seligman & Csikszentmihalyi, 2000). Positive emoting is associated with multiple nervous systems. Their function can be negatively impacted by life events such as trauma as well as by genetic vulnerability to developing post-traumatic stress disorders (Skelton et al., 2012).

Fredrickson's broaden-and-build theory of positive emotion explains the evolutionarily different roles served by positive versus negative emotions (Fredrickson & Levenson, 1998). Negative emotions serve the purpose of perpetuating adaptive traits when one is threatened by fear. In contrast, positive emotions establish themselves during times when there is no threat to one's life, so that one is able to build physical, psychological, and social resources. Recurring positive emotions play a key role in developing and maintaining resiliency, because they allow for a widening of the range of people's positive feelings and cognitions. Over time, this broadening can become habitual and contribute to adaptive responding. Indeed, higher trait-resilience was correlated with higher experiences of positive emotions (Tugade & Fredrickson, 2007).

In this vein, positive emotions build psychological resources that resilient individuals use to adapt to stress (Fredrickson et al., 2003; Tugade & Fredrickson, 2007). For example, a trajectory of coping was predicted for police officers who demonstrated positive emotive traits during training versus those who exhibited a negative emotion profile (Galatzer-Levy et al., 2013). The presence of positive emotions in moderation is instrumental for coping processes (Bonanno, 2008; Folkman & Moskowitz, 2000). Additional research on social joy and laughter suggests that happiness is mediated by the amount of time people experience positive emotions and not the strength at which they experience it (Lyubomirsky et al., 2005).

Therapeutically, positive emotions have been associated with self-mastery, pride, gratitude, and love. Happiness and pleasure are supported by attitudes and behaviors such as curiosity and playfulness (Gallagher & Lopez, 2007). The authors describe curiosity as a combination of two elements: exploration of new situations and absorption. The latter represents the inclination to become fully immersed in life experiences and situations. These therapeutic elements are innately supported through art therapy creative endeavors. Engaging in creative curiosity represents a resilient shift from negative to positive responses.

Perhaps this move results in a shift from neuroendocrine-mediated feelings of loss of control to sympathetic nervous system feelings of acceptance or being in control (Henry & Wang, 1998). Affective neuroscience research has solidly demonstrated that negativity and positivity, meaning approach and avoidance are cortically differentiated: The left hemisphere which holds the highly evolved language centers of the brain is biased toward approach-based action and positive rewarding feelings whereas the right hemisphere is associated with negativity and avoidance (Demaree et al., 2005; Roesmann et al., 2019). These cortical functions, aptly named as "sword and shield hypothesis" have been correlated with handedness and with the way hands' motor activity executes approach and avoidance actions (Brookshire & Casasanto, 2018). This research and hypothesis sheds light on art therapy processes. As avoidant processes are activated, the client is encouraged to explore and become absorbed in art making, while language processes involved in talking about the art likely modulate feelings of control and can support emotional approach. Furthermore, neuropathways between the right hemisphere and the subcortical limbic system associated with both fear and joy contribute (Styliadis et al. 2014) to therapeutic integration. For example, executive action, playfulness, and pleasure in the art making likely support the experiencing of positive feelings, expanding perceptions, and the range of action and social possibilities (Hass-Cohen & Clyde Findlay, 2015). Further art therapy research is needed to translate the extensive research on the distribution of emotions in the brain (Alexander et al., 2021).

5.7 TRANSFORMATIVE INTEGRATION

Autobiographical Processing

From this perspective, functions of autobiographical memory, self, social, and prospection represent personally experienced information, whereas mentalizing and intersubjectivity are functions of one's imagination and creativity (Summerfield et al., 2009). Autobiographical memories represent a coherent integration of pleasant, unpleasant, and neutral experiences.

From a neurobiological perspective, positivity and negativity can coexist, which contributes to an understanding that positive and negative emotions are discrete phenomena that can be worked on simultaneously in therapy. An important frontal area involved in the processing of clues to positive emotion and autobiographical memories is the orbital-frontal cortex (OFC) (Panksepp, & Burgdorf, 2006). Discrete OFC regions, process visuospatial and somatosensory rewarding and or aversive stimuli (Figure 5.5). For example, pleasant odors activate the medial OFC; unpleasant odors activate the dorsal ACC and mid OFC (Grabenhorst et al., 2007).

The human brain is adept at simultaneously representing the positive and negative values of a complex stimulus, contributing to effective decision making. This process of allowing and accepting both the good and the bad hones the ability to examine, consider, and act upon emotional responses and make up the autobiographical sense

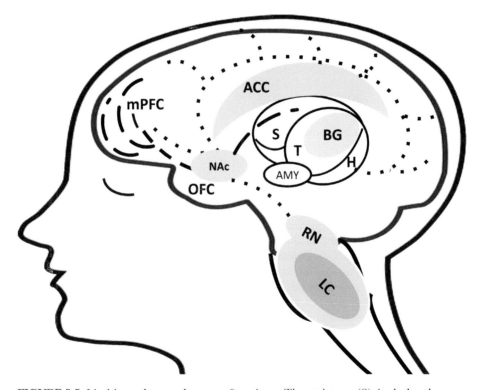

FIGURE 5.5 Limbic and reward system functions. The striatum (S) includes the caudate nucleus and putamen part of the basal ganglia (BG) and the nucleus accumbens (NAc), an area associated with the reward system that includes the locus coeruleus (LC). Dotted lines represent the dispersion of serotonin in the brain. A main source of serotonin in the brain is the raphe nucleus (RN). Note that dopamine is heavily dispersed in the frontal lobe, specifically the medial prefrontal cortex (mPFC) Also shown is the orbital frontal cortex (OFC) (Noah Hass-Cohen)

of self. Therapeutic art making provides opportunities to practice tolerance of the simultaneous arousal of joy and pleasure as well as judgment and pain. This unique quality of art therapy expands clients' ability to self-regulate and use both positive and negative emotions to make prospective autobiographical decisions.

Retrieval of any positive memories can build upon a sense of self. This may require the assistance of third parties, such as family members, who can provide positive and supportive memories. In therapy, the art therapist might also suggest that the client add some positive features to a dark drawing. First engaging a client in a neutral or positive experience is a useful tactic because it has proven helpful in obtaining a more detailed recollection of the traumatic experience (Coan et al., 2006). In the short term, this "silver lining" may decrease the effect of negative emotions and throughout therapy provides opportunities for the practice of positive emotional regulation and creativity and resiliency. Thus, integrated creativity (Default Mode Network and Central Executive Network functions) can support imagining solutions to problems. The art making likely allows action that may mitigate not only right hemispheric anxiety but also left hemispheric dissociation, which has been associated with lack of action in face of trauma (Lanius et al., 2003). Art therapy is particularly suited for this work as the vivid creative positive experiences that it advances have the potential to interfere with traumatic memories. Through spontaneous and structured art therapy and dramatic interventions, the imagination provides clues to what is happening and to the needed solutions (Lahad, 1993; Lahad at al., 2000).

Empathizing and Compassion

Even after traumatic memory extinction, areas in the amygdala seem to remember the trigger and can be easily re-sensitized to react. This suggests that art therapy interventions, which target in-vivo responses, positive cognitive-emotive appraisals, as well as experiences of mastery and control, may not be sufficiently effective. There is a high remission of chronic traumatic stress (CTS) even when people are treated with empirical approaches. In addition, some survivors may not be able to tolerate any trauma processing. Others may have some amnesia for the event. For example, childhood sole survivors of airplane crashes may little recollect the event yet still suffer debilitating consequences, although, for the most part, they do not have a specific memory that they can process (Dickens, 2014). Therefore, it may be necessary to attempt reconsolidation of autobiographical memories by actively aiming to update them with information that may seem a mismatch with the client's expectations (Barreiro et al., 2013).

As discussed throughout this chapter, art making, and expressive communication insert novelty into trauma processing and may offer an opportunity for such a mismatch. Often the arts allow for non-integrated sensory representations to integrate with contextualized implicit expressions in surprising ways. This quality of art therapy can be helpful because the reconsolidation of memories involves the function of three brain areas that are all sensitive to novel information: the amygdala, hippocampus, and prefrontal cortex areas (Yamsaki & Takeuchi, 2017). Pertinent to memory reconsolidation and resiliency, it is now becoming clear that neurogenesis assists in coping with stress (Iordanova et al., 2011; Ming & Song, 2011).

Under the auspices of a traumatology-trained art therapist, creative art making can lead to previously unknown personal strengths and meaning. Two additional treatment avenues reduce risk for relapse prevention: connecting to new social networks and developing the capacity for self-compassion (Neff et al., 2007). Therapists may consider mentoring trauma survivors to develop a network of people who have had similar experiences. In addition, the arts can be used to imagine and explore such give and take support (Hass-Cohen & Ziegler, 2014).

Development of self- and other compassion can further lay the foundation for such social connectivity. Empathy and compassion are supported through an increased ability to successfully put oneself in one's mind and in another's shoes. Self-compassion skills also help clients accept and forgive themselves for any recurring symptoms, an important step since a one-time triggering of symptoms often spirals into relapse. Providing clients with information on the likelihood of relapse and how to practice self-compassion can soften this reaction and reduce the probability of relapse (Scaer, 2007). Self-acceptance and affect tolerance can also be achieved through mindfulness meditation (Kabat-Zinn, 2005). Non-judgmental attention provides a gateway to compassion, kindness, and the desire to relieve another's suffering. However, this indirect pathway, possibly requiring many hours of practice and meditating, may be threatening, and activating for trauma survivors (Briere & Scott, 2015; Segal et al., 2012). Additional therapy approaches that incorporate acceptance – Dialectical-Behavior Therapy and Mindfulness-Based Cognitive Therapy – have proven effective with conditions difficult to treat. These approaches share interventions that focus on disentangling from thinking and learning to stay with an unpleasant experience. However, a more direct pathway to empathy may be available through mindfulness self-compassion (MSC) interventions (Germer & Neff, 2013). There are three MSC components: mindfulness versus over-identification with hurtful painful experiences, self-kindness versus self-judgment, and common humanity versus isolation. All the interventions focus on the self, which is critical as CTS survivors often carry a tremendous amount of guilt and self-intolerance, or even self-hate (Rothschild & Wolf, 2013).

In therapy, the development of self-compassion and empathy starts with the art therapist's sensitivity to embedded relational media transactions, his or her unconditional acceptance of the art product, and transmission of genuine interest, caring, and respect. The art therapist, who then functions as the client's "third hand," "third eye," and "second mind," overtly and symbolically senses what the client needs. The client also has the opportunity to mimic the therapist's resonance, forming a language that conveys understanding and empathy. Such reciprocal dialogue moves the client toward experiences of felt and anticipated aid. In art therapy, neurobiological activations in response to implied and actual movement, in particular mirror neurons and mirroring systems, evoke empathizing compassion, pleasure, and joy. Understanding these mirroring responses embodies empathic reactions to art. Other involved systems include the integration of right and left hemispheric functions, bottom-up arousal and top-down regulation, and balanced activation of positive reward system activation (Siegel, 2006).

Explicit MSC interventions, such as the "self-compassion break," entail the person saying specific mindful, humane, and kindness-oriented phrases (Germer

& Neff, 2013) and can easily translate to art therapy. An example would be "ask yourself what you need right now and draw it." Asking a question and engaging in this self-compassion cultivates goodwill toward oneself. An ATR-N protocol, the autobiographical compassionate timeline incorporates social support and a vision of the future (Hass-Cohen & Clyde Findlay, 2015). The timeline request is to "draw your past, present, and future, as they would be seen by someone who loves or cares for you or from a kind and supportive self-perspective." For a traumatized person, it is often more culturally acceptable or easier to care for another person than for the self. As it is often easier to start with caring for another, a necessary preliminary step might be needed, for example, "imagine and draw a future for someone you love or care for." Different directives might be needed for individuals with disruptive attachment or trauma histories as they may have a foreshortened sense of the future. Depending on the client's situation, directive wording or sequencing might be further adapted, such as "Draw your future, as it would be foreseen by someone who loved or cared for you in the past." A very isolated individual may be unable to identify a current or past caring relationship. Then the caring person could be a pet, a beloved person who has passed, or a therapist. When shared, the art process promotes social connectivity and empathy. There is also a sense of universality, because discussing the art raises a presumed, shared understanding of what is meaningful and beautiful (Ramachandran & Hirstein, 1999). Thought to be mediated by the activation of mirror neuron systems, such confident aesthetic experiences have also been associated with activating reward-related brain circuitry (Kawabata & Zeki, 2004). These directives help reconsolidate the self, other, and prospective functions of memory.

5.8   SUMMARY

Therapeutic experiences happen through the continued process of reactivation, re-encoding, and reconsolidation of memories. Through this process, new rules or schemas will be updated, allowing clients more flexible ways of engaging with autobiographical narratives. The degree to which change is lasting will vary, based on how generalized the reconsolidation of memory is or how wide or narrow a context the new memory applies to. The changes to traumatic memories being made in art psychotherapy are not only new memories being created or new semantic structures being established. The changes represent a transformative integration of the autobiographical mind and body and social self. Art therapy practices directly contribute to reconsolidating and updating new memories. As stated earlier, essential components of transformative integration and creating therapeutic change include reactivating old memories, engaging in new emotional experiences that are incorporated in these reactivated memories, and reinforcing the change. The more contexts in which this new way of experiencing the world is practiced, the stronger the change (Lane et al., 2015). Research has suggested that the ATR-N CREATE memory reconsolidation factors described in this chapter need to be continued to be incorporated into sequential protocols and procedures (Hass-Cohen et al., 2022b; Hass-Cohen et al., 2021; Hass-Cohen, & Clyde Findlay, 2019; Hass-Cohen et al., 2018).

REFERENCES

Agarwal, V. (2021). Mimetic self-reflexivity and intersubjectivity in complementary and alternative medicine practices: The mirror neuron system in breast cancer survivorship. *Frontiers in Integrative Neuroscience, 15,* 641219.

Alexander, R., Aragón, O. R., Bookwala, J., Cherbuin, N., Gatt, J. M., Kahrilas, I. J., Kästner, N., Lawrence, A., Lowe, L., Morrison, R. G., Mueller, S. C., Nusslock, R., Papadelis, C., Polnaszek, K. L., Helene Richter, S., Silton, R. L., & Styliadis, C. (2021). The neuroscience of positive emotions and affect: Implications for cultivating happiness and wellbeing. *Neuroscience and biobehavioral reviews, 121,* 220–249.

Ammaniti, M., & Gallese, V. (2014). *The birth of intersubjectivity: psychodynamics, neurobiology, and the self.* W.W. Norton.

Astill Wright, L., Horstmann, L., Holmes, E. A., & Bisson, J. I. (2021). Consolidation/reconsolidation therapies for the prevention and treatment of PTSD and re-experiencing: a systematic review and meta-analysis. *Translational Psychiatry, 11*(1), 453. https://doi.org/10.1038/s41398-021-01570-w

Barreiro, K. A., Suárez, L. D., Lynch, V. M., Molina, V. A., & Delorenzi, A. (2013). Memory expression is independent of memory labialization/reconsolidation. *Neurobiology of Learning and Memory, 106,* 283–291.

Bat-Or, M. (2010). Clay sculpting of mother and child figures encourages mentalization. *The Arts in Psychotherapy, 37*(4), 319–327.

Bonanno, G. A. (2008). Loss, trauma, and human resilience: Have we underestimated the human capacity to thrive after extremely aversive events? *American Psychologist, 1,* 101–113.

Brewin, C. R., Gregory, J. D., Lipton, M., & Burgess, N. (2010). Intrusive images in psychological disorders: Characteristics, neural mechanisms, and treatment implications. *Psychological Review, 117*(1), 210–232.

Briere, J., & Scott, C. (2015). *Principles of trauma therapy: A guide to symptoms, evaluation, and treatment* (2nd ed.). Sage Publications.

Brookshire, G., & Casasanto, D. (2018). Approach motivation in human cerebral cortex. *Philosophical transactions of the Royal Society of London. Series B, Biological sciences, 373*(1752), 20170141.

Chapman, L. (2014). *Neurobiologically informed trauma therapy with children and adolescents: Understanding mechanisms of change.* W.W. Norton.

Chapman, L., Morabito, D., Ladakakos, C., Schreier, H., & Knudson, M. (2001). The effectiveness of art therapy interventions in reducing posttraumatic stress disorder (PTSD) symptoms in pediatric trauma patients. *Art Therapy: Journal of the American Art Therapy Association, 18*(2), 100–104.

Coan, J. A., Schaefer, H. S., & Davidson, R. J. (2006) Lending a hand: Social regulation of the neural response to threat. *Psychological Science, 17,* 1032–1039.

Deblinger, E., Mannarino, A. P., Cohen, J. A., & Steer, R. A. (2006). A follow-up study of a multisite, randomized, controlled trial for children with sexual abuse-related PTSD symptoms. *Journal of the American Academy of Child & Adolescent Psychiatry, 45*(12), 1474–1484.

Dekel, S., Mandl, C., & Solomon, Z. (2011). Shared and unique predictors of post-traumatic growth and distress. *Journal of Clinical Psychology, 67,* 241–252.

de Kloet, E., Joëls, M., & Holsboer, F. (2005). Stress and the brain: From adaptation to disease. *Nature Reviews Neuroscience, 6*(6), 463–475.

Demaree, H. A., Everhart, D., Youngstrom, E. A., & Harrison, D. W. (2005). Brain lateralization of emotional processing: Historical roots and a future incorporating "dominance." *Behavioral and cognitive neuroscience reviews, 4*(1), 3–20. https://doi.org/10.1177/1534582305276837

de Oliveira Alvares, L., & Do-Monte, F. H. (2021). Understanding the dynamic and destiny of memories. *Neuroscience and Biobehavioral Reviews, 125,* 592–607.

Dickens, K., producer, & Stanley, P., director. (2014). *Sole survivor* (Film). Yellow Wing Productions.

Duax, J. M., Bohnert, K. M., Rauch, S. A., & Defever, A. M. (2014). Posttraumatic stress disorder symptoms, levels of social support, and emotional hiding in returning veterans. *Journal of Rehabilitation Research & Development, 51*(4), 571–578.

Duschek, S., Nassauer, L., Montoro, C. I., Bair, A., & Montoya, P. (2019). Dispositional empathy is associated with experimental pain reduction during provision of social support by romantic partners. *Scandinavian Journal of Pain, 20*(1), 205–209.

Ehlers, A., & Clark, D. M. (2000). A cognitive model of posttraumatic stress disorder. *Behavior Research and Therapy, 38*(4), 319–345.

Ekman, P. (1992). An argument for basic emotions. *Cognition and Emotion, 6*(3–4), 169–200.

Ellingsen, D. M., Isenburg, K., Jung, C., Lee, J., Gerber, J., Mawla, I., Sclocco, R., Jensen, K. B., Edwards, R. R., Kelley, J. M., Kirsch, I., Kaptchuk, T. J., & Napadow, V. (2020). Dynamic brain-to-brain concordance and behavioral mirroring as a mechanism of the patient-clinician interaction. *Science advances, 6*(43), eabc1304.

Emerson, D. (2015). *Trauma-sensitive yoga in therapy bringing the body into treatment.* W.W. Norton.

Feng, H., Zeng, Y., & Lu, E. (2022). Brain-inspired affective empathy computational model and its application on altruistic rescue task. *Frontiers in Computational Neuroscience, 16,* 784967.

Ferrari, P. F., Gerbella, M., Coudé, G., & Rozzi, S. (2017). Two different mirror neuron networks: The sensorimotor (hand) and limbic (face) pathways. *Neuroscience, 358,* 300–315. https://doi.org/10.1016/j.neuroscience.2017.06.052

Fish, B. (2012). Art response art: The art of the art therapist. *Art Therapy: Journal of the American Art therapy Association, 29*(3), 138–143.

Folkman, S., & Moskowitz, J. (2000). Positive affect and the other side of coping. *American Psychologist, 55*(6), 647–654.

Franklin, M. (2010). Affect regulation, mirror neurons and the 3rd hand: Formulating mindful empathic art interventions. *Art Therapy: Journal of the American Art therapy Association, 27*(4), 160–167.

Fredrickson, B. L., & Levenson, R. W. (1998). Positive emotions speed recovery from the cardiovascular sequelae of negative emotions. *Cognition and Emotion, 12*(2), 191–220.

Fredrickson, B. L., Mancuso, R. A., Branigan, C., & Tugade, M. M. (2000). The undoing effect of positive emotions. *Motivation and Emotion, 24*(4), 237–258.

Fredrickson, B. L., Tugade, M. M., Waugh, C. E., & Larkin, G. R. (2003). What good are positive emotions in crisis? A prospective study of resilience and emotions following the terrorist attacks on the United States on September 11th, 2001. *Journal of Personality and Social Psychology, 84*(2), 365.

Galatzer-Levy, I. R., Brown, A. D., Henn-Haase, C., Metzler, T. J., Neylan, T. C., & Marmar, C. R. (2013). Positive and negative emotion prospectively predict trajectories of resilience and distress among high-exposure police officers. *Emotion, 13*(3), 545–553.

Gallagher, M. W., & Lopez, S. J. (2007). Curiosity and well-being. *The Journal of Positive Psychology, 2*(4), 236–248.

Gavron, T. (2013). Meeting on common ground: Assessing parent–child relationships through the joint painting procedure. *Art Therapy, 30*(1), 12–19.

Germer, C. K., & Neff, D. (2013). Self-compassion in clinical practice. *Journal of Clinical Psychology: In Session, 69*(8), 856–867.

Gil, E. (2010). *Working with children to heal interpersonal trauma: The power of play.* Guilford Press.

Godoy, L. D., Rossignoli, M. T., Delfino-Pereira, P., Garcia-Cairasco, N., & de Lima Umeoka, E. H. (2018). A Comprehensive Overview on Stress Neurobiology: Basic Concepts and Clinical Implications. *Frontiers in behavioral neuroscience, 12,* 127.

Gold, S. N. (2008). Benefits of a contextual approach to understanding and treating complex trauma. *Journal of Trauma & Dissociation, 9*(2), 269–292.

Grabenhorst, F., Rolls, E. T., Margot, C., Da Silva, M. P., & Velazco, M. (2007). How pleasant and unpleasant stimuli combine in different brain regions: Odor mixtures. *Journal of Neuroscience, 27*(49), 13532–13540.

Gray, A. E. L. (2011). Expressive arts therapies: Working with survivors of torture. *Torture*, (*21*), 1, 40–47.

Hartley, C. A., Gorun, A., Reddan, M. C., Ramirez, F., & Phelps, E. A. (2014). Stressor controllability modulates fear extinction in humans. *Neurobiology of Learning and Memory*, *113*, 149–156.

Hass-Cohen, N., & Clyde Findlay, J. (2009). Pain, attachment, and meaning making: Report on an Art Therapy Relational Neuroscience assessment protocol (a case study). *Arts in Psychotherapy*, *36*(4), 175–184.

Hass-Cohen, N., & Clyde Findlay, J. (2015). *Art therapy & the neuroscience of relationships, creativity, and resiliency: Skills and practices* (Illustrated edition). The Interpersonal Neurobiology Series. W.W. Norton.

Hass-Cohen, N., & Clyde Findlay, J. (2019). The art therapy relational neuroscience and memory reconsolidation four drawing protocol. *The Arts in Psychotherapy*, *63*, 51–59.

Hass-Cohen, N., & Ziegler, K. A (2014). Vicarious trauma and resiliency focused supervision and expressive writing activity. In R. Bean, S. Davis, & Davey (Eds.), *Clinical supervision activities for increasing competence and self-awareness*. John Wiley & Sons.

Hass-Cohen, N., Bokoch, R., & Fowler, G. (2022a). The Compassionate Arts Psychotherapy Program: Benefits of a compassionate arts media continuum. *Art Therapy: Journal of the American Art Therapy Association*, *0*(1), 5–14. https://doi.org/10.1080/07421656.2022.2100690

Hass-Cohen, N., Bokoch, R., & McAnuff, J. (2022b). A year later: The pain protocol study findings and memory reconsolidation factors. *The Arts in Psychotherapy*, *80*, 101949.

Hass-Cohen, N., Bokoch, R., Clyde Findlay, J., & Banford, A. (2018). A four-drawing art therapy trauma and resiliency protocol study. *The Arts in Psychotherapy*, *61*, 44–56.

Hass-Cohen, N, Bokoch, R., Goodman, K., & Conover, K. J. (2021). Art therapy drawing protocols for chronic pain: Quantitative results from a mixed methods pilot study. *The Arts in Psychotherapy*, *73*, 101749.

Hass-Cohen, N., Bokoch, R., Goodman, K., & McAnuff, J. (2022c). Art therapy drawing protocols for chronic pain: Qualitative findings from a mixed method pilot study. *Art Therapy: Journal of the American Art Therapy Association*, 39(4), 182–193. https://doi.org/10.1080/07421656.2022.2085491

Hass-Cohen, N., & Findlay, J. C. (2015). *Art therapy and the neuroscience of relationships, creativity, and resiliency: Skills and practices* (Norton series on Interpersonal Neurobiology). WW Norton.

Hass-Cohen, N., Clyde Findlay, J., Carr, R., & Vanderlan, J. (2014). "CHECK, change and/or keep what you need": An art therapy relational neurobiological (ATR-N) trauma intervention. *Art Therapy: Journal of the American Art Therapy Association*, *31*(2) 69–78.

Hass-Cohen, N. (2008). CREATE art therapy relational neuroscience principles (ATR-N). In N. Hass-Cohen & R. Carr (Eds.), *Art therapy and clinical neuroscience* (pp. 283–309). New York: Jessica Kingsley Publishers.

Hass-Cohen, N. (2007). Cultural arts in action, musings on empathy. *GAINS Summer Quarterly*, 41–48.

Hass-Cohen, N., Kim, S. H., & Mangassarian, M. (2015). Art mediated interpersonal touch and space: A phenomenological study with Korean female art therapy students. *The Arts in Psychotherapy*, *46*, 1–8, https://doi.org/10.1016/j.aip.2015.07.001

Henry, J. P., & Wang, S. (1998). Effects of early stress on adult affiliative behavior. *Psychoneuroendocrinology*, *23*(8), 863–875.

Herman, J. (1997). *Trauma and recovery: The aftermath of violence – from domestic abuse to political terror*. Basic Books.

Herry, C, Ferraguti, F., Singewald, N., Letzkus, J. J., Ehrlich, I., & Lu, A. (2010). Neuronal circuits of fear extinction. *European Journal of Neuroscience*, *31*, 599–612.

Heyes, C., & Catmur, C. (2022). What happened to mirror neurons? *Perspectives on Psychological Science*, 17(1), 153–168.

Iordanova, M. D., Good, M., & Honey, R. C. (2011). Retrieval-mediated learning involving episodes requires synaptic plasticity in the hippocampus. *The Journal of Neuroscience*, *31*(19), 7156–7162.

Jung, R. E., Mead, B. S., Carrasco, J., & Flores, R. A. (2013). The structure of creative cognition in the human brain. *Frontiers in Human Neuroscience*, *7*, 330.

Kabat-Zinn, J. (2005). *Full catastrophe living: Using the wisdom of your body and mind to face stress, pain, and illness* (15th anniversary ed.). Bantam Dell.

Kaiser, D. H., & Deaver, S. (2009). Assessing attachment with the Bird's Nest Drawing: A review of the research. *Art Therapy: Journal of the American Art Therapy Association, 26*(1), 26–33.

Kashdan, T. B., Rose, P., & Fincham, F. D. (2004). Curiosity and exploration: Facilitating positive subjective experiences and personal growth opportunities. *Journal of Personality Assessment, 82*, 291–305.

Kawabata, H., & Zeki, S. (2004). Neural correlates of beauty. *Journal of Neurophysiology, 91*(4), 1699–1705.

Kindt, M., Soeter, M., & Vervliet, B. (2009). Beyond extinction: Erasing human fear responses and preventing the return of fear. *Nature Neuroscience, 12*(3), 256–258.

King, A. P., Erickson, T. M., Giardino, N. D., Favorite, T., Rauch, S. A., Robinson, E., … Liberzon, I. (2013). A pilot study of group mindfulness-based cognitive therapy (MBCT) for combat veterans with posttraumatic stress disorder (PTSD). *Depression & Anxiety (10914269), 30*(7), 638–645.

King-West, E., & Hass-Cohen, N., (2008). Art therapy, neuroscience and complex PTSD. In N. Hass-Cohen & R. Carr (Eds.), *Art therapy and clinical neuroscience* (pp. 223–253). Jessica Kingsley.

Klorer, P. G. (2005). Expressive therapy with severely maltreated children: Neuroscience contributions. *Art Therapy: Journal of the American Art Therapy Association, 22*(4), 213–220. https://doi.org/10.1080/07421656.2005.10129523

Knol, A. S. L., Huiskes, M., Koole, T., Meganck, R., Loeys, T., & Desmet, M. (2020). Reformulating and mirroring in psychotherapy: A conversation analytic perspective. *Frontiers in Psychology, 11*, 318.

Konarski, J. Z., McIntyre, R. S., Grupp, L. A., & Kennedy, S. H. (2005). Is the cerebellum relevant in the circuitry of neuropsychiatric disorders? *Journal of Psychiatry & Neuroscience, 30*(3), 178–186.

Kozlowska, K., Walker, P., McLean, L., & Carrive, P. (2015). Fear and the defense cascade: Clinical implications and management. *Harvard Review of Psychiatry, 23*(4), 263–287.

Kramer, E. (1990). *Art therapy in a children's community.* Schocken Books.

Lahad, S., Shacham, Y., & Niv, S. (2000). Coping and community resources in children facing disaster. In *International handbook of human response to trauma* (pp. 389–395). Springer.

Lahad, S. (1993). Tracing coping resources through a story in six parts – The "BASIC PH" model. In S. Levinson (ed.), *Psychology at school and the community during peaceful and emergency times* (pp. 55–70). Levinson-Hadar (in Hebrew).

Lane, R. D., Ryan, L., Nadel, L., & Greenberg, L. (2015). Memory reconsolidation, emotional arousal, and the process of change in psychotherapy: New insights from brain science. *The Behavioral and Brain Sciences.* http://dx.doi.org/10.1017/S0140525X14000041 (Published online. 19 pages.)

Lanius, R. A., Bluhm, R. L., Coupland, N. J., Hegadoren, K. M., Rowe, B., Théberge, J., Neufeld, R. W., Williamson, P. C., & Brimson, M. (2010). Default mode network connectivity as a predictor of post-traumatic stress disorder symptom severity in acutely traumatized subjects. *Acta Psychiatrica Scandinavica, 121*(1), 33–40.

Lanius, R. A., Bluhm, R. L., & Frewen, P. A. (2011). How understanding the neurobiology of complex post-traumatic stress disorder can inform clinical practice: A social cognitive and affective neuroscience approach. *Acta Psychiatrica Scandinavica, 124*, 331–348.

Lanius, R. A., Hopper, J. W., & Menon, R. S. (2003). Individual differences in a husband and wife who developed PTSD after a motor vehicle accident: A functional MRI case study. *American Journal of Psychiatry, 160*(4), 667–669.

Lanius, R. A., Vermetten, E., Loewenstein, R. J., Brand, B., Schmahl, C., Bremner, J., & Spiegel, D. (2010). Emotion modulation in PTSD: Clinical and neurobiological evidence for a dissociative subtype. *The American Journal of Psychiatry, 167*(6), 640–647.

LeDoux, J. (2003). The emotional brain, fear, and the amygdala. *Cellular and molecular neurobiology, 23*, 727–738.

Lee, J. L. C., Nader, K., & Schiller, D. (2017). An update on memory reconsolidation updating. *Trends in Cognitive Sciences, 21*(7), 531–545.

Lonergan, M. H., Olivera-Figueroa, L. A., Pitman, R. K., & Brunet, A. (2013). Propranolol's effects on the consolidation and reconsolidation of long-term emotional memory in healthy partici-pants: a meta-analysis. *Journal of Psychiatry and Neuroscience, 38*(4), 222–231.

Lucre, K., & Clapton, N. (2021). The Compassionate Kitbag: A creative and integrative approach to compassion-focused therapy. *Psychology and Psychotherapy: Theory, Research and Practice, 94*(S2), e12291.

Lyubomirsky, S., King, L., & Diener, E. (2005). The benefits of frequent positive affect: Does happi-ness lead to success?. *Psychological Bulletin, 131*(6), 803.

Malchiodi, C. A. (2017). Art therapy approaches to facilitate verbal expression: Getting past the impasse. In C. A. Malchiodi & D. A. Crenshaw (Eds.), *What to do when children clam up in psychother-apy: Interventions to facilitate communication* (pp. 197–216). The Guilford Press.

Markowitz, J. C., Milrod, B., Bleiberg, K., & Marshall, R. D. (2009). Interpersonal factors in under-standing and treating posttraumatic stress disorder. *Journal of Psychiatric Practice, 15*(2), 133–140.

McEwen, B. S. (2007). Physiology and neurobiology of stress and adaptation: Central role of the brain. *Physiological Reviews, 87*(3), 873–904.

McEwen, B. S. (2012). Brain on stress: How the social environment gets under the skin. *Proceed-ings of the National Academy of Sciences,* 109(Suppl 2), 17180–17185. https://doi.org/10.1073/pnas.1121254109

McGaugh, J. L., & Roozendaal, B. (2002). Role of adrenal stress hormones in forming lasting mem-ories in the brain. *Current Opinion in Neurobiology, 12*(2), 205–210.

Meekums, B. (1999). A creative model for recovery from child sexual abuse trauma. *The Arts in Psy-chotherapy, 26*(4), 247–259.

Ming, G. L., & Song, H. (2011). Adult neurogenesis in the mammalian brain: Significant answers and significant questions. *Neuron, 70*(4), 687–702.

Missirlian, T. M., Toukmanian, S. G., Warwar, S. H., & Greenberg, L. S. (2005). Emotional arousal, client perceptual processing, and the working alliance in experiential psychotherapy for depres-sion. *Journal of Consulting and Clinical Psychology, 73,* 861–871.

Moon, C. H. (2001). *Studio art therapy: Cultivating the artist identity in the art therapist.* Jessica Kingsley.

Moscovitch, M., & Gilboa, A. (2022). Has the concept of systems consolidation outlived its useful-ness? Identification and evaluation of premises underlying systems consolidation. *Faculty Reviews, 11,* 33. https://doi.org/10.12703/r/11-33. Jessica Kingsley.

Mukamel, R., Ekstrom, A.D., Kaplan, J., Iacoboni, M., & Fried, I. (2010). Single-neuron responses in humans during execution and observation of actions. *Current Biology, 20,* 750–756.

Nader, K., Schafe, G. E., & LeDoux, J. E. (2000). The labile nature of consolidation theory. *Biological Psychiatry, 15,* 76(4), 274–280.

Neff, K., D., Kirkpatrick, K. L., & Rude, S. S. (2007). Self-compassion and adaptive psychological functioning. *Journal of Research in Personality, 41,* 139–154.

Panksepp, J., & Burgdorf, J. (2006). The neurobiology of positive emotions. *Neuroscience and Biobe-havioral Reviews, 30*(2), 173–187.

Perry, B. D. (2006). Applying principles of neurodevelopment to clinical work with maltreated and traumatized children. The neurosequential model of therapeutics. In N. Boyd Webb (Ed.), *Work-ing with child abuse in welfare.* Guildford Press.

Perry, B. D., Pollard, R. A., Blakely, T. L., Baker, W. L., & Vigilante, D. (1995). Childhood trauma, the neurobiology of adaptation and "use-dependent" development of the brain: How "states" become "traits." *Infant Mental Health Journal, 16*(4), 271–291.

Pessoa, L., & Adolphs, R. (2010). Emotion processing and the amygdala: from a 'low road' to 'many roads' of evaluating biological significance. *Nature Reviews Neuroscience, 11*(11), 773–783.

Peterson, C., Ruch, W., Beerman, U., Park, N., & Seligman, M. E. P. (2007). Strengths of character, orientations to happiness, and life satisfaction. *Journal of Positive Psychology, 2,* 149–156.

Phelps, E. A., & Ledoux, J. E. (2005). Contributions of the amygdala to emotions processing; From animal models to human behavior. *Neuron,* 175–187.

Porges, S. W. (2022). Polyvagal theory: A science of safety. *Frontiers in Integrative Neuroscience, 16*, 27.

Porges, S. W. (2001). The polyvagal theory: Phylogenetic substrates of a social nervous system. *International Journal of Psychophysiology, 42*, 123–146.

Porges S. W. (2009). The polyvagal theory: New insights into adaptive reactions of the autonomic nervous system. *Cleveland Clinic journal of medicine, 76* (Suppl 2), S86–S90. https://doi.org/10.3949/ccjm.76.s2.17

Porges, S. W. (2013). A psychophysiology of developmental disabilities: A personal and historical perspective. *American Journal on Intellectual and Developmental Disabilities, 118*(6), 416–418.

Qin, L. D., Wang, Z., Sun, Y. W., Wan, J. Q., Su, S. S., Zhou, Y., & Xu, J. R. (2012). A preliminary study of alterations in default network connectivity in post-traumatic stress disorder patients following recent trauma. *Brain Research, 12*(1484), 50–56.

Ramachandran, V. S., & Hirstein, W. (1999). The science of art: A neurological theory of aesthetic experience. *Journal of Consciousness Studies, 6*(6–7), 15–51.

Rizzolatti, G., Fogassi, L., & Gallese, V. (2001). Neurophysiological mechanisms underlying the understanding and imitation of action. *Nature Reviews Neuroscience, 2*(9), 661–670

Roesmann, K., Dellert, T., Junghoefer, M., Kissler, J., Zwitserlood, P., Zwanzger, P., & Dobel, C. (2019). The causal role of prefrontal hemispheric asymmetry in valence processing of words: Insights from a combined cTBS-MEG study. *NeuroImage, 191*, 367–379.

Rothschild, B., & Wolf, C. (2013). *Mindfulness and trauma: Theory and tools to enhance client healing and therapist self-care.* Presented at InsightLA, Los Angeles, CA.

Sapolsky, R. M. (2004). *Why zebras don't get ulcers: An updated guide to stress, stress-related diseases, and coping* (3rd ed.). W.H. Freeman & Co.

Scaer, R. C. (2007). *The body bears the burden: Trauma, dissociation, and disease* (2nd ed.). The Haworth Medical Press/The Haworth Press.

Schelling, G., Roozendaal, B., Krauseneck, T., Schmoelz, M., De Quervain, D., & Briegel, J. (2006). Efficacy of hydrocortisone in preventing posttraumatic stress disorder following critical illness and major surgery. In R. Yehuda (Ed.), *Psychobiology of posttraumatic stress disorders: A decade of progress* (Vol. 1071) (pp. 46–53). Blackwell Publishing.

Schiller, D., Monfils, M. H., Raio, C. M., Johnson, D. C., Ledoux, J. E., & Phelps, E. A. (2010). Preventing the return of fear in humans using reconsolidation update mechanisms. *Nature, 7*(7277), 49–53.

Schulkin, J. (2003). *Rethinking homeostasis: Allostatic regulation in physiology and pathophysiology.* MIT Press.

Schulkin, J. (2011). Social allostasis: Anticipatory regulation of the internal milieu. *Frontiers in Evolutionary Neuroscience, 2*(111), 1–15.

Schwabe, L., Nader, K., & Pruessner, J. C. (2014). Reconsolidation of human memory: Brain mechanisms and clinical relevance. *Biological Psychiatry, 76*(4), 274–280.

Seeman, T. E., Singer, B.H., Ryff, C. D., Dienberg Love, G., Levy-Storms, L. (2002). Social relationships, gender, and allostatic load across two age cohorts. *Psychosomatic Medicine, 64*(3), 395–406.

Segal, Z. V., Williams, J. M. G., & Teasdale, J. D. (2012). *Mindfulness-based cognitive therapy for depression.* Guilford Press.

Seligman, M. P., & Csikszentmihalyi, M. (2000). Positive psychology: An introduction. *American Psychologist, 55*(1), 5–14.

Shahar, G., Elad-Strenger, J., & Henrich, C. C. (2012). Risky resilience and resilient risk: The key role of intentionality in an emerging dialectics. *Journal of Social & Clinical Psychology, 31*(6), 618–640.

Siegel, D. J. (2006). An interpersonal neurobiology approach to psychotherapy: Awareness, mirror neurons, and neural plasticity in the development of well-being. *Psychiatric Annals, 36*(4), 248–256. https://doi.org/10.3928/00485713-20060401-06

Singer, J. A. (2004). Narrative identity and meaning making across the adult lifespan: An introduction. *Journal of Personality, 72*, 437–459.

Skelton, K., Ressler, K. J., Norrholm, S. D., Jovanovic, T., & Bradley-Davino, B. (2012). PTSD and gene variants: New pathways and new thinking. *Neuropharmacology*, *62*(2), 628–637.

Sorrells, S. F., & Sapolsky, R. M. (2007). An inflammatory review of glucocorticoid actions in the CNS. *Brain, Behavior, and Immunity*, *21*(3), 259–272.

Spreng, R. N., & Grady, C. L. (2010). Patterns of brain activity supporting autobiographical memory, prospection, and theory of mind, and their relationship to the default mode network. *Journal of Cognitive Neuroscience*, *22*(6), 1112–1123.

Stephen, G., Muldoon Orla, T., & Bennett Kate, M. (2021). Multiple group membership, social network size, allostatic load and well-being: A mediation analysis. *Journal of Psychosomatic Research*, *151*, 110636.

Sterling, P., & Eyer, J. (1988). Allostasis: A new paradigm to explain arousal pathology. In S. Fisher & J. T. Reason (Eds.), *Handbook of life stress, cognition, and health* (pp. 629–640). John Wiley & Sons.

St. Jacques, P. L. (2012). Functional neuroimaging of autobiographical memory. In D. Bernsten & D. C. Rubin (Eds.), *Understanding autobiographical memory: Theories and approaches* (pp. 114–138). Cambridge University Press.

Strouse, S., Hass-Cohen, N. & Bokoch, R. (2021). Benefits of an open art studio to military suicide survivors. *The Arts in Psychotherapy*, *72*(1), 101722. https://doi.org/10.1016/j.aip.2020.101722.

Styliadis, C., Ioannides, A. A., Bamidis, P. D., & Papadelis, C. (2014). Amygdala responses to Valence and its interaction by arousal revealed by MEG. *International Journal of Psychophysiology: Official Journal of the International Organization of Psychophysiology*, *93*(1), 121–133.

Summerfield, J. J., Hassabis, D., & Maguire, E. A. (2009). Cortical midline involvement in autobiographical memory. *Neuroimage*, *44*(3), 1188–1200.

Sutherland, K., & Bryant, R. A. (2005). Self-defining memories in post-traumatic stress disorder. *British Journal of Clinical Psychology*, *44*(4), 591–598.

Tronson, N. C., & Taylor, J. R. (2007). Molecular mechanisms of memory reconsolidation. *Nature Reviews Neuroscience*, *8*(4), 262–275.

Tsai, J., El-Gabalawy, R., Sledge, W. H., Southwick, S. M., & Pietrzak, R. H. (2014). Post-traumatic growth among veterans in the USA: Results from the National Health and Resilience in Veterans Study. *Psychological Medicine*, *2*, 1–15.

Tugade, M. M., & Fredrickson, B. L. (2007). Regulation of positive emotions: Emotion regulation strategies that promote resilience. *Journal of Happiness Studies*, *8*(3), 311–333.

Villanueva, C. M., Silton, R. L., Heller, W., Barch, D. M., & Gruber, J. (2021). Change is on the horizon: call to action for the study of positive emotion and reward in psychopathology. *Current Opinion in Behavioral Sciences*, *39*, 34–40.

Walsh, J. J., Christoffel, D. J., Wu, X., Pomrenze, M. B., & Malenka, R. C. (2021). Dissecting neural mechanisms of prosocial behaviors. *Current Opinion in Neurobiology*, *68*, 9–14.

Wood, S. K., Walker, H. E., Valentino, R. J., & Bhatnagar, S. (2010). Individual differences in reactivity to social stress predict susceptibility and resilience to a depressive phenotype: Role of corticotropin-releasing factor. *Endocrinology*, *151*(4), 1795–1805.

Yamasaki, M., & Takeuchi, T. (2017). Locus coeruleus and dopamine-dependent memory consolidation. *Neural Plasticity*. https://doi.org/10.1155/2017/8602690

Yehuda, R., & LeDoux, J. (2007). Response variation following trauma: A translational neuroscience approach to understanding PTSD. *Neuron*, *56*(1), 19–32.

CHAPTER 6

NEUROSCIENCE AND ART THERAPY WITH SEVERELY TRAUMATIZED CHILDREN

The Art is the Evidence

P. Gussie Klorer

*I had not heard him enter the waiting room, but I anticipated that 12-year-old Jack (a pseud-
onym*¹) would be hiding either under the beanbag chair or behind the door in my waiting room
when I went in to pick him up at exactly 2:00, his regularly scheduled appointment time. It was
a ritual repeated every week, reminiscent of a much younger child playing peek-a-boo. I found
Jack, and as we walked into the inner office he said: "I didn't want to come here today. They
made me come." I caught his eyes fleetingly, smiled, and told him I was happy to see him. Before
sitting down, he took a clock off the shelf and placed it on the table facing his chair so that he
could monitor the time. He claimed this attention was so I didn't get a single extra minute out
of him, but I believed he wanted to feel a sense of control. Jack's history was not unlike many
children in state custody. The abuse and long-term neglect during his crucial developmental
years left him with few inner resources. Jack was 4 and his brothers were 2 and 3 when they were
found abandoned in an impoverished home, untended for days. Jack attempted to change his
brothers' diapers and gave them water and Cheerios. The children were put in separate foster
homes, and ultimately his brothers were adopted by a family member who severed all contact with
Jack. Jack spent his childhood in foster homes, abusive environments, and residential treatment
centers. He had poor social skills, no manners, terrible hygiene, and avoided eye contact. When
he perceived an injustice, his behavior escalated into physical aggression. Jack was referred to
art therapy because he was not making progress in his verbal processing group or individual
therapy provided by his residential treatment program. Although there were varied goals in
therapy, the most important initial treatment goal was to form a therapeutic relationship based
upon safety and trust. Jack's first picture in art therapy, a lone wolf (Figure 6.1), was one his
foster mother told me he had painted many times before, suggesting that on some level it was an
unconscious self-portrait. He repeatedly painted this image during the nine years I worked with
him. Jack intended the wolf to look angry and menacing and, it showed Jack's ability to lash
out offensively and push people away. Yet the wolf appeared to be young, defensive, and scared.
This painting coincided with other drawings Jack did, such as an aggressive knife-wielding
male figure, facing backwards so that he could not see (Figure 6.2). The lack of facial features
in this figure, preventing genuine contact with others, echoed Jack's avoidant approach to all
relationships and was metaphorically repeated every time he hid in my waiting room.*

I continued to see Jack weekly for the next several years. To supplement
our work, at age 14 he was referred to a Trauma Focused Cognitive Behavioral
Therapy (TF-CBT) experimental trial, which was not effective. Developments in
evidence-based practice (EBP) research recognize the difficulty for children like
Jack to assimilate into a trauma protocol that requires them to provide a narrative when there is not a discrete traumatic event, they have incomplete recall of

DOI: 10.4324/9781003348207-6

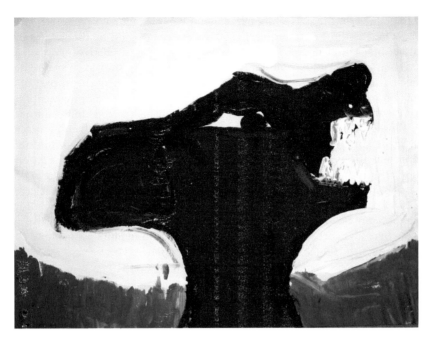

FIGURE 6.1 Jack, age 12. Painting of a wolf

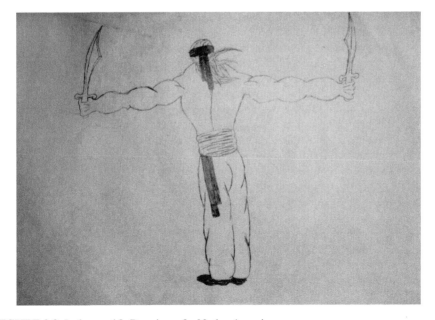

FIGURE 6.2 Jack, age 13. Drawing of a Native American

what happened, or their attachment issues are complex (Amaya-Jackson & deRosa, 2007). Whereas the 1990s and early 2000s were dominated by the favorability of cognitive behavioral, manualized approaches as the desired treatment protocol for trauma, Johnson (2009) noted that EBP is now being overtaken by the neuro-science paradigm. Neuroscience offers a new understanding of the impact of early trauma on brain development, requiring adjustments to treatment conceptualiza-tion. This chapter will focus on therapy with severely maltreated children who have been abused and neglected at an early age by their principal attachment figures. The very person upon whom the child relied for basic needs, such as holding and feeding, was the person who hurt and neglected the child. This population can include children whose behaviors suggest severe disturbance even if the reported abuse does not seem severe, because the extent of what these children have expe-rienced can be completely unknown (Haugaard, 2004). This is a population for whom there are no easy answers or cookbook approaches. Through this case exam-ple couched in neuroscience theory, I will demonstrate how in evidence-based practice, the art produced in art therapy *is* the evidence.

The term *evidence-based practice* is often misunderstood. The American Psycho-logical Association Presidential Task Force on Evidence-Based Practice defined the term as "the integration of the best available research with clinical expertise in the context of patient characteristics and preferences" (American Psychological Associa-tion, 2006, p. 273). EBP is *not* necessarily equivalent to randomized controlled trials or brief, manualized approaches. Clinical expertise is an important component of this broad definition, as is current research.

A trauma narrative, as would be expected in a TF-CBT approach to therapy, doesn't work for the child who was abused at a pre-verbal stage of development (Finn et al., 2018; Gantt & Tripp, 2016), nor for the child whose abuse necessitated a dis-sociative response (Goren, 2020), nor the child who cannot tolerate the memory due to a complex attachment to an abusive caregiver. Treatment interventions that bypass the severely maltreated child's habitual or defensive modes of response are needed, and these kinds of interventions are often expressively based (Coleman & Macintosh, 2015). Expressive therapy supports the client's coping skills at his or her emotional-developmental level, and helps the child express that which is impossible to verbalize. At a later developmental stage (typically late adolescence or possibly not until adulthood), it is possible to work more directly with the trauma, both through art and cognitive behavioral approaches. The clinical implication is that pressing too hard for verbal therapy with a child who has severe parental abuse issues can be counterproductive and counter therapeutic (Klorer, 2017).

Best practice when working with this population is a neuroscience approach that takes into account current research about brain functioning, traumatic responses, attachment issues, and accessing therapeutic issues through expressive means (Chapman, 2002, 2014; Cox et al., 2021; Klorer, 2005, 2017). Best practice requires individualizing treatment and developing a genuine therapeutic relation-ship over a longer period of time than a 12–16 week manualized trauma protocol. It entails following the child or adolescent's path of creative expression, and trusting the importance of safety and relationship building through the use of metaphor and connection. Relation-based therapy recognizes that children who have been harmed within relationships have to be healed through the child's social networks

(Cox et al., 2021; Schore & Schore, 2008). Children with early relational deprivation can develop self-awareness and social neural plasticity through positive interactions in a therapeutic milieu (Cozolino, 2014).

6.1   NEUROSCIENCE CONTRIBUTIONS TO UNDERSTANDING TRAUMA

Neuroscience provides important information for therapists working with severely maltreated children. This research presents solid evidence for the observations that Bowlby (1969) made over forty years ago when developing ideas for object relations and attachment theory (Schore, 2001; Cox et al., 2021). We now know that severe maltreatment and a lack of significant attachment figures in the crucial early years is associated with adverse brain development including decreased hippocampal volume (Bremner, 2001; Chugani et al., 2002; De Bellis, 2001; De Bellis et al., 1999; Perry, 1997; Rutter & O'Connor, 2004). Brain-imaging studies have greatly increased our capacity to understand changes in brain structure, though they cannot always predict causality. The brain's plasticity allows for rewiring and recovery, and imaging allows us to observe change and continually revise our interventions (Konopka, 2014, 2016). As will be discussed throughout this chapter, the brain's neuroplasticity contributes to the resilience that is seen in clients whose histories might indicate a more hopeless outcome.

Feldman (2020) noted that the quality of the mother/child bond leads to either resiliency or high risk, unregulated behavior. Feldman's three longitudinal studies looked at resilience factors based upon the neurobiology of affiliation. Mothers and children from three cohorts (maternal depression, pre-mature birth, or war trauma) were studied from the child's infancy through early adulthood. Feldman noted that the maternal bond creates endocrine, genetic, and molecular synchrony that has a continuous biological external-regulatory impact over time. We can assume by his history that Jack missed the early holding and stimulation from his mother that was so necessary for affiliation and affect regulation. He did not learn to self-regulate, which may be one reason external physical restraint was required to contain his anger.

The flawed attachment itself affects brain development. During the early years the human brain depends upon both genetic information and external stimulation for growth. During the first two years of life the basic circuits of the brain are being established (Balbernie, 2001; De Bellis, 2001; Schore, 2002; Schore & Schore, 2008). The child's brain develops in what Perry (2001) termed a use-dependent fashion, meaning that the more any neural system is activated, the more likely it is to become imbedded, although we know now that the brain is malleable and capable of forming new pathways as situations and relationships change. For children born into an environment where external stimulation such as holding and talking is lacking, neuropathways devoted to language do not form, and the children will develop language slower than usual. Communication delays result because those parts of the brain were not stimulated at a crucial developmental time. Holding and talking to a child are crucial components of normal cognitive and emotional development. Schore (2002; Schore & Schore, 2008) described the neurobiology of a secure attachment: early in the relationship the primary caretaker comforts the distressed baby by holding and feeding. In order to form a complete and healthy attachment, the mother must be able to create psycho-biological attunement with the infant, developing what Schore defined as affect synchrony. When the infant cries, the mother creates attunement by holding and rocking so that the child becomes synchronized with the mother's rhythmic struc-ture. This begins as an external regulator for the child, and neuropathways in the brain are stimulated each time this happens. With repetition, the neuropathways become fortified and stronger, and ultimately the child learns to self-regulate. When the maternal figure does not provide this comforting stimulation, the child suf-fers greatly. According to Schore (2002), a lack of stimulation affects the develop-ment of the frontolimbic regions of the brain, especially the right cortical areas that are prospectively involved in affect-regulating functions. Therefore, the child operates at a much lower socio-emotional developmental level than normal in terms of affect regulation and behavior management. Schore suggested that the early attachment relationship shapes the neurobiology of the core of the individual's right brain systems involved in affect and self-regulation and attach-ment theory is more aptly termed regulation theory, as this becomes the focus of treatment (Schore & Schore, 2008). In neurobiologically informed therapy, the relational aspect of the work facilitates the plasticity of the right brain to improve emotional self-regulatory processes, which often happens in non-verbal interac-tions. Schore (2014) stated,

> the psychobiologically attuned clinician tracks not just the verbal content but the nonverbal moment-to-moment rhythmic structures of the patient's internal states, and is flexibly and fluidly modifying his or her own behavior to synchronize with that structure, thereby co-creating with the patient a growth-facilitating context for the organization of the therapeutic alliance.
>
> (p. 390)

For a child such as Jack, re-experiencing early relational interactions can help to re-wire the brain. Neuroplasticity allows the brain to continue to adapt and change (positively or negatively) throughout the lifespan (Leitch, 2017). Harvey (1990, 1991) suggested that expressive modalities can define and assist change in the devel-opment and construction of new attachment communication, vital for the child's success in a foster care or pre-adoptive family. Cox and Perry (Cox et al., 2021) noted that prioritizing a relational model of intervention and a system of therapeutic rela-tionships promoted statistically significant resilience and positive sense of self in chil-dren with severe trauma.

The therapist's role is to provide structure, safety, coregulation, exploration, and boundaries necessary for the child to experiment with new roles and relation-ships. Sometimes this takes the form of physical and sensory activities, such as swing-ing, climbing, or spinning to help the child feel regulated (Goren, 2020). Klorer (2017) found a large elastic Co-operBand created by a dance therapist to be an exceptional tool for creating boundaries and movement exploration with young attachment-challenged children. Jernberg developed "Theraplay," a therapeutic technique designed to repeat those games and interactions that normally occur in a parent's relationship with a young child but are now re-experienced in a healthier, more secure situation. According to Jernberg (1979), work with abused children may not need to focus so much on the trauma itself, but rather on engaging children in situations that make them feel lovable, helping the caretaker or parent to recreate missed positive parent/infant interactions, and encouraging the child to abandon abuse-evoking behaviors. In a neuro-informed child centered play therapy model called SECURE, Conroy (Conroy & Perryman, 2022) proposed offering regulatory experiences and adaptive functioning through Safety, Engagement, Co-regulation, Understanding, Regulatory Expansion, and Exploration. By actively participating with the child and often the foster or adoptive parent, the therapist allows the child to choreograph scenarios that echo the child's attachment dilemma. Some of these play therapy techniques articulated above actually encourage regression to an infant or toddler developmental stage, allowing the child to fulfill some of these unmet needs. Jack's version of play was to hide from me, a developmentally regressed game that he continued to adapt as he grew older. The goal of therapy is to provide the child with a new repertoire of positive experiences from which to draw. Through repetition, new relational neuropathways are formed.

During the next few years of therapy, around age 13–14, Jack was too big to hide under the beanbag chair in the waiting room. His new hiding place was in the larger hallway leading to the office. He would open and shut the outer door so that I would think he had come in, and then he would stay in the hallway so that I had to pursue him further. He liked being "found." Although our relationship was firmly established, he still wanted me to believe that he came to see me only under coercion. In his residential treatment center, Jack engaged in fits of uncontrollable rage over the slightest perceived injustice. He was a large adolescent, and his aggressive outbursts were so intense they resulted in physical restraints requiring four adult men to contain him. His emotional instability challenged his teachers and caregivers, and his triggers for emotional upheaval were unpredictable. His psychiatrist frequently adjusted Jack's medication. In art therapy, another side of Jack emerged. He began making pillows, those wonderful soft objects that comfort us in our beds at night. He made pillows of varying sizes and shapes for his bed. He entrusted me to hand sew the seams with him, one of us working on each side of the pillow in an intimate sharing of space. He was just beginning to learn to self-soothe, an important component of behavioral regulation.

6.2   THE COMPLEXITY OF ATTACHMENT ISSUES

There are tremendous psychological complications for treatment when the abuser was the person upon whom the child must rely for meeting basic needs. This layer of complexity is reminiscent of Cairns' (1966a, 1966b) experiments of attachment behavior between species, in particular the pairing of lambs with dogs in a cage. Punishments did not affect the attachment, and in fact even in cases where the dog bit and mauled the lamb, after separation the lamb sought out the dog for companionship. Though we cannot make direct comparison between children and animals, professionals who work with abused children note that when a child is removed from an abusive parent, there is often an overwhelming desire to be reunited, no matter how intense the abuse was. This habitual response, described by van der Kolk (1989), reflects a longing for the original attachment figure and a loss of conscious memory of the trauma. Corwin and Olafson's (1997) study of Jane Doe, a client initially interviewed at age 6 disclosing sexual abuse, and then again 11 years later at age 17, demonstrated how a child's ability to recall events changes over time and is particularly impacted by the child's desire to reconnect to the parent, even years after a seemingly good adjustment in a foster or adoptive home.

Jack had unexplained scars, the source of which he could not remember. It was very clear in therapy that Jack needed to remember his mother as good. He longed for her. He could not remember what she looked like, but he said he missed her all the time. He made excuses for her, saying that perhaps she was in an accident, and that's why she never came back. Jack once said, "She was the best thing that ever happened to me." He did not want to hear the facts of his case when they were presented by his social worker. Although his early abuse and trauma were important parts of Jack, trying to focus therapy on what happened at an earlier age would be counterproductive at this stage of treatment because he could not talk about the abuse and he could not betray his need to protect his mother.

Often we find that the child who could disclose enough detail to assist in substantiating abuse during the acute trauma stage (in Jack's case, when the children were found alone in the house) will stop using words about the trauma during the treatment phase. Some children will "forget" that it was the parent who elicited the trauma or will simply deny the trauma (Corwin & Olafson, 1997).

Workers in residential children's homes can describe numerous examples of severely maltreated children who desperately want to return home. According to Fairbairn, there is a critical need to preserve and protect an image of a good parent, because if the parent isn't good, there is a startling reality that the child could die (1941). In order to preserve the image of a loving parent, children who are victims of severe parental abuse and neglect deny that the abuse happened or justify it as being deserved. The child assimilates the qualities of the bad object and preserves the abusing parent as the good object, rather than risk losing the parent (Fairbairn, 1941; Seinfeld, 1989; St. Clair, 1986, van der Kolk, 1989). While these children verbally protect and defend the abuser, in art they sometimes depict deeper feelings that they cannot possibly articulate or understand. We often see family pictures reflective of chaos and anger: a child draws her mother with such aggression that she tears holes in the picture; a young boy draws his parents and then scribbles them out repeatedly. The art allows for expression of unconscious feelings that are too unbearably painful to articulate, but are contained within the metaphor of the picture. The art doesn't lie. In the two examples above, at the time the child made the artwork the child vigorously defended the abusive parent and could not tolerate that the parent was anything less than loving toward him or her.

How does the art capture feelings that the client cannot access? These early memories of abuse and neglect, stored in the unconscious and kept at bay by coping skills and defenses, are like sleeping volcanoes. The hallmark of the traumatic response is physiologic hyperarousal to current stimuli reminiscent of the original trauma (Perry, 1995). Victims of trauma respond to contemporary stimuli as if they were back in the traumatic moment, with the same physiologic emergency response (van der Kolk, 1989). So when a child is asked to draw a picture that stimulates the original trauma (for example, a family picture), he or she is likely to immediately be propelled back to that physiologic hyperaroused state, and the artwork will reflect the chaos and feelings of that point in time rather than the usual defended self. This may explain why, in my own practice with abused and neglected children, the family drawing is the most often refused drawing in an art evaluation, or is drawn at a regressed developmental stage.

6.3   TREATMENT IMPLICATIONS

As Jack became more comfortable in his residential treatment center, he began making animal-shaped pillows for the staff. The pillows were a sought-after commodity; all the staff wanted one. Giving away his pillows was his safe way of being relational, and the staff responded to this childlike gesture in a nurturing way. He began to enjoy these safe relationships and started teasing with the staff, similar to his teasing me about not wanting to come to therapy.

In trauma cases there has been a paradigm shift away from conscious, explicit left-brain discourse to the nonverbal, body-based approaches. (Chapman, 2014; Cox et al., 2021; Perry, 2009; Schore, 2012). These latter approaches rely less on verbalization and more on expressive output. Treatment should be targeted at the child's emotional–developmental age, not chronological age. There should be an implicit understanding that later, perhaps not until adulthood, the client will be able to approach issues of severe parental maltreatment at a more sophisticated level of understanding than is currently possible. Perry (2001) suggested that children exposed to violence or trauma at young ages spend a large amount of time in a low-level state of fear, mediated by brainstem and midbrain areas, and their cognition is dominated by the sub-cortical and limbic areas. In a state of hypervigilence, they tend to focus on non-verbal clues and often misinterpret them, reacting impulsively without cognitively processing actual events. For example, when Jack caught some-one giving his shoes a funny look, he assumed he was being criticized and pounced on the child, quickly escalating the interaction into a physical fight. This hypervig-ilence did not lead to sensitivity to others' feelings, however. In fact, the opposite occurred. Jack would be the first to make fun of someone else's shoes or to say "Your mama" to a child who also had maternal issues, so fights in his cottage and classroom were frequent. His lack of empathy harkens back to his early developmental losses.

Perry (2009; Cox et al., 2021; Hambrick et al., 2018) developed the neurose-quential model of therapeutics (NMT) to conceptualize treatment with severely maltreated children. He suggested conceptualizing the beginning of treatment as working with the brainstem, the area associated with self-regulation, attention, arousal, and impulsivity. At this stage Perry recommended patterned, repetitive, and sensory activities, such as music, movement, yoga, or drumming. These activities are associated with pre-verbal neuro input to the brainstem, and the repetitions would provide the regulating input that would help to alleviate anxiety and impulsivity.

Chapman (2014) compiled a variety of sensory motor art techniques and games based upon neuroscience principles designed to facilitate cortical development. Her techniques provide the opportunity for relational exchanges between the child and therapist or child and caregiver that mimic early parent/child interactions and facil-itate neurodevelopment, including visual development, tactile development, gross and fine motor development, auditory development, vestibular development, and proprioceptive development.

Whereas Chapman uses directives to lead clients to relational exchanges, chil-dren often develop these types of games on their own. Jack's repeated desire to hide in the waiting room was his own invention and demonstrated that he was operating at a developmental stage much younger than his chronological age. "Finding" him always resulted in smiles, very similar to when a two-year-old hides and is found. One of the games Jack and other children like to play early in therapy is hiding jewels or animals in the sandtray and taking turns sifting through the sand to find them. Older children often invent games that seem age-inappropriate. They tend to repeat the game until they have worked through that earlier stage of development. The therapist doesn't have to search for these kinds of games; children invent what they need. Jack's hide-and-seek game was relational and speaks to his resiliency. The importance of following the relational rituals a child invents cannot be overstated. Jack's affectionate gesture of making pillows as gifts reflected a slightly later developmental progression in relationships, similar to kindergarten or elementary aged children making presents for their mothers. Children and adolescents gravitate towards materials and themes that resonate with their issues. Sewing is an unusual activity for a large adolescent male, and certainly not something I would have chosen for Jack. The activity began when he brought in a pair of pants and asked if I would help to mend them. I showed him how to thread a needle and sew. This progressed into his idea of making pillows. What Jack may have discovered in the process of learning to sew was what women for thousands of years have discovered in the process of textile arts: that the experience can be calming and helps them to feel grounded (Collier, 2011). Additionally, the tactile nature of the arts helps individuals relax, lower stress levels and achieve what is termed a flow state, where time disappears amid a seemingly effortless activity that ultimately brings pleasure (Huotilainen et al., 2018). For Jack, sewing presented an opportunity for new neuropathways of calm, focused attention and fine motor movements to be expressed and solidified. It also allowed for new relational neuropathways to be experienced, as we were working in close proximity, in a non-verbal, non-threatening shared experience.

Through these relational experiences of making and giving pillows, Jack gained confidence in relationships. He started asking his caseworker for a foster family and began talking about adoption, indicating he was getting ready to relinquish the idealized image of his biological mother and possibly acknowledge that she was never going to come back and get him. At age 15 in art therapy he made his first sculpture of a bear family (Figure 6.3). As is often the case, at the time I did not realize the significance of this sculpture, but he would make similar sculptures three times over the next four years, which suggested that he was working through something important with this sculpture. The first version looked hauntingly un-nurturing because the characters lacked facial features. Although he yearned for a family, it was apparent that he really did not understand how families should work. The three bears faced outward, and without facial features they could not interact. He did not notice anything unusual about the bears and glazed the sculpture to finish it.

According to Perry's (2009) neurosequential model, "Once there is improvement in self-regulation, the therapeutic work can move to more relational-related problems (limbic) using more traditional play or arts therapies" (p. 252). It was not an accident that Jack's artwork took on a more relational tone in content when he began exploring the relational aspects of his own life through practicing what it meant to be in relationship with staff. His developmental level had progressed beyond the most primitive brain stem levels; he was progressing on his behavioral level system in his treatment center, to the point that he was moved to a less restrictive unit.

Jack made progress on his behavioral level system, although he still had many challenges. At age 15 Jack got his wish and moved into a foster home with a wonderful woman who considered teenaged boys her specialty. I could be the best therapist in the world, but nothing I did

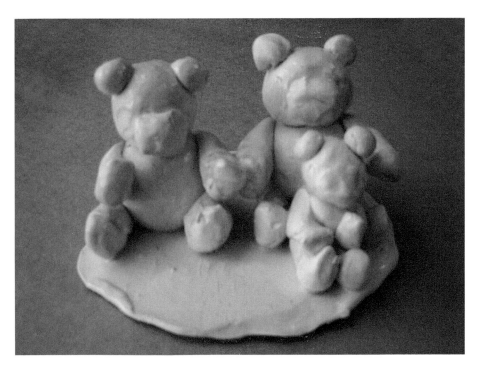

FIGURE 6.3 Jack, age 15. First Bear Sculpture

in 50 minutes per week compared to the fact that the foster mother wanted Jack and made a long-term commitment to his care. Jack did a lot of testing of this relationship. The foster mother learned early on that consequences devastated Jack and he was hypersensitive to rejection. If he got into trouble, he assumed that his foster mother no longer wanted him and he would become violent or run away.

One of the difficulties in work with institutionalized children is the lack of consistency in caregivers. Foster homes are not usually long term, nor is consistency in therapists typical. Children in state custody lose therapists as frequently as they change placements, and they change social workers, schools, psychiatrists, and house parents continually. Somehow through all of this I became one of only two long-term relationships in Jack's life. Once I started working with Jack, my ability to follow him from residential treatment to a foster home, through two more hospitalizations, two more residential placements, another group home, and back to his foster mother, was partially my insistence and partially luck. Many children with attachment issues end up with multiple placements because the system does not value relationships. Others end up with multiple placements because the children actively push away the very people who are trying to love and help them (Hughes, 1997, 1998). Foster parents become frustrated by a child's inability to bond, and thus a cycle of failed placements continues. Family therapy with the foster parent and child, even if it is not a pre-adoptive home, becomes a crucial intervention to safeguard the placement and break this pattern (Klorer, 2017). Family therapy with Jack and his foster mother was imperative in order for Jack to learn how to be in a family, and we alternated family and individual sessions. The most important treatment goal for Jack at age 15 was to form an attachment with his foster mother.

Jack began making presents for his foster family. He made pillows for everyone, including a stuffed animal pillow with an imbedded squeaky toy for the family dog. He made an origami person for the college-aged daughter (Figure 6.4) and a doll for his 17-year-old foster brother (Figure 6.5). As was typical of his art, faces were devoid of features. We needed to help Jack get to the point that he could look people in the eye and not be afraid of their faces. Jack had a number of explosive incidents during the next few years, several with police involvement, and he had to leave the foster home for hospitalizations. Twice he returned to residential treatment centers, but his foster parents genuinely cared about him and always took him back. Jack made his bear sculpture again at age 16 (Figure 6.6). He was still trying to understand what it meant to live in a family. His foster mother reported that he was most comfortable spending time alone in his room rather than interacting with others in the house. Yet he was reaching out to family members and expressing affection through his art. During this same time period he tried to "fire" me as his therapist several times, claiming that I tortured him. I teased him and told him I wanted to work with him until he was at least 21, and maybe even an old man. He would smile.

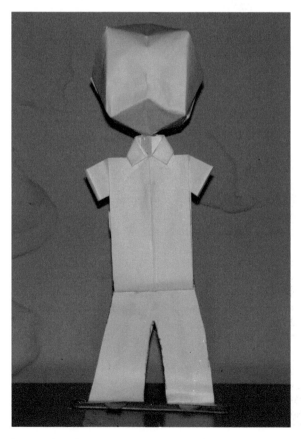

FIGURE 6.4 Jack, age 15. Origami person made for his foster sister

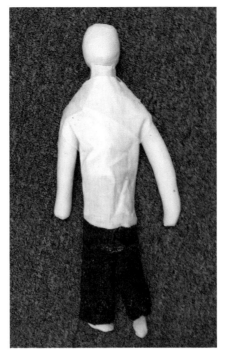

FIGURE 6.5 Jack, age 16. Doll made for his foster brother

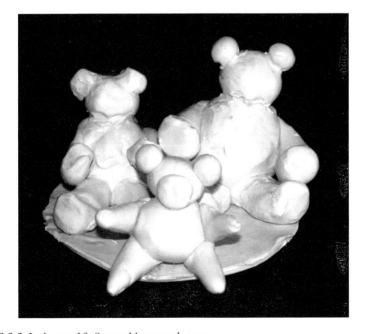

FIGURE 6.6 Jack, age 16. Second bear sculpture

In her Neuro-developmental Art Therapy model, Chapman (2014) identified the "Problem Phase" as when the child is exploring non-verbal emotions through art and play. As Jack was becoming more secure in his attachment with his foster mother, which suggested that relational neuropathways were being formulated, he could experiment with pushing me away. The fact that I wouldn't leave was another testament to the power of a secure attachment and would help strengthen those pathways

Perry (2009) noted in his neurosequential model that "once fundamental dyadic relational skills have improved, the therapeutic techniques can be more verbal and insight oriented (cortical) using any variety of cognitive-behavioral or psychodynamic approach" (p. 252). This was evidenced by Jack's ability in the following years to take advantage of verbal therapy, not possible until his neurodevelopmental functioning reached the cortex and further demonstrating the plasticity of the brain.

At ages 17–18 Jack sat in the waiting room with his hooded sweatshirt pulled so far over his head that only the bottom third of his face showed. At 225 pounds he didn't fit under the beanbag chair or behind the door anymore, and he felt foolish hiding in the hallway, but he still wanted me to find him. Jack still had difficulty making eye contact unless I asked him to, with the exception of when he was lying; then he looked directly into my eyes and smiled. Then we would both laugh knowingly. The trust and security of our relationship was firm enough that we could joke around and then focus on a real problem. Once he unconvincingly told me that he hadn't had any problems in school that week, he could start talking about the problems he had had in school. His foster mother continued to attend sessions and assisted him in behavior regulation. Cognitive behavioral approaches were now more successful, so we utilized positive self-talk to de-escalate his anger before an outburst, relaxation techniques, and role playing for social problem solving. However, Jack's primary treatment goals continued to focus on that which he had missed in his early developmental years: emotional regulation through attachment with a maternal figure. At age 19 Jack had a crucial turning point in his life when his foster mother discovered that in a fit of anger he had destroyed all of the family photos she had given him. Although she told him she understood why he did it, she wanted him to know it hurt her feelings. Perceiving this as another rejection, he became very angry, began yelling, threw some of his things in a bag, and said he was going back to the group home to live. Although the foster mother thought he was going to bolt, she kept talking to him calmly. Finally, he started crying, she started crying, and they hugged. She told him she loved him with all her heart. Through tears he said he wanted to stay. The next few months of therapy Jack opened up in therapy as he never had before about painful recollections of his biological mother and other abusive people in his life. With the security of his foster mother's love, he could finally face these feelings. Jack stopped hiding in my waiting room at about that same time.

Later that year, Jack began making another bear sculpture. The sculpture took more than a month to complete, as he started and then abandoned it several times. An amazing thing about this sculpture, when it was finally finished, was that the bears (2 bears instead of 3) had facial features (Figure 6.7). Jack finally understood what it was like to make a genuine connection with his foster mother.

A secure attachment is a necessary ingredient to face early developmental trauma. In Jack's case, the facial features, which for him represented the

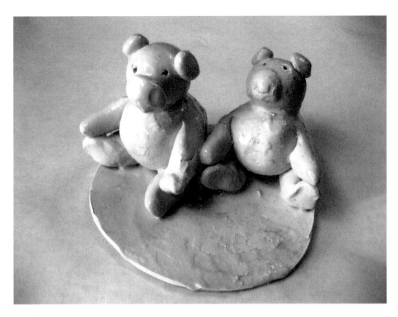

FIGURE 6.7 Jack, age 19. Third bear sculpture

emotional center of the figure, could not be incorporated in the family figures until he had experienced such connections first hand in a relationship and in the higher cortical function of the brain. The neuroplasticity of the brain allowed him to change and grow in relationship. His resiliency is beautifully evidenced in the art.

6.4   SUMMARY: NEUROSCIENCE INFORMED APPROACHES TO ATTACHMENT RELATED TRAUMA

A neuroscience approach to therapy with children severely traumatized by their principle attachment figures takes in to account the psychological and physiological effects of abuse. This approach entails working at the child's socio-emotional level rather than chronological age (Perry, 2009), recognizing that the child may be functioning at a much lower developmental level than anticipated. Early relational games and interactions, some that might appear on the surface to be too young for the client, may actually hold his or her interest for quite a while. The therapist will want to provide opportunities for the child to experiment with new modes of interactive responses with the therapist and primary support group. Aligning therapeutic support with the treatment center, foster parent, or pre-adoptive family is imperative, as those relationships can be where the most important work happens. Helping caregivers to understand the meaning behind the behavior can sometimes save a placement. Although it is beyond the scope of this chapter to discuss medication regimens, medication evaluation and adjustments may also be a necessary component of treatment. One should postpone cognitive-based therapies in favor of expressive and relational work until the child is able to form an attachment (Perry, 2009). Later, cognitive approaches for symptom reduction and acquisition of coping skills may be used.

Using expressive methods in a relational way enables the child or adolescent to make emotional connections. The child will create imagery reflective of his or her relationships. Hass-Cohen (2016) described art therapy as contributing to a transformative reintegration of autobiographical data. Old memories are reactivated and consolidated with new emotional experiences creating therapeutic change, which is evidenced and reinforced through the art created.

It is an idiosyncratic process, in that what is an important symbol for one client is irrelevant for another. A lack of facial features was an important symbol for Jack, but one could not generalize this to another client. For the same reason that artwork alone cannot be used to diagnose sexual or physical abuse, there is no defined set of graphic indicators that will indicate success of treatment. Rather, the therapist has to track the changes in the client's own imagery in comparison to changes in behaviors. Jack's art reflected his attachment issues, although we did not talk about that interpretation directly. We lived the attachment issues through a genuine relationship.

To summarize, Jack's first attempts in art were well defended and his beginning art reflected his fear of closeness (Figures 6.1 and 6.2). As he began to trust his staff, his art became more relational, as if he were in the practicing phase of attachment/separation/individuation. At the same time, he invited me to assist him in sewing, which brought us into an intimate, shared space as an important relational connection was being formed. When he moved to a foster home, he continued to use art relationally. His fear of closeness was apparent in the lack of facial features on the people and animals that he made as gifts (Figures 6.3, 6.4, 6.5, and 6.6). As those relationships were forged and he engaged in a genuine familial relationship, Jack's art changed. His final sculpture (Figure 6.7) demonstrated this relational progression. At termination, Jack understood, on a deep, molecular, neuronal level related to the changes that occurred in the brain (Feldman, 2020), what it meant to be in a family. The art is the evidence.

What made these changes in art possible? The brain is malleable and the early relational stimulation that happens between a primary caretaker and child is instrumental in forming relational neuro pathways which assist a child in making an attachment and learning affect regulation (Perry, 2001; Schore, 2002, 2014). Jack could not have made that last sculpture until he had experienced a positive connection with another. It began in a practicing-stage while in residential treatment, and was solidified through therapy and his foster mother. New neuropathways developed when he was able to experience those aspects of the mother/child bond that he missed as a child. Art therapy and the therapeutic alliance provided an avenue for Jack to explore these themes.

At age 21, Jack and I terminated therapy. He signed release forms so that I could photograph his artwork and possibly share his story someday. He took all the artwork that had been left in the office over the nine years of our work together, and he moved into a semi-independent living program for adults. Although Jack continued to have challenges, in our last communication the foster mother reported she was still seeing Jack for occasional outings and dinner.

6.5   PRACTICAL APPLICATIONS FOR CLIENTS WITH SEVERE EARLY RELATIONAL TRAUMA

How does one take a neuroscience-informed treatment approach when working with severe early relational trauma? The following suggestions will assist in creating new relational neuropathways for optimal change and developmental progression through missed stages. These suggestions may seem too elementary or anti-climactic to mention, yet even seasoned therapists often miss these very basic foundational tenets. Going back to the basics of good therapy results in good therapy.

First and foremost, establish trust with your client. When a child's early relationships have been fraught with chaos, creating trust means the therapeutic space needs to be predictable and consistent. Incorporate simple "Therapy 101" things, like establishing a specific day and time to meet. If the session is at 2:00 on Tuesdays, begin the session at *exactly* 2:00 because every minute you are late is perceived as a potential abandonment. Consistency in every aspect of the therapy builds security. Tables, chairs and office contents should all be in place upon the client's arrival. Cleaning up art materials used and restoring the space back to its original state at the end of sessions contributes to creating safety and predictability and the client should be part of that. Create trust by encouraging the creation of soothing rituals, like beginning and ending sessions the same way and giving the child as much control as possible within the safe boundaries of the session.

Begin the work at the child's emotional level of function rather than chronological age. This means being receptive to the child's interest in materials and methods that may appear age-inappropriate. Let the client lead. The most powerful work in art therapy often comes from non-directive, client-centered work. When provided with psychological safety in the art room and a trusting relationship with a therapist, children and adolescents find their own paths. Pay particular attention to a child's repeated themes, which suggest that new neuronal links are being established, practiced, and in time will be incorporated into new learning and change (King et al., 2019).

Acknowledge that the work is going to be long term, with accompanying boundaries insuring that the client understands and is not confused by the nature of the relationship. The transference can be complicated in cases of maternal abuse and neglect, so healthy therapeutic boundaries are crucial. There should be no therapist-self-disclosure; it is a one-way relationship. And yet, the relationship needs to be genuine. Ultimately, it comes down to a very basic tenet: the child needs to *feel* loved, without the therapist *saying* love. Keep in mind that, in a meta-analysis of hundreds of psychological studies of therapeutic effectiveness, by far the most important factor of successful treatment is the alliance between therapist and client (Norcross & Lambert, 2006, 2019). In therapy with this population, the relationship is paramount.

Track the changes in the client's own imagery in comparison to changes in behaviors. Bear in mind that we seldom know what the artwork "means" during the process of doing therapy, and a therapist has to be comfortable with not knowing. As we get to know the client's themes, we get to know the client. Changes in themes track therapeutic progression. *The art is the evidence.*

> **Practical Suggestions for Clients with Severe Relational Trauma**
>
> 1 Postpone cognitive-based therapies in favor of expressive and relational work until the child is able to form an attachment.
> 2 Establish trust by consistency in day and time of treatment, safety, and predictability.
> 3 Begin the work at the child's emotional, not chronological, age.
> 4 Let the client lead.
> 5 Acknowledge that the work will be long term.
> 6 Provide firm boundaries to insure that the client is not confused by the nature of the relationship.
> 7 Track the changes in the client's own imagery in comparison to changes in behaviors.

NOTE

1 Although details of this case have been changed to protect confidentiality, the essence of the case and the artwork are real.

REFERENCES

Amaya-Jackson, L., & deRosa, R. R. (2007). Treatment considerations for clinicians in applying evidence-based practice to complex presentations in child trauma. *Journal of Traumatic Stress, 20*(4), 379–390. https://doi.org/10.1002/jts.20266

American Psychological Association, APA Presidential Task Force on Evidence-Based Practice (2006). Evidence-based practice in psychology. *American Psychologist, 61*(4), 271–285. https://doi.org/10.1037/0003-066X.61.4.271

Balbernie, R. (2001). Circuits and circumstances: The neurobiological consequences of early relationship experiences and how they shape later behavior. *Journal of Child Psychotherapy, 27*(3), 237–255. https://doi.org/10.1080/00754170110087531

Bowlby, J. (1969). *Attachment* (2nd ed., Vol. I). Basic Books.

Bremner, J. D. (2001). A biological model for delayed recall of childhood abuse. *Journal of Aggression, Maltreatment and Trauma, 4*(2), 165–183.

Cairns, R. B. (1966a). Attachment behavior of mammals. *Psychological Review, 73*(5), 409–426. https://doi.org/10.1037/h0023691

Cairns, R. B. (1966b). Development, maintenance, and extinction of social attachment behavior in sheep. *Journal of Comparative Physiological Psychology, 62*(2), 298–306. https://doi.org/10.1037/h0023692

Chapman, L. (2002, November). *A neuro-developmental approach to treating post-traumatic stress disorder and symptoms.* Paper presented at the American Art Therapy Association's 33rd Annual Conference, Washington, DC.

Chapman, L. (2014). *Neurobiologically informed trauma therapy with children and adolescents.* New York, NY: Norton.

Chugani, H. T., Behen, M. E., Muzik, O., Juhasz, C., Nagy, F., & Chugani, D. C. (2002). Local brain functional activity following early deprivation: A study of postinstitutionalized Romanian orphans. *Neuroimage, 14*(6), 1290–1301. http://dx.doi.org/10.1006/nimg.2001.0917

Coleman, K., & Macintosh, H. B. (2015). Art and evidence: Balancing the discussion on arts- and evidence-based practices with traumatized children. *Journal of Child & Adolescent Trauma*, 8(1), 21–31. https://doi.org/10.1007/s40653-015-0036-1

Collier, A. F. (2011). The well-being of women who create with textiles: Implications for art therapy. *Art Therapy*, 28(3), 104–112. https://doi.org/10.1080/07421656.2011.597025

Conroy, J., & Perryman, K. (2022). Treating trauma with child-centered play therapy through the SECURE lens of polyvagal theory. *International Journal of Play Therapy*, 31(3), 143–152. https://doi.org/10.1037/pla0000172

Corwin, D., & Olafson, E. (1997). Videotaped discovery of a reportedly unrecallable memory of child sexual abuse: Comparison with a childhood interview videotaped 11 years before. *Child Maltreatment*, 2(2), 91–112. https://doi.org/10.1177/1077559597002002001

Cox, A., Perry, B., D., & Frederico, M. (2021). Resourcing the system and enhancing relationships: Pathways to positive outcomes for children impacted by abuse and neglect. *Child Welfare*, 98(6), 177–202.

Cozolino, L. (2014). *The neuroscience of human relationships: Attachment and the developing social brain.* W.W. Norton.

De Bellis, M. (2001). Developmental traumatology: The psychobiological development of maltreated children and its implications for research, treatment, and policy. *Development and Psychopathology*, 13(3) 539–564.

De Bellis, M., Keshavan, M., Clark, D., Dasey, B., Giedd, J., Boring, A., … Ryan, N. (1999). Developmental traumatology Part II: Brain development. *Biological Psychiatry*, 45(10), 1271–1284. https://doi.org/10.1016/S0006-3223(99)00045-1

Fairbairn, W. R. D. (1941). *An object-relations theory of the personality.* Basic Books.

Feldman, R. (2020). What is resilience: An affiliative neuroscience approach. *World Psychiatry*, 19(2), 132–150. https://doi.org/10.1002/wps.20729

Finn, H., Warner, E., Price, M., & Spinazzola, J. (2018, September). The boy who was hit in the face: Somatic regulation and processing of preverbal complex trauma. *Journal of Child & Adolescent Trauma*, 11(3), 277–288. https://doi.org/10.1007/s40653-017-0165-9

Gantt, L., & Tripp, T. (2016). The image comes first: Treating preverbal trauma with art therapy. In J. King (Ed.), *Art therapy, trauma, and neuroscience: Theoretical and practical perspectives* (pp. 67–99). Routledge.

Goren, A. (2020). "Something else" in child psychotherapy with traumatised adopted children. *Journal of Child Psychotherapy*, 46(2), 152–167. https://doi.org/10.1080/0075417X.2020.1791228

Hambrick, E. P., Brawner, T. W., Perry, B. D., Wang, E. Y., Griffin, G., DeMarco, T., Capparelli, C., Grove, T., Maikoetter, M., O'Malley, D., Paxton, D., Freedle, L., Friedman, J., Mackenzie, J., Perry, K. M., Cudney, P., Hartman, J., Kuh, E., Morris, J., Polales, C., & Strother, M. (2018). Restraint and critical incident reduction following introduction of the neurosequential model of therapeutics (NMT). *Residential Treatment for Children & Youth*, 35(1), 2–23. https://doi.org/10.1080/08865 71X.2018.1425651

Harvey, S. (1990). Dynamic play therapy: An integrative expressive arts approach to the family therapy of young children. *The Arts in Psychotherapy*, 17(3), 239–246. https://doi.org/10.1016/0197-4556(90)90007-D

Harvey, S. (1991). Creating a family: An integrated expressive approach to adoption. *The Arts in Psychotherapy*, 18(3), 213–222. http://dx.doi.org/10.1016/0197-4556(91)90115-Q

Hass-Cohen, N. (2016). Secure resiliency: Art therapy relational neuroscience trauma treatment prinicples and guildelines. In J. King (Ed.), *Art therapy, trauma, and neuroscience: Theoretical and practical perspectives* (pp. 100–138). Routledge. https://doi.org/10.4324/9781003196242-5

Haugaard, J. (2004). Recognizing and treating uncommon behavioral and emotional disorders in children and adolescents who have been severely maltreated: Introduction. *Child Maltreatment*, 9(2), 123–130. https://doi.org/10.1177/1077559504264305

Hughes, D. (1997). *Facilitating developmental attachment.* Jason Aronson.

Hughes, D. (1998). *Building the bonds of attachment*. Jason Aronson.

Huotilainen, M., Rankanen, M., Groth, C., Seitamaa-Hakkarainen, P., & Mäkelä, M. (2018). Why our brains love arts and crafts Implications of creative practices on psychophysical well-being. *FORMakademisk*, *11*(2), 1–17. https://doi.org/10.7577/formakademisk.1908

Jernberg, A. (1979). *Theraplay: A new treatment using structured play for problem children and their families*. Jossey-Bass.

Johnson, D. R. (2009). Commentary: Examining underlying paradigms in the creative arts therapies of trauma. *The Arts in Psychotherapy*, *36*(2), 114–120. http://dx.doi.org/10.1016/j.aip.2009.01.011

King, J. L., Kaimal, G., Konopka, L., Belkofer, C., & Strang, C. E. (2019). Practical applications of neuroscience-informed art therapy. *Art Therapy*, *36*(3), 149–156. https://doi.org/10.1080/0742 1656.2019.1649549

Klorer, P. G. (2005). Expressive therapy with severely maltreated children: Neuroscience contributions. *Art Therapy: Journal of the American Art Therapy Association*, *22*(4), 213–220. https://doi.org/10.1080/07421656.2005.10129523

Klorer, P. G. (2017). *Expressive therapy with traumatized children*. Rowman & Littlefield.

Konopka, L. (2014, Feb). Where art meets neuroscience: a new horizon of art therapy. *Croatian Medical Journal*, *55*(1), 73–74. https://doi.org/10.3325/cmj.2014.55.73

Konopka, L. (2016). Neuroscience concepts in clinical practice. In J. King (Ed.), *Art therapy, trauma, and neuroscience* (pp. 11–41). Routledge.

Leitch, L. (2017). Action steps using ACEs and trauma-informed care: A resilience model. *Health & justice*, *5*(1), 5–5. https://doi.org/10.1186/s40352-017-0050-5

Norcross, J., & Lambert, M. (2006). The therapy relationship. In J. Norcross, L. Beutler, & R. Levant (Eds.), *Evidence-based practices in mental health* (pp. 208–218). American Psychological Association.

Norcross, J., & Lambert, M. (2019). Evidence-based psychotherapy relationship: The third task force. In *Psychotherapy Relationships that Work. Vol 1: Evidence-Based Therapist Contributions* (pp. 1–23). Oxford Academic. https://doi.org/10.1093/med-psych/9780190843953.003.0001

Perry, B. (1995). Childhood trauma, the neurobiology of adaptation, and "use dependent" development of the brain: How "states" become "traits." *Infant Mental Health Journal*, *16*(4), 271–291.

Perry, B. (1997). Incubated in terror: Neurodevelopmental factors in the "Cycle of Violence." In J. Osofsky (Ed.), *Children in a violent society* (pp. 124–148). Guilford.

Perry, B. (2001). *Violence and childhood: How persisting fear can alter the developing child's brain* (October 25, 2001). www.ChildTrauma.org

Perry, B. (2009). Examining child maltreatment through a neurodevelopmental lens: Clinical applications of the neurosequential model of therapeutics. *Journal of Loss & Trauma*, *14*(4), 240–255. https://doi.org/10.1080/15325020903004350

Rutter, M., & O'Connor, T. (2004). Are there biological programming effects for psychological development? Findings from a study of Romanian orphans. *Developmental Psychology*, *40*(1), 81–94. https://doi.org/10.1037/0012-1649.40.1.81

Schore, A. (2001). The effects of a secure attachment relationship on right brain development, affect regulation, and infant mental health. *Infant Mental Health Journal*, *22*(1/2), 7–66. https://doi.org/10.1002/1097-0355(200101/04)22:1<7::AID-IMHJ2>3.0.CO;2-N

Schore, A. (2002). Dysregulation of the right brain: a fundamental mechanism of traumatic attachment and the psychopathogenesis of posttraumatic stress disorder. *Australian and New Zealand Journal of Psychiatry*, *36*(1), 9–30.

Schore, A. N. (2012). *The science of the art of psychotherapy*. W.W. Norton.

Schore, A. N. (2014). The right brain is dominant in psychotherapy. *Psychotherapy*, *51*(3), 388–397. https://doi.org/10.1037/a0037083

Schore, J. R., & Schore, A. N. (2008). Modern attachment theory: The central role of affect regulation in development and treatment. *Clinical Social Work Journal, 36*(1), 9–20. https://doi.org/10.1007/s10615-007-0111-7

Seinfeld, J. (1989). Therapy with severely abused child: An object relations perspective. *Clinical Social Work Journal, 17*(1), 40–49.

St. Clair, M. (1986). *Object relations and self psychology: An introduction.* Brooks/Cole Publishing.

van der Kolk, B. (1989). The compulsion to repeat the trauma. *Psychiatric Clinics of North America, 12*(2), 389–411.

CHAPTER 7

PRACTICAL APPLICATIONS OF NEUROSCIENCE IN ART THERAPY

A Holistic Approach to Treating Trauma in Children

Christopher M. Belkofer and Emily Nolan

When working with children who have experienced trauma it is common for relatively small stimuli such as perceived rejection, an authority figure saying "no," or a redirection of behavior to result in outbursts of defiance, anger, sadness, despair, disconnection, and often aggression. These extreme reactions can be described as low input–high output responses. A mild stimulus (low input) often evokes an extreme response (high output). Encountering such "meltdowns" proposes a series of challenges and complexities for the therapist, support staff, and/or primary caregiver. Moreover, because of their neurodevelopment, children, traumatized or not, lack the verbal processing skills necessary to discuss their feelings and emotions (Siegel & Bryson, 2012). This chapter explores how the practice of art therapy has unique characteristics that can address these challenges. In the following pages we will explore the assertion that process-oriented art therapy approaches to treatment may help clients practice self-regulation by increasing their awareness of their own bodies (Hass-Cohen, 2008; Hass-Cohen & Findlay, 2015; Malchiodi, 2020). The physical properties of art media used in art therapy are done in the service of the therapeutic relationship and can target the underlying components of trauma in a way that language often cannot.

The collective impact of childhood trauma can result in numerous maladaptive coping strategies that range from avoiding interpersonal connections to impaired cognitive functioning, to severe negative bias, to rapidly fluctuating emotional responses (Doba et al., 2022). It is essential to conceptualize these challenging behaviors as rooted in the individual's damaged biological systems as opposed to a lack of will or a refusal to "try." For example, repeated exposure to real or perceived threats, such as those that are associated with psychological and physical trauma, can result in changes in neurophysiology such as variations in hormones (Sherin & Nemeroff, 2011), breathing patterns (Salah et al, 2021), and levels of cortical arousal (Howells et al., 2012). Psychological trauma may result in lingering fatigue and chronic pain (Van Houdenhove et al., 2009). These physical manifestations, which are "real" in a bodily sense, are typically presented as products of the mind and manifested in behaviors as opposed to being understood as symptoms of trauma.

Perception of one's reality and own felt sense of the world is influenced by one's neurophysiology (Siegel, 2020). Variations in the systems of the brain and other related parts of the body influence perception and mood, as well as thoughts and feelings. The communication between cells, the flow of blood and oxygen, and the secretion of hormones directly constitute how one experiences one's realities (Levine, 2010). Trauma disrupts these bodily systems, which correlates with a rupture

DOI: 10.4324/9781003348207-7

in how people experience the world. This estrangement in how a person feels in and about the world impacts the self. To understand how trauma disrupts the mind – or, if we prefer, the self – we must also appreciate how trauma impacts the body.

7.1   TRAUMA AND THE BODY

In many ways, people who have experienced trauma often struggle within their own bodies (van der Kolk, 2006). To escape and survive a person may ignore, numb, deny, and suppress their awareness of their inner feelings, sensations, and intuitions. During this time, they struggle to access what is called interoceptive awareness (Carvalho & Damasio, 2021). As survivors lose touch with their bodies, they grow increasingly distant from a connection with their own sense of self. Compounding the issue, the loss of access to one's inner world leads to significant challenges experiencing and attuning to the inner world of others. As clients shut down connection and communication from their bodies, they also sever connections to other humans and the world around them. To conceptualize this image, imagine that a person who has experienced trauma observes themself on the opposite shore of a river. What they see across from them is disconnected from what they feel. The self is ruptured by the ripples of trauma, and relationships with others become distant, and dangerous.

Scientists and researchers are garnering evidence that the impacts of psychological trauma from verbal abuse and emotional neglect last far beyond the duration of the event (Glaser, 2000). Researchers have shown that early life trauma leads not only to long-term mental health problems well into adulthood, such as depression and suicidal thoughts, but also diseases including cancer and diabetes (Anda et al., 2006). Although a full review of the literature on the impact of psychological trauma on the body and the mind is beyond the scope of this chapter, there are arching implications of these findings for mental health. There is a need for greater understanding of the development of psychiatric symptoms as related to "stress-induced changes in neurobiology" (Bremner & Vermetten, 2001, p. 481).

Clinical neuroscience and interpersonal neurobiology (Siegel, 2020; Siegel et al., 2021) have built upon seminal attachment theory (Schore, 2001) to work toward addressing mental health as an interpersonally influenced mind/body holistic experience (Hass-Cohen & Clyde Findlay, 2015; Kain & Terrell, 2018; Poole Heller, 2019). We understand how the relational bond between mother and child, or child client and therapist, for example, impacts the structure and function of brain development (Chapman, 2014; Kravits, 2008). This era of increased appreciation of the brain has led to paradigm shifts in how mental health is conceptualized and treated (Cozolino, 2002; Damasio, 1994, 1999; Perry; 1996; Schore, 1994, 2001; Siegel, 2020; Siegel & Bryson, 2012; van der Kolk 2003, 2006). While a full summary of the emergent research and theories that can be gleaned from neuroscience-informed approaches to mental health is far beyond the scope of this chapter, for the sake of simplicity and with a potential for reduction, the collective influence of these shifts as pertinent to our writing can be broadly summarized as follows:

- Interpersonal relationships directly influence the development and performance of structures and systems within the brain.

- Our thoughts, feelings, and behaviors are made up of dynamic processes that directly relate to the whole self.
- Traumatic memories are difficult to access and process exclusively with language.
- Mental health disorders associated with trauma relate directly to physiological processes such as levels of hyper- and hypo-arousal.
- Neuroplasticity: our brains are not fixed and can change throughout the life span.
- Interpersonal relationships are a mechanism that may help to rewire the brain.

The implication of these influences is that effective mental health models no longer conceptualize the brain as distinct from the body. The brain and the body "are intimately linked together" in the formation of the mind (Newberg & d'Aquili, 2000, p. 54).

Newberg and d'Aquili (2000) clarify:

> Perhaps the easiest way to understand the relationship between the mind and the brain is to regard the brain as the structure that performs all of the functions and the mind as the product of these functions. Thus, the mind and brain may be considered two ways of looking at the same thing. The brain refers more to the structural components, and the mind refers more to the functional components.
>
> (p. 54)

The implications of these assertions have widespread applications for art therapy. It is not surprising that a field that was once ambivalent toward scientific paradigms (Kaplan, 2000) has enthusiastically looked toward neuroscience for greater understanding and at times legitimization (Johnson, 2009). In addition to the development of brain-based art therapy clinical models (Buk, 2009; Chapman, 2014; Collie et al., 2006; Hass-Cohen, 2008; Hass-Cohen & Clyde Findlay, 2015; Malchiodi, 2020) and exploratory brain imaging studies (Belkofer & Konopka, 2008; Belkofer et al., 2014; King et al., 2017; Kruk et al., 2014) that consider how media impacts the brain, an entire special issue of *Art Therapy: Journal of the American Art Therapy Association* was dedicated to the topic of art therapy and neuroscience (Kapitan, 2014). Johnson (2009) asserted that "the fact that the brain is involved is not evidence that the creative arts therapies are effective" and that applications of neuroscience in art therapy remain primarily "metaphorical" (pp. 116–117). These observations do not take away from the significant advancements that have led us past a conceptualization of art therapy as a right-brained profession and toward an increasing appreciation that visual "art making" takes place all over the brain (Belkofer, 2012).

The emphasis of this chapter is on how the brain-based knowledge has informed our work as art therapists. We hope to illustrate through two case vignettes how the therapeutic use of the visual arts is an effective means for working with children who either cannot or will not express themselves in traditional verbal narratives. To illustrate this we build from two primary foundational assertions: (i) art engages the body (Belkofer, 2014; Malchiodi, 2006; 2020; Kossak, 2009), (ii) the seminal work of van der Kolk (2006, 2014) that emphasizes the body in treating the psychological impacts of trauma. Even through in the early part of the 20th century, Adler's theory of holism posited that there is no separation between the brain and the body (as cited in Mosak & Maniacci, 1999), bodily elements of psychotherapy treatment have remained largely understated in comparison to the emphasis on cognitive processing and behavior modification. As noted by Malchiodi (2020), "expressive arts therapy, however, adds something uniquely important to work with traumatized individuals by naturally bringing implicit sensory and body-based elements to psychotherapeutic dynamics that are not always available through even the most skilled verbal exchanges" (p. 100). For our purposes, we assert that although targeting the body has been a longstanding feature of expressive therapies (of which art therapy is often classified as a form of) such as dance movement therapy, drama therapy, and music therapy (Pearson & Wilson, 2009), the bodily characteristics of art therapy have remained less explicit. We do not intend to diminish the significant emphasis on the physical elements of art-based approaches to art therapy (McNiff, 1992; B. L. Moon, 2009; B. L. Moon & Belkofer, 2014), yet traditionally these theories have overtly attempted to differentiate art therapy from traditional scientific models. Regardless of these differences, contemporary views of art therapy are no longer bound to the old models of "art psychotherapy" (Naumburg, 1987) versus "art as therapy" (Cane, 1983; Kramer, 1958), but rather view the work as existing on a continuum. The ability of art therapists to work from a variety of approaches as determined by the needs of the client as well as the suitability of the setting is a basic expectation of art therapy training today.

Lending support to this expanding view, the development of the Expressive Therapies Continuum (ETC) has helped to provide a conceptual framework for the therapeutic potential of process-oriented and non-verbal art making as well as more traditional models of verbal insight (Hinz, 2020). The ETC categorizes engagement with art media on three levels that posit a set of continuums: kinesthetic/sensory (K/S), perceptual/affective (P/A), and cognitive/symbolic (C/Sy). For example, an individual that repeatedly smooths out pieces of earthen clay would be working on the K/S level of the continuum. By contrast a client creating a self-portrait in colored pencil exploring their professional identity would be working on a more C/Sy level.

Lusebrink (2010) theorized that the differing levels of the continuum correspond with discernable brain structures and brain functioning. In this view, changes within the levels of the continuum reflect variations in the brain. The K/S level, for example, hypothetically would involve brain functioning associated with movement and somatosensory functioning. By contrast, working on the C/Sy level would reflect cognitive functioning such as abstraction, metaphor, and "concept formation" (Lusebrink, 2010, p. 171). Although art therapy is not necessarily sequential or bound to one level or another, art therapists can use the ETC to appreciate the range of dynamic brain structures and processes broadly associated with the therapeutic applications of the creation of visual imagery. More empirical support is needed to support this theory, but the varied responses of art making afforded by the ETC model may be well suited for initially conceptualizing a rationale for how divergent ways of working as an art therapist correspond to divergent processes within the client's brain.

The brain is a creative system. Rather than mirroring the environment around it, as an engineered information processing device would, each brain constructs maps of that environment using its own parameters and internal design, and thus creates a world unique to the class of brains comparably designed (Damasio, 1999, p. 322).

The action-oriented use of the body and perceptual and sensory processing associated with the ETC aligns art therapy with conceptual models of neuroscience-informed approaches to trauma that emphasize learning how to feel feelings in a safe way and also the practice of self-regulation (Perry, 2009; van der Kolk, 2006). The bodily awareness afforded by the K/S and P/A levels of the continuum is a foundational step toward effectively working with clients who have experienced complex trauma to conceptualize their emotions in a metaphoric and insightful way. A solid rationale that is based upon empirical research for the nonverbal, kinesthetic, and sensory elements of art therapy is helpful not only to the profession but also for art therapy clients. The neuroscience-informed ETC model allows for approaches that are clinically grounded but inclusive of diverse ways of practicing art therapy as well as the diverse ways of knowing that our clients exhibit. As noted by Pearson and Wilson (2009), "an inclusive emotional healing process offers combined cognitive, somatic, kinesthetic and intra-personal reconnection with sources of past and present experiences" (p. 49). In our own art therapy work we have identified the importance of including how our clients experience the world with our own clinical agenda.

7.2   VOLCANOES AND ICE CREAM CONES: CHRISTOPHER'S CASE VIGNETTE

I, Christopher (first author), previously worked as an art therapist at a residential treatment center for troubled youth. One evening a young girl, Kristy (pseudonym), was on the way to a movie group, a standard part of our evening programming for the residents. To go to the movie group, she had to pass through the gym. As excited children often do, she entered the gym without stopping at the door, a standard procedure. She was directed to walk through the gym again. Instantly becoming upset and refusing, she became verbally aggressive to staff, which quickly escalated into physical aggression. This required the staff to place her in a therapeutic hold, which led to her being held on the ground of the gym floor. There she attempted to bang her head on the hard tiles, screamed, and cried. This behavior lasted for 45 minutes; stages of emotions would subside only to return again with reattempted head banging (which staff prevented with a pillow, a mat, and therapeutic holds). Kristy had a history of abuse. Touch – even if designed to be nurturing and caring – was confusing, painful, and frightening from her perspective.

After her intense emotions subsided and she returned to the unit, I met Kristy in her room. I brought paper and oil pastels and gave them to her with no instructions.

"Wow," I said. "I was really worried about you earlier." I picked up the pastels and began a scribble drawing. "That was pretty scary." I breathed in and sighed. She picked up the oil pastels and started a drawing.

"What do you think about when that happens?" I asked.

"Nothing" she said. "I actually don't even remember it happening."

"I wonder how that feels."

"Like this," she said, showing me her drawing. "When I get angry I feel like a volcano."

"I see," I said. "Volcanoes are powerful. I wonder if there is something you can do to stop the volcano from exploding."

"I don't know," she said.

"When I feel like a volcano, sometimes I breathe like this," I said, taking a big breath. "Can you breathe like this too?" I asked.

"Oh, you mean like in yoga!"

"Yes, like in yoga," I said. Together we breathed.

After taking a few deep breaths, Kristy turned her picture over and drew a pink bubbly cloud at what once was the base of the volcano.

"I like the colors there," I said.

"This is an ice cream cone," she replied. "Even though I can be like a volcano, I am a sweet girl too."

"Yes, you are," I said.

"Can I go back to my room now?" she asked, letting me know she was finished.

"I think so," I said. "But first, what can you do next time when you feel like a volcano?"

"Breathe," she said, exaggeratedly drawing the word out.

"How are you going to be the rest of the night?" I asked. "I don't want to hear that you turned into a volcano again. Can you be an ice cream cone?"

"Yes, I can be an ice cream cone," Kristy said.

This vignette offers an example of how a minor redirection from staff (being told to walk though the gym as opposed to running) triggered a powerful emotional and physical response. When asked later, the client did not remember an almost hour-long regression into crying, kicking, and self-harming. The small stimulus led her to relive her previous trauma in the moment. Luckily, Kristy was supported by trained professionals who were able to identify this regression as a product of her PTSD. As part of the treatment team, I was able to use art therapy to help assess her current psychological state. Through the use of visual imagery, we were able to identify a means of communication. This communication, which occurred primarily through visual imagery, inherently involves the brain. For example, the experience of the color of the images as well the process of recognizing one object as a volcano and another as an ice cream are reliant upon structures, cells, and synaptic transmission of the visual system (for more detailed descriptions of how visual art is processed in the brain see, Livingstone, 2002; Lusebrink 2004; Zeki, 1999). In the language of art, we found the metaphor of the ice cream cone and the volcano. Yet, the language of visual art references "the grammar of the brain" (Belkofer & Konopka, 2008).

Ice cream cones are cool and sweet. Volcanoes are hot and explosive. Through the sensory characteristics of the visual objects Kristy created on the page, she was able to describe the sensory characteristics of herself. It is the sensory nature of artistic expression that helps the client and the therapist bridge the limitations of language and communicates concepts that would be difficult to express otherwise. Although our entire encounter lasted no more than 10 minutes, the metaphor of the imagery gave Kristy a reference for expressing and understanding herself and her behaviors that extended beyond the time of our meeting. This reference was visual and bodily. She could see the volcano cone in her head and feel the molten lava boil in her stomach. For the remainder of the evening I was able to check up with her while she was on the unit with the simple question/prompt: "Ice cream cone or volcano?" In future encounters I was able to assess her affect through the same imagery.

In this vignette I made art alongside my client. We both had pieces of paper and oil pastels. As I scribbled, she scribbled. Through these motions there was a sense of synchronicity that occurred. As I made a mark, she made a mark. In this synchronized kinesthetic action, a rhythm emerged. In this rhythm of shared visual art making, it is possible that Kristy and I reached a state of interpersonal connection called "therapeutic attunement" (Kossak, 2009). This sensory-based exchange of energy need not be conceptualized as made up of some kind of abstract cosmic "stuff" that floats all around us. Rather, as conceptualized by Siegel (2020) the shared energy was a resonance occurring in our brain and our minds. As noted by Hass-Cohen (2008), art therapy can promote an interpersonal resonance related to "expressing, experiencing and learning how to regulate affects ... through sensory integration activities and kinesthetic movement associated with art therapy activities" (p. 35).

One way to conceptualize this connection is through the act of *entrainment*, which is "a felt inner sense of deep shared connectivity or merging in the moment" (Kossak, 2009, p. 16). The therapeutic use of the arts (as in art therapy, dance/movement therapy, poetry therapy, drama therapy, and music therapy) helps therapists tune in to the inner reality of their clients through creative expression, improvisation, movement, and rhythm (Kossak, 2009). The felt sense of interpersonal connection associated with entrainment involves dynamic changes in the brain and other parts of the body. Although it is essential that art therapists and other mental health providers do not reduce complex behaviors to a single brain function and/or system and refrain from reaching overly enthusiastic conclusions from a science that is still emerging (Heyes & Catmur, 2022; Kilner, & Lemon, 2013; Napolitano, 2021), the "bodily resonances" (Freedberg & Gallese, 2007, p. 197) often associated with witnessing and making art may be associated with the activation of cells, called mirror neurons, identified by a team of Italian researchers (Gallese et al., 1996). Art therapists have explored the theoretical potential of these cells, which are found in the motor cortex of the brain, as possibly playing an important role in the bodily experience of empathy and the felt aesthetic responses associated with the therapeutic applications of the arts (Belkofer, 2014; Buk, 2009; Franklin, 2010; Hass-Cohen & Clyde-Findlay, 2015). Though there are data (Mukamel et al., 2010) to indicate that humans have populations of neurons that respond to observing behaviors as well as to enacting behaviors, evidence expanding beyond the data is indirect at best. Yet, the act of shared art making affords opportunities for strong personal interconnections (B. L. Moon, 2010) and art therapists may benefit from studying growing research that explores the biological systems involved in such interpersonal potentials. Working side-by-side with a client or on the same art piece may allow for a sense of connection that may be non-verbal, embodied, and related to, as yet to be fully researched, brain functioning.

The act of shared art making affords opportunities for strong personal interconnections (B. L. Moon, 2010). Working side-by-side or on the same art piece opens a door for entrainment. Where my mark making resulted in nonobjective imagery, my client's work referenced the imagery of volcanoes and ice cream cones. I did not provide a directive for Kristy to draw a specific object or image. This is consistent with Klorer's (2005) assertion that:

> For true transformative work to happen in expressive work with a severely maltreated child, it appears that imagery has the most potential for therapy when it comes from the child and is not imposed by the therapist. Directives aimed at certain issues are not nearly as effective as the metaphors brought by the client.
>
> (p. 218)

7.3   THE STORY OF NATE: EMILY'S CASE VIGNETTE

Much like Christopher's experience with Kristy, I, Emily (second author), also had a revelatory experience when working with a young boy named Nate (pseudonym) who opened my eyes to the integrative potential of art therapy. Nate began therapy after having been severely sexually abused by an older adopted sibling in his foster home. The sexual abuse occurred on a nearly daily basis from the age of 6 weeks to 8 years old. The following vignette shows how Nate was able to use his art making to develop his own nonverbal method of self-soothing.

When Nate first began therapy with me, it took a long time to build trust between us. For the first three years of therapy, he would only play board games. Art didn't seem important or interesting to him. As Nate slowly began to show signs of trusting me, he would experiment with the art materials that I provided for him. Nate was nonverbal. I think he would listen to me talk, but he hardly ever answered with words, and he rarely made eye contact. I relied on reports from his adoptive mother and teachers, and I attempted to interpret his behaviors and actions to understand his experience.

Nate used the media and materials in the art therapy studio in a way that was uniquely therapeutic for him. I typically did not give him directives. I purposefully gave him limited choices, and once he discovered what materials felt good to work with, he continued to experiment with that medium. In my mind, this was my way of addressing Nate's complex feelings related to control and his perception of authority figures. Having experienced sexual abuse – something outside of his control – he often engaged in power struggles with important adults in his life. Art therapy offered Nate a different experience: a new way to rework his previous emotional and behavioral patterns that resulted from feeling powerless.

After nearly four years in session, Nate had developed a regular routine in the art therapy studio. He would gather his own paints and brushes, begin painting, and make significant progress on several pieces during each session. I noticed that he worked in a very kinesthetic way, building up the surface of the canvas with paint to create peaks and texture. He worked on one painting, over and over, for almost three years (Figure 7.1). Most weeks he simply added a new layer to continue building the texture of the surface. I told him that the spikey peaks reminded me of armor that could be used to protect him, perhaps similar to his outbursts of angry, defensive

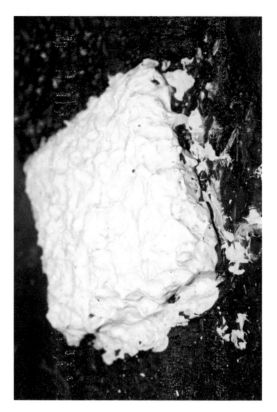

FIGURE 7.1 Client process painting

behavior at home with his mom and at school with his teachers. He listened intently and made eye contact as I shared my own response drawing of a figure with spikes with him. (Figure 7.2).

Our work continued this way; Nate used the materials in the studio to paint, and I made connections to how his art-making behaviors might relate to what had happened to him and how these experiences were affecting him currently. At one point I asked him to do an experiential task that I often asked other clients to do close to the beginning of treatment. I asked him to write a list of emotions down on paper. I usually expect that a typical emotionally regulated child in his age range can name at least six. Nate had difficulty naming any emotion words, so I helped him with a few. When I asked him to try and conjure up each feeling within himself and imagine it was traveling down his arm and onto the paper as an extension of the emotion, he used all the colors and scribbled them together. He covered the entire paper and not one mark or color stood out from the others.

At first, I was frustrated that he didn't seem to be following my directions. I took a minute to think about what he was really communicating to me through his art actions. Then it dawned on me that this was a kinesthetic and sensory way of working. Nate was practicing his ability to self-soothe, not only with the paint and his paintings, but also with the scribble drawings. I also wondered if he was not able to

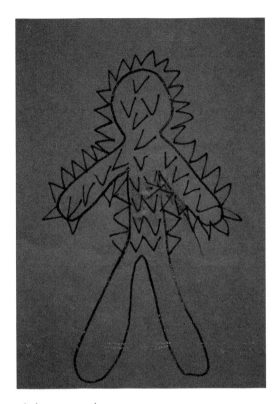

FIGURE 7.2 Therapist's response image

differentiate his emotions. I hypothesized that when a feeling arose, he might often be feeling a complicated, mixed-up jumble of emotions. If this were true, I imagined it would be very hard for Nate to discern what he was feeling, except for the overall sense that it was bad. Did every emotional state just feel the same? In our next session I asked Nate about it to test out my hypothesis. He nodded "yes" when I suggested that "he felt it all at once," and "the feelings were all over his body."

Nate continued his regular routine of painting, but I noticed that he began to leave time at the end of each session to organize the art room. He would pull out materials, like stamps and other cans of odds and ends, and put them in order. Over the next few months, I noticed that although he continued to work on his paintings and organize materials in the studio, he also began new paintings in which forms were beginning to emerge. He started to use modeling paste to paint waves and a beach. His paintings incorporated sculptural elements such as three-dimensional shapes. Nate also started to paint egg case palettes. He mixed colors and painted each color in a rainbow succession. He seemed to be organizing the palettes (Figure 7.3), one color in each well where each color of the rainbow should go. He took a break from the paintings and each week he would paint the palettes. I wondered if Nate's pattern of creating the egg cases meant that he had increased his ability to differentiate some of his emotions. I could see he was beginning to self-organize, and then my clinical understanding was confirmed.

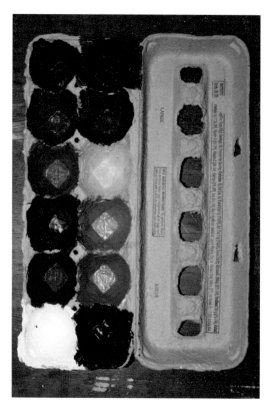

FIGURE 7.3 Egg create palette

At one session in particular, Nate's mother came in exasperated, reporting that he had stolen a movie and money from his aunt. Stealing was not uncommon behavior for Nate. As a result of the complex trauma he had endured and his resulting attention deficit and hyperactivity symptoms, Nate struggled with impulse control. Because we had been working on a foundation of understanding and articulating emotions, I used a direct verbal approach to address the emotions underneath the stealing behaviors. While Nate was painting, I asked him several questions about his feelings, his thoughts, and the circumstances that had led up to the act of stealing. Nate eventually revealed that he had been anxious about a missing homework assignment at school right before he went to his aunt's house. With troubling feelings of anxiety swirling through his body, Nate swiped the movie and the money. I asked Nate to go home that week and think about where he felt anxiety in his body and proposed that next week we could develop a plan to prevent the stealing behavior when he felt the impulse.

When Nate returned the following week, he told me that he felt the anxiety in his stomach. He acknowledged that there was usually something that precipitated his feeling anxious. When the anxiety hit, Nate felt desperate to alleviate the uncomfortable, tight, and swirling feeling in his stomach. His first resort was to steal something, but he would immediately feel guilty and ashamed. It was a painful cycle: one bad feeling led to an action that led back to a bad feeling. However, Nate was now able to understand his emotions better, and he created a plan for when this feeling emerged in his stomach again. Instead of immediately acting on his impulse to soothe his bad feelings, he could talk to his trusted sister or he could make art, and, since then Nate has refrained from stealing.

When children feel upset, caregivers validating their feelings can help the children practice self-regulating their emotions (Siegel & Bryson, 2012). Validation can be difficult for parents and caregivers, especially if the child is annoying or frustrating the adult with the behavior. Children also learn to tolerate the ambiguity that life often brings; they learn that many times there are no precise right answers. The process of self-regulation can be learned and practiced, by both the child and the caregiver. Art therapy can be an effective way for children to learn about their bodies and their brains through sensory, perceptual, action-oriented means that aid self-regulation. In the case examples above, both clients used art therapy to communicate, understand their bodily sensations, and develop positive plans of action when they felt stressed. Enacting their plans appropriately in those times of stress demonstrated evidence of their brain's neuroplasticity, or ability to change (Siegel, 2020).

7.4   SUMMARY

In this chapter we have reviewed how the negative bodily impacts of psychological trauma can disrupt an individuals' abilities to connect with their own emotions (van der Kolk, 2006). This loss of bodily awareness can be associated with a loss of a sense of the self. As a result of this disconnection, clients suffering from trauma often become removed from their own internal realities. As they lose touch with their emotions, they have a harder time connecting to the world and the people around them in vibrant and positive ways. The cumulative effect of these impacts may render verbal and insight-based approaches ineffective. Clients first "need to learn that it is safe to have feelings and sensations" (van der Kolk, 2006, p. 287). The goal of treatment shifts to a more experiential base aimed at emotional regulation of the body. Without these basic building blocks clients can become trapped in a reactionary state of helplessness. Unable to organize their emotions they live in a chronic state of "physical immobilization" (van der Kolk, 2006, p. 283). They become trapped in a body that erupts like a volcano or feels like an undifferentiated mix of color.

Psychological trauma primes one's emotional system to be highly reactive and can negatively impact a person's ability to effectively practice emotional regulation (Ehring & Quack, 2010). Mental health practitioners, who are often trained to focus primarily on matters of the mind such as cognition and behavior, may benefit from conceptualizing treatment as grounded in the premise that persons who have experienced psychological trauma reside in bodies that may have been profoundly altered. Neuroscience research shows that the high output behavioral responses often seen in children who have experienced severe trauma are related to dysregulated systems within the brain and other parts of the body (Glaser, 2000; Klorer, 2005; Perry, 2009). As noted by Malchiodi (2020), "there is now a general agreement that traumatic memory is also a somatic experience, one held not in the brain and the mind, but also expressed by the body" (p. 202).

This work impacts individuals who have experienced trauma and outlines how the authors fostered neuroplasticity that leads to resilience. Neuroplasticity offers hope that one's brain and body functions can be positively influenced through targeted artistic endeavors. Although the inherent action-oriented kinesthetic and sensory foundations of visual art making are a natural quality of the work of art therapy that also "naturally shifts individuals from being 'in their mind' to being more fully in their bodies" (Malchiodi, 2020, p. 27), the practice of art therapy does not occur in isolation. When art therapists work with individuals, those individuals are a part of a larger community, and so any individual change impacts that larger community. The felt sense of one's own body is essential to healthy interpersonal communication between individuals and within communities. As detailed in their descriptions of the CREATE framework, Hass-Cohen and Clyde Findlay (2015) emphasize the phenomenon of "Relational Resonating" as essential to effective applications of neuroscience informed approaches to art therapy practice (pp. 10–11). Hass-Cohen and Clyde Findlay operationally define Relational Resonating as grounded in "co-creation, co-consciousness, co-regulation and co-meaning making" (p. 68). In other words, although directives and/or interventions that are designed to target the flow of energy within the brain are a part of the process, the dynamic exchange of energy within and between the client and the therapist is essential for fully using the arts to address trauma. These phenomena, which are often difficult to plan, are "propelled by the additional support of non-verbal communication" (p. 68) and essential to the client's self-regulation and combating the cumulative effects of trauma.

People are created, gestated in, and born in connection; people need positive interactions and feelings of belonging with others to thrive. Our work happens in the here and now, but is also future oriented, and anchored to hope. One important goal the authors work toward with clients is to help them develop the resilience and then feel secure to engage in the larger community. When working with children, seeding positive community interactions is incredibly important as they will continue to trust and rely on their community and surroundings. The relationship between the client and therapist, which is informed by creative process and structures within the brain, remains central in effective arts-based trauma approaches.

REFERENCES

Anda, R. F., Vincent, F.J., Bremner, J. D., Walker, J. D., Whitfield, C., Perry, B. D., ... Giles, W. H. (2006). The enduring effects of abuse and related adverse experiences in childhood: A convergence of evidence from neurobiology and epidemiology. *European Archives of Psychiatry and Clinical Neuroscience, 256,* 174–186. https://doi.org/10.1007/s00406-005-0624-4

Belkofer, C. M. (2014). Mind, body, brain, and art: A rationale for the therapeutic use of the arts. *Yellowbrick Journal of Emerging Adulthood, 4,* 20–22.

Belkofer, C. M., & Konopka, L. M. (2008). Conducting art therapy research using quantitative EEG measures. *Art Therapy: Journal of the American Art Therapy Association, 25*(2), 56–63. https://doi.org/10.1080/07421656.2008.10129412

Belkofer, C. M. (2012). *The impact of visual art making on the brain.* (Doctoral dissertation). https://digitalcommons.lesley.edu/expressive_dissertations/110/

Belkofer, C. M., Vaughan Van Hecke, A., & Konopka, L. M. (2014) Effects of drawing on alpha activity: A quantitative EEG study with implications for art therapy. *Art Therapy: Journal of the American Art Therapy Association, 31*(2), 61–68.

Bremner, J. D., & Vermetten, E. (2001). Stress and development: Behavioral and biological consequences. *Development and Psychopathology, 13*, 473–489.

Buk, A. (2009). The mirror neuron system and embodied simulation: Clinical implications for art therapists working with trauma survivors. *The Arts in Psychotherapy, 36*, 61–74.

Cane, F. (1983). *The artist in each of us* (2nd ed.). Art Therapy Publications.

Chapman, L. (2014). *Neurobiologically informed trauma therapy with children and adolescents: Understanding mechanisms of change.* W. W. Norton & Company.

Collie, K., Backos, A., Malchiodi, C., & Spiegel, D. (2006). Art therapy for combat-related PTSD: Recommendations for research and practice. *Art Therapy: Journal of the American Art Therapy Association, 23*(4), 157–164.

Cozolino, L. (2002). *The neuroscience of psychotherapy: Building and rebuilding the human brain.* W.W. Norton.

Carvalho, G.B. & Damasio, A. (2021). Interoception and the origin of feelings: A new synthesis. *BioEssays: News and Reviews in Molecular, Cellular and Developmental Biology, 43*(6), e2000261.

Damasio, A. R., (1994). *Descarte's error: Emotion, reason, and the human brain.* Putnam.

Damasio, A. R. (1999). *The feeling of what happens: Body and emotion in the making of consciousness.* Harcourt.

Doba, K., Saloppé, X., Choukri, F., & Nandrino, J. L. (2022). Childhood trauma posttraumatic stress symptoms in adolescents and young adults: The mediating role of mentalizing and emotion regulation strategies. *Child Abuse & Neglect, 132*, 105815. https://doi.org/10.1016/j.chiabu.2022.105815

Ehring, T., & Quack, D. (2010). Emotion regulation difficulties in trauma survivors: the role of trauma type and PTSD symptom severity. *Behavior therapy, 41*(4), 587–598. https://doi.org/10.1016/j.beth.2010.04.004

Franklin, M. (2010). Affect regulation, mirror neurons, and the third hand: Formulating mindful empathic art interventions. *Art Therapy: Journal of the American Art Therapy Association, 27*(4), 160–167.

Freedberg, D. & Gallese, V. (2007). *Motion, emotion, and empathy in esthetic experience Trends in Cognitive Sciences, 11*(5), 197–203.

Gallese, V., Fadiga, L., Fogassi, L., & Rizzolatti, G. (1996). Action recognition in the premotor cortex. *Brain, 119*(2), 593–609.

Glaser, D. (2000). Child abuse and neglect and the brain: A review. *Journal of Child Psychology and Psychiatry, 41*(1), 99–116.

Hass-Cohen, N. (2008). CREATE: Art therapy relational neuroscience principles. In N. Hass-Cohen & R. Carr (Eds.), *Art Therapy and Clinical Neuroscience* (pp. 283–309). Jessica Kingsley.

Hass-Cohen, N. & Clyde Findlay, J. (2015). *Art therapy & the neuroscience of relationships, creativity, and resiliency.* W.W. Norton.

Heyes, C., & Catmur, C. (2022). What happened to mirror neurons? *Perspectives on Psychological Science, 17*(1), 153–168. https://doi.org/10.1177/1745691621990638

Hinz, L. (2020). *Expressive Therapies Continuum: A framework for using art in therapy* (2nd ed.). Routledge.

Howells, M. F., Stein, D. J., Vivienne, A. R. (2012). Childhood trauma is associated with altered cortical arousal: Insights from an EEG study. *Frontiers in Integrative Neuroscience, 6*(120), 119. https://doi.org/10.3389/fnint.2012.00120

Johnson, D. R. (2009). Commentary: Examining the underlying paradigms in the creative arts therapies of trauma. *The Arts in Psychotherapy, 36*, 114–120.

Kain, K., and Terrell, S. (2018). *Nurturing resilience: Helping clients move forward from developmental trauma.* North Atlantic Books.

Kapitan, L. (Ed.) (2014). The neuroscience of art therapy and trauma. [Special Issue]. *Art Therapy: Journal of the American Art Therapy Association, 31*(2). https://doi.org/10.1080/07421656.2014.911027

Kaplan, F. F. (2000). *Art, science and art therapy: Repainting the picture.* Jessica Kingsley.

Kilner, J. M., & Lemon, R. N. (2013). What We Know Currently about Mirror Neurons. *Current Biology, 23*(23), R1057–R1062. https://doi.org/10.1016/j.cub.2013.10.051

King, J. L., Knapp, K. E., Shaikh, A., Li, F., Sabau, D., Pascuzzi, R. M., & Osburn, L. L. (2017). Cortical activity changes after art making and rote motor movement as measured by EEG: A preliminary study. *Biomedical Journal of Scientific & Technical Research, 1,* 1–21.

Klorer, G. P. (2005). Expressive therapy with severely maltreated children: Neuroscience contributions. *Art Therapy: Journal of the American Art Therapy Association, 22*(4), 213–219.

Kossak, M. (2009). Therapeutic attunement: A transpersonal view of expressive arts therapy. *The Arts in Psychotherapy, 36,* 13–18.

Kramer, E. (1958.) *Art in a children's community.* Charles C Thomas.

Kravits, K. (2008). The neurobiology of relatedness: Attachment. In N. Hass-Cohen & R. Carr (Eds.), *Art therapy and clinical neuroscience* (pp. 131–146). Jessica Kingsley.

Kruk, K. A., Aravich, P. F., Deaver, S. P., & deBeus, R. (2014). Comparison of brain activity during drawing and clay sculpture: A preliminary qEEG study. *Art Therapy: Journal of the American Art Therapy Association, 31*(2), 52–60.

Levine, P. (2010). *In an unspoken voice: How the body releases trauma and restores goodness.* North Atlantic Books.

Livingstone, M. (2002). *Vision and art: The biology of seeing.* Harry N. Abrams.

Lusebrink, V. B. (2004). Art therapy and the brain: An attempt to understand the underlying processes of art expression in therapy. *Art Therapy: Journal of the American Art Therapy Association, 21*(3), 125–135.

Lusebrink, V. B. (2010). Assessment and therapeutic application of the Expressive Therapies Continuum: Implications for brain structures and functions. *Art Therapy: Journal of the American Art Therapy Association, 27*(4), 168–177.

Malchiodi, C. A. (2006). Expressive therapies: History, theory, and practice. In C. A. Malchiodi (Ed.), Expressive therapies (pp. 1–15). Guilford Press.

Malchiodi, C. A. (2020). *Trauma and Expressive Arts Therapy: Brain, body, and imagination in the healing process.* New York: The Guilford Press.

McNiff, S. (1992). *Art as medicine: Creating a therapy of the imagination.* Shambhala.

Moon, B. L. (2009). *Existential art therapy: The canvas mirror* (3rd ed.). Charles C Thomas.

Moon, B. L. (2010). *Art-based group therapy: Theory and practice.* Charles C Thomas.

Moon, B. L., & Belkofer, C. (2014). *Artist, therapist, and teacher: Selected writings by Bruce L. Moon.* Charles C Thomas.

Mosak, H., & Maniacci, M. (1999). *Primer of Adlerian psychology: The analytic-behavioural-cognitive psychology of Alfred Adler.* Routledge.

Mukamel, R., Ekstrom, A. D., Kaplan, J., Iacoboni, M., & Fried, I. (2010). Single neuron responses in humans during execution and observation of actions. *Current Biology: CB, 20*(8), 750–756.

Napolitano, A. (2021). Study casts new light on mirror neurons. *Nature Italy.* https://doi.org/10.1038/d43978-021-00101-x

Naumburg, M. (1987.) *Dynamically oriented art therapy: Its principals and practice.* Magnolia Street.

Newberg, A. B., & d'Aquili, E. G. (2000). The creative brain/the creative mind. *Zygon, 35*(1), 53–68.

Pearson, M., & Wilson, H. (2009). *Using expressive arts to work with mind, body and emotions: Theory and practice.* Jessica Kingsley.

Perry, B. D. (1996). *Maltreated children: Experience, brain development and the next generation.* W.W. Norton.

Perry, B. D. (2009). Examining child maltreatment through a neurodevelopmental lens: Clinical applications of the neurosequential model of therapeutics. *Journal of Loss and Trauma, 14*(240), 240–255.

Poole Heller, D. (2019). *The power of attachment: How to create deep and lasting intimate relationships.* Sounds True.

Salah, A.A., Salah, A.A., Kaya, H., Doyran, M., Kavcar, E. (2021). The sound of silence: Breathing analysis for finding traces of trauma and depression in oral history archives. *Digital Scholarship in the Humanities, 36*(2), ii2–ii8. https://doi.org/10.1093/llc/fqaa056

Schore, A. N. (1994). *Affect regulation and the origin of the self: The neurobiology of emotional development.* Erlbaum.

Schore, A. N. (2001). Effects of secure attachment relationships on right brain development, affect regulation, and infant mental health. *Infant Mental Health Journal, 22*, 7–66.

Sherin J. E. & Nemeroff, C. B. (2011) Post-traumatic stress disorder: The neurobiological impact of psychological trauma. *Dialogues in Clinical Neuroscience, 13* (3), 263–278. https://doi.org/10.31887/DCNS.2011.13.2/jsherin

Siegel, D. J. (2020). *The developing mind: How relationships and the brain interact to shape who we are* (3rd ed.). Guilford Press.

Siegel, D.J., & Bryson, T. (2012). *The whole brain child: 12 revolutionary strategies to nurture your child's developing mind.* Bantam.

Siegel, D.J., Schore, A. N., & Cozolino, L. (Eds.) (2021). *Interpersonal neurobiology and clinical practice.* W.W. Norton.

van der Kolk, B. A. (2003). The neurobiology of childhood trauma and abuse. *Child and Adolescent Psychiatric Clinics of North America, 12*(2), 293–317.

van der Kolk, B. A. (2006). Clinical implications of neuroscience research in PTSD. *Annals of the New York Academy of Sciences, 1071*, 277–293.

van der Kolk, B. A. (2014). *The body keeps the score.* Penguin.

Van Houdenhove, B., Luyten, P., & Tiber Eagle, U. (2009). The role of childhood trauma in chronic pain and fatigue. In V. L. Banyard, V. J. Edwards, & K. Kendall-Tackett (Eds.), *Trauma and physical health: Understanding the effect of extreme stress and of psychological harm* (pp. 37–64). Routledge.

Zeki, S. (1999). *Inner vision: An exploration of art and the brain.* Oxford University Press.

CHAPTER 8

NEA CREATIVE FORCES® ADVANCES ART THERAPY RESEARCH WITH MILITARY-CONNECTED POPULATIONS

Gioia Chilton, Janell S. Payano Sosa, Chandler Sours Rhodes, and Melissa Walker

The views expressed in this chapter are those of the authors and do not necessarily reflect the official policy or position of the Department of the Navy, Army, or Air Force, the Department of Defense, nor the U.S. Government.

In the following chapter, we describe the use of art therapy for United States military-connected populations to address trauma and discuss promising new research in this area using neuroscience theory, tools, and methods. To begin, we briefly trace the history of the profession of art therapy, which arose in part to aid veterans, then turn to outlining the current implementation of art therapy services for the military, focusing on highlighting work with those on active duty. First providing the context of the neurobiology of the trauma response, we will then share clinical vignettes to provide concrete examples of this work, illuminated by the patient's own visual voice, their artwork. Pointing to variables unique to art therapy, we review the current literature and briefly offer suggestions for future directions in researching these variables. We then outline several art therapy interventions that have been standardized and used across military settings, then turn to describing the current art therapy research being conducted within the U.S. Department of Defense (DoD) and the use of neuroscience theory and retrospective neuroimaging metrics in these studies. To conclude this robust chapter, we provide a list of cultural considerations art therapists may find useful when working in military and veteran care settings. As art therapists and neuroscientists, we are grateful for the opportunity to share this work with the intention of supporting art therapists and researchers working with military populations, and ultimately improving the health and well-being of our service members, veterans, their families, and caregivers. Indeed, we hope and expect that findings stemming from art therapy research in the military will ultimately benefit health outcomes for many, advancing care for both service personnel and civilian communities alike (Rasmussen et al., 2014).

Historically, the profession of art therapy has roots in local arts cultural experiences, formal art educational programs, and in medical and psychiatric facilities, as various communities have discovered (and re-discovered, over the years) the healing benefits of the arts. Following WWII, efforts were made to address the health needs of military veterans experiencing what was then called "soldier's heart" or "shell shock" but what we now refer to as post-traumatic stress (Crocq & Crocq, 2000). While working with WWII veterans, artists and art educators Adrian Hill and Mary Huntoon, in Great Britain and the United States respectively, started to develop group art therapy which included art making within a supportive and psychologically safe art studio setting, noting it to be beneficial to the veterans (Howie, 2017; Wix, 2000). Art therapy

DOI: 10.4324/9781003348207-8

was then established as a formal profession in the 1950s and 1960s, during which the first government-funded art therapy research studies were conducted at the National Institutes of Health in Bethesda, Maryland (Robb, 2012). In the years since, art therapists employed within military and civilian medical facilities have continued to support military-connected individuals in their efforts to recover from trauma and reintegrate into civilian communities. Art therapy is thought to enable service members to express the invisible wounds of combat trauma through art making, and the power of visual imagery was found to be a useful tool to overcome the culture of silence so prevalent in military communities (Lobban & Murphy, 2019; Walker, 2017). Many veterans and service members who have participated in art therapy now champion its value and effectiveness (DeLucia & Kennedy, 2021; Ramirez et al., 2016).

8.1   NATIONAL ENDOWMENT FOR THE ARTS ESTABLISHES CREATIVE FORCES

In 2004, the National Endowment for the Arts (NEA) created the *Operation Homecoming: Writing the Wartime Experience* initiative with the goal of helping U.S. troops and their families write about their wartime experiences in Afghanistan, Iraq, and stateside (Operation Homecoming, n.d.). To accomplish this, NEA partnered with the DoD to provide writing workshops to active-duty troops and veterans at military installations, military hospitals, Department of Veterans Affairs (VA) medical centers, and affiliated centers in communities around the country. In 2011, the NEA again partnered with the DoD to bring in creative arts and therapeutic writing resources to expand upon the National Intrepid Center of Excellence (NICoE)'s Healing Arts Program at Walter Reed National Military Medical Center, which had already integrated art therapy into their treatment model. NEA eventually expanded support to include additional clinicians from the distinct professions of art therapy, music therapy, and dance/movement therapy, collectively known as creative arts therapies (CATs).

In 2016, due to the success of the NEA/DoD partnership, Congress specifically allocated a $1.928 million budget increase for the NEA to expand the reach and impact of the program, now officially known as Creative Forces®: NEA Military Healing Arts Network (NEA and DOD Launch, 2016; 2022). Creative Forces is a partnership with the U.S. Departments of Defense and Veterans Affairs and state and local arts agencies, with administrative support provided by Americans for the Arts, the Henry M. Jackson Foundation for the Advancement of Military Medicine, Inc., and Mid-America Arts Alliance. Over the next few years additional DoD and VA clinical sites, research, program analytics and evaluation, an online National Resource Center, and a community arts grant program were launched (Our Impact, 2022). Additionally, at many VA sites, telehealth creative arts therapies services are now being provided through a partnership between the VA Office of Rural Health and Creative Forces to overcome barriers to care such as stigma, distance, and disability through the Rural Veterans TeleRehabilitation Initiative (RVTRI; Spooner et al., 2019). Within the DoD, Creative Forces supports creative arts therapies across various specialty clinics including the NICoE and many of the Intrepid Spirit Centers, who provide care to service members suffering from traumatic brain injury (TBI) and associated psychological health conditions through an interdisciplinary treatment model (Degraba et al., 2021).

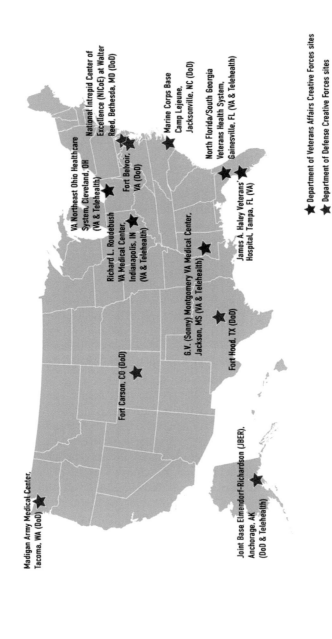

FIGURE 8.1 Creative Forces clinical sites

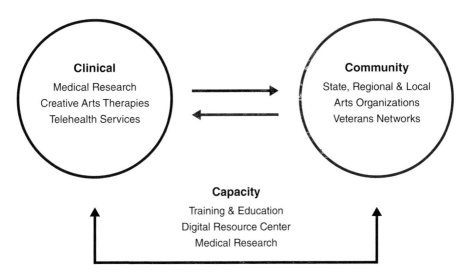

FIGURE 8.2 Pillars of Creative Forces

As of this writing, there are approximately 30 CAT positions across the Creative Forces Network who are funded by either the NEA, DoD, or the VA. They are embedded into clinical interdisciplinary teams nationwide across VA and DoD sites (see Figure 8.1). As part of these teams, art therapists must be well equipped to communicate with a variety of medical experts such as physical therapists, psychiatrists, and social workers, in order to provide the best patient care (Nancarrow et al., 2013). Recent studies indicate that interdisciplinary care programs often benefit from improved patient retention when art therapists are included as part of the team (Campbell et al., 2016; Decker et al., 2018).

Creative Forces operates in three distinct areas – clinical, community, and capacity – which function multi-directionally to support efforts in a broad range of areas (see Figure 8.2). For more information, please view the robust website, the Creative Forces National Resource Center (n.d., www.creativeforcesnrc.arts.gov/) that includes the clinical research studies published in peer reviewed journals since 2016. While the pillars of Creative Forces work together synergistically, in this chapter, our focus is on the clinical art therapy practice and research being done within the Creative Forces network.

8.2   OUR CLINICAL POPULATION

Similar to the civilian healthcare system, the U.S. DoD and VA healthcare systems are treating high rates of mental and behavioral disorders that likely result from the cumulative military-related and non-military related traumatic stress that occurs throughout the lifespan of active-duty service members and veterans (Crum-Cianflone et al., 2016). Creative Forces personnel focus on supporting these military-connected populations both within healthcare systems and in the community. Each of the clinical and community sites supports sub-populations that vary due to their various locations and missions which can include active duty, National Guard, reservist, and veteran populations. Initially, Creative Forces focused on service members seeking treatment for TBI and associated psychological health conditions at the NICoE. There, a highly effective patient-centered, holistic interdisciplinary program was developed to provide a national model of care that now includes art therapy, dance/ movement therapy, and music therapy (DeGraba et al., 2021). The NICoE as well as affiliated programs across additional Intrepid Spirit Center sites integrate these creative arts therapies treatments into this interdisciplinary model. Patients receive care through individual and group sessions in both intensive outpatient program (IOP) and traditional outpatient program settings, although each location has adapted this model of care to meet the unique needs of the individuals they serve. Recent research indicates there is a need to increase access to these Intrepid Spirit Centers to serve additional active duty, active and inactive National Guard and reservists, as well as retired military personnel (Banaag et al., 2022).

Art therapy services in particular were highlighted in the February 2015 edition of the *National Geographic* magazine headlined "Healing Our Soldiers." This issue displayed art created by active-duty service members of the conflicts in Iraq and Afghanistan during their art therapy sessions at the NICoE (Alexander, 2015). Portraits expertly photographed by Lynn Johnson showed service members in their homes, and with their families and military teammates, holding the expressive masks they had made in art therapy to vividly illustrate physical and psychological injures and experiences in ways words alone could not emphasize. Mask-making is an art therapy directive used to help individuals to reveal – and conceal – their identity and depict self-image transformations (Dunn-Snow, & Joy-Smellie, 2000; Joseph, et al., 2017). The iconic photography in the *National Geographic* issue made an impact as the public was educated on the effect of TBI and post-traumatic stress disorder (PTSD) on the brains and bodies of service members and their families. All could now see the formerly invisible suffering of those impacted in new light. This *National Geographic* issue also helped the featured service members tell their personal stories of how art therapy helped them heal, thus providing opportunity to center their voices in the public eye.

8.3   NEUROIMAGING OF PTSD

For active-duty service members and veterans, traumatic events are often marked by a threat to life through both military-related stressors such as exposure to explosive devices, incoming fire, and non-military related stressors including motor vehicle accidents or sexual violence (Ramchand et al., 2010; Judkins et al., 2020; World Health Organization, 2015). In the aftermath of trauma, survivors are more susceptible to chronic disease, anxiety disorders, depression, addiction, and suicide (Mancini, 2020). A prevalent anxiety disorder found in service members and veterans exposed to traumatic events is PTSD (Kong et al., 2022; Judkins et al., 2020; World Health Organization, 2015; Tanielian & Jaycox, 2008). PTSD symptoms may include flashbacks of unwanted memories, severe mistrust, emotional detachment, helplessness, fear, agitation, irritability, hypervigilance, insomnia, and nightmares. Because of such a wide range of symptoms, PTSD is considered to be a complex, heterogeneous disorder. These symptoms impact a person's health, well-being, social relationships and overall ability to function in their lives. This has created an interest in integrative mental health services that incorporate cost effective non-pharmaco-logical approaches (Peterson et al., 2021; Philips & Wang, 2014).

Through the use of neuroimaging, researchers have found a range of brain alter-ations associated with post-traumatic stress (PTS) symptoms (Hughes & Shin, 2011; Sheynin et al., 2020; Hayes et al., 2011; Sripada et al., 2012; Ross and Cisler, 2020; Miller et al., 2017; Dunkley et al., 2014). As noted elsewhere in this book, functional magnetic resonance imaging (fMRI) is a neuroimaging modality that is used to indirectly mea-sure brain function based on changes in blood oxygenation dependent level (BOLD) signal in the brain (Damoiseaux et al., 2006; Rubinov & Sporns, 2010). How BOLD signal is correlated across brain regions is termed functional connectivity, which can be calculated during both resting and task-based conditions (Chen & Glover, 2015). The amygdala is a subcortical brain region associated with emotion processing that is often theorized to be overactive in PTSD, potentially leading to an exaggerated response to fear (Shin et al., 2005; Bryant et al., 2008; Badura-Brack et al., 2018; Forster et al., 2017; Sripada et al., 2012; Dunkley et al., 2014). The ventral medial prefrontal cortex sup-ports decision-making processes in the brain and has been shown to be under-active in individuals with PTSD (Shin et al., 2005; Bryant et al., 2008). This has been shown to be associated with a failure to inhibit the amygdala and therefore may impair the ability to extinguish fear memories when the threat is no longer present. The hippocampus is a memory processing region that has been shown to be functionally abnormal in PTSD and believed to lead to deficits in identifying safe contexts and memory impairments (Hughes & Shin, 2011; Leite et al., 2022). In addition to the regions noted above, altered neural communication across various networks including the central executive network, default mode network, and salience network have also been hypothesized to lead to the PTS-related cognitive dysfunction, altered self-referential processing, and dysregulated arousal and interoceptive processing, respectively (Nicholson et al., 2018). However, the degree to which these brain regions and networks are involved in PTSD varies according to the specific PTS symptoms, individual experiences, and variation in neuroimaging methods across studies (Leite et al., 2022; Hughes & Shin, 2011) implying that further research in this area is needed. Additionally, due to the cor-relative nature of fMRI studies, whether the origin of these functional brain abnormal-ities found in PTSD are caused by a pre-existing increased risk to develop PTSD after trauma or developed post PTSD onset have yet to be explored (Hughes & Shin, 2011).

8.4   ASSOCIATIONS BETWEEN PTSD AND TBI

According to the National Institute of Neurological and Stroke Disorders, "trau-matic brain injury (TBI) occurs when external physical forces cause damage to the brain, whether from impact, penetrating objects, blast waves or rapid movement of the brain within the skull" (Focus on Traumatic Brain, 2022). TBIs have been con-sidered the signature wound of recent military conflicts and may have long-lasting impacts on service member's readiness through reducing training and deployment capabilities (Military Health System, 2022). TBIs are classified as mild, moderate, or severe; however, mild TBI (mTBI), also referred to as a concussion, is the most com-monly found among service members and has been defined as "a transient alteration of brain function after exposure to external physical forces" (Focus on Traumatic Brain, 2022). Recent clinical and preclinical research has made many advances in our understanding of the secondary injury cascade associated with TBI including inflammatory, neurochemical and metabolic alterations to the neurons and glia of the brain (Khatri et al., 2021; Ng & Lee, 2019; Ray et al., 2002). Symptoms associated with TBI include dizziness, irritability, headache, memory and attention deficits, sleep disturbances, and others (Hoover et al., 2022; Cicerone & Kalmar, 1995; Andrews et al., 2018). Furthermore, especially within military cohorts, where comorbid TBI and PTS (post-traumatic stress) is common, the significant overlap in symptoms between the two make diagnosis and treatment difficult. Patients experience a very challenging cluster of symptoms: dizziness, vision issues, headache, sleep disturbance, attention and memory challenges, fatigue, poor concentration, impaired self-regulation and emotional processing, leading to re-experiencing (Lee et al., 2019). Furthermore, chronic stress such as those seen in active-duty service members who are tasked with multiple deployments, may manifest as long-lasting symptoms and persistent neural network dysfunction (Lee et al., 2019).

8.5   CLINICAL ILLUSTRATIONS: THE ART TELLS THE STORY

In conjunction with managing chronic stress, service members and veterans engaging in art therapy services may be processing complex combat-related trauma. While military training is designed to support resiliency to the effects of living through combat – being shot at, attacked, receiving rocket or mortar fire, killing others, or knowing someone killed or seriously injured – combat exposure may still result in post-traumatic stress, complicated grief responses and moral injury (Jones, 2017; Combat Exposure, 2022). Complicated grief happens when a typical grief response becomes intractable and results in prolonged experience of sadness and an inability to accept the reality of loss, be it loss of one's sense of self, innocence, trust, or relationships (Shear, 2015). Moral injury involves violations of deeply held moral beliefs resulting in guilt, shame, self-condemnation, and/or loss of meaning and purpose in life, and spiritual conflict (Hall et al., 2022, Litz et al. 2009; Shay, 1994). As Molendijk, Kramer, and Verweij (2018) write:

> [M]oral injury does not always entail the experience of straightforward transgression. In cases of clashing values, soldiers may grapple with the question whether the acts they witnessed or committed were good or bad. Such a struggle may also engender moral conflict with regard to the overall purpose and righteousness of the mission in which they were deployed, which, in turn, may hinder the process of coming to terms with particular deployment events.
>
> (p. 50)

Figures 8.3a and 8.3b present the art product of a service member processing moral injury and complicated grief through art therapy. The front of his mask was painted to look like a steel slab which covered the mouth area, mirrors were placed behind the eyes, and the inside of the mask was painted to show inner tears. The phrase, "let them see what they want to see," was written in the inside of the forehead area of the mask, while "hide your feelings" was written sideways on the inside. He chose to frame the piece in a recycled oval gold frame, allowing a small opening in the back so that the work on the inside could be seen, when he chose to view it to show it to others. This service member had served in combat as well as part of the

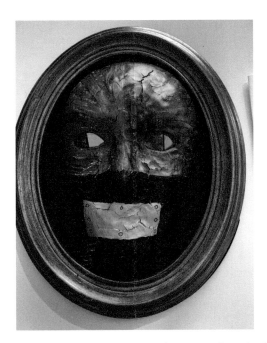

FIGURE 8.3A Mask created by army member of the Honor Guard, with "hide your feelings" written on the inside

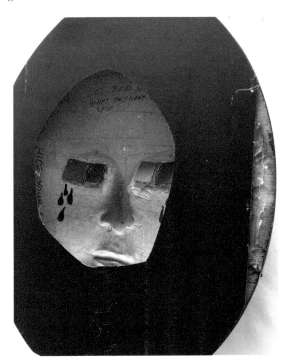

FIGURE 8.3B Interior detail of the framed mask

Honor Guard, which is a special duty for selected esteemed military to represent the U.S. military at funerals and other ceremonies, where any show of emotions is discouraged (see Text Box: Military Cultural Considerations for Art Therapists).

An additional example of PTS and complicated grief is shown in artwork created by a female service member processing combat trauma through art therapy prior to her retirement (Figure 8.4a and 8.4b). She stated that she suffered remembering the traumatized children she had seen in combat zones. Although previous to art therapy treatment she had not identified as an artist, with the art therapist's assistance she created a series of pour paintings. This activity was design to help her circumvent inhibitions, and was experienced as fun, freeing, and may have boosted her artistic self-confidence. With the therapeutic alliance well established, she then spent several sessions to create a detailed lift-the flap, folded page collage. She found a magazine image of a helmeted female soldier with a dull, sad stare to represent herself, and added a flap that vividly showed what trauma felt like: eyes wide, face aflame, mouth screaming. This face could be folded up (incidentally protecting the brain area) to present the face of the numb soldier, or flipped down to express how it really felt to witness the horror of children (and adults) suffering in wartime. The entire collage could also be folded to shut the page, providing containment and control of when and how she would view these images (Chilton, 2007). In this collage, the interactive features allowed the retiring service member opportunities to externalize imagery representing her traumatic experiences and thus make sense of it.

While these clinical examples may look shocking to bystanders, service members working within the therapeutic relationship with an art therapist often find

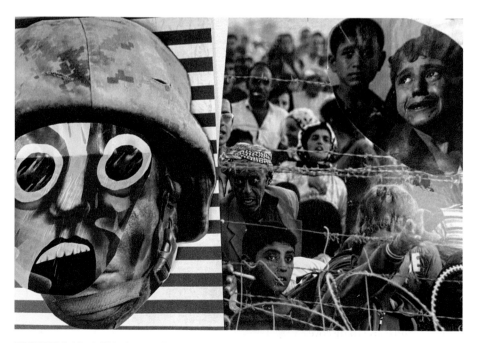

FIGURE 8.4A A "lift the flap" collage by a female solider showing what combat trauma felt like internally

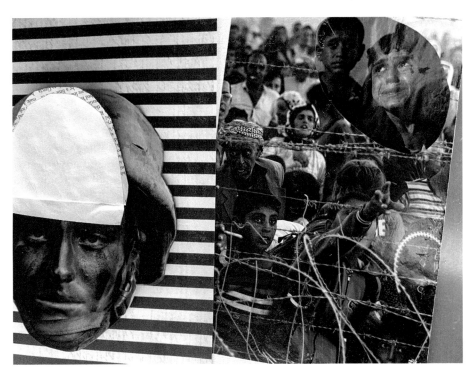

FIGURE 8.4B A "lift the flap" collage by a female solider showing what combat trauma looked like externally

these images quite satisfying to produce, as finally they can *art it out* to communicate extremely difficult emotions and thoughts which may have disturbed them for years, turning shame into shared pain which lessens in the light of day. Yet as Walker (2019) remarks, use of art psychotherapy with traumatized individuals "can conjure traumatic content, feelings, and emotions which are difficult to process and contain safely if an individual is not adequately trained," therefore the employment of trauma-informed, competent, trained professional art therapists is a requirement for this work (p.117).

In addition to the programming to provide professional art therapy to service members, family art therapy is also offered across various Creative Forces sites. Military families often face challenges associated with the many stressors of military life. Art therapy engages military families in a developmentally appropriate manner and can be a strength-based intervention to support improved family functioning (Chilton et al, 2021). Art therapy interventions are designed with attention to the unique cultural considerations and needs of military families to improve intrafamilial interaction and build attachment bonds (Howie & Sobol, 2013). For example, Creative Forces developed a protocolized intervention, *The Animal Strengths and Family Environment Directive*, in which the family comes together to illustrate character strengths through animal metaphors (see Table 8.1 for details). The family then jointly creates a visual landscape to discover and express familial roles, strengths, safety, and needs, in the process creating a map of family dynamics which can increase communication and foster family resiliency (Herman & Chilton, 2022). Additional program evaluations and research are needed to further explore the possible outcomes of such art therapy interventions with military families.

8.6 ART THERAPY IS A COMPLEX PROCESS

As illuminated by the clinical examples, there are many variables in art therapy we can research using the tools of neuroscience (King, 2016). In the following section, we sketch areas of research interest, and touch on some of the academic literature which explores process variables. These variables include engagement and flow, the therapeutic alliance with the art therapist, and the use of different art media and materials in art therapy.

Put simply, art therapists help people engage in a creative process using various art materials. If successful, art therapy participants will enter a state of optimal attention, in which one is deeply absorbed and engaged, termed, *flow* (Csíkszentmihályi, 1996). This experience was named flow because, like color flowing from a watercolor brush, the experience of being so deeply engaged in life's activities *flows*, as one's attention feels effortless. When one is in flow, there is a distorted sense of time, lack of worry, reduced self-awareness, a boost in concentration, creativity, and increased sense of playfulness (Csíkszentmihályi, 1996; Gold & Ciorciari, 2020). Flow pioneer psychologist Csíkszentmihályi explained that during flow an individual's skill level is optimally balanced with the challenging task at hand leading to an overall rewarding experience (Csíkszentmihályi, 2004). For example, as a patient spends more time in art therapy, their skill level with both art making and self-expression may improve, leading to an overall rewarding experience when met with the challenging task of expressing trauma with art materials. At the level of the brain, Dietrich (2004) hypothesized that flow takes place when the explicit information processing system in the prefrontal cortex, in particular, the anterior cingulate cortex, shifts to an implicit, automatic, nonverbal, skill-based processing system. During flow, executive attention is the only prefrontal cortex function still active as there is a selective disengagement of other higher order cognitive functions while the person focuses resources on the task at hand, thus we have the sense of concentrating without trying hard (Dietrich, 2004). Outside of the context of art therapy, neuroimagers have found that during flow there is a decrease in activity in the amygdala potentially representative of negative thought suppression, a decrease in activity of the default mode network's medial prefrontal cortex associated with reduced attention to the self, along with an increase in communication between brain networks associated with reward and cognitive control (Weber et al., 2009; Ulrich et al., 2014; Huskey et al., 2018). While research and theory in the neuroscience of flow is ongoing, theorists agree that the implicit system is not accessible to conscious awareness, while during conscious awareness the brain is mainly communicating with the dorsolateral prefrontal cortex which is a brain region that plays an important role in higher cognitive processing and self-reflective consciousness (Gold & Ciorciari, 2020). Theoretically, engaging in states of flow may give art therapy participants the ability to visually express and ultimately contextualize past traumatic memories with more ease, as illustrated in the vignettes described above and the case studied by Walker et al. (2016) which we will describe shortly.

If engagement and flow produce increased communication between brain networks, the effectiveness of art therapy could be due in part to the ability of the art therapist to attune with their patients and assist them in reaching the artistic skill balance that allows entry into flow states (Chilton, 2013). As part of the therapeutic alliance, the ability to use empathy to exchange conscious and unconscious thoughts and feelings between two or more people, called intersubjectivity, is important for trust to be established between the art therapist and their patient (Cooper-White, 2014). Theoretically, the ability to co-regulate emotions with their art therapists allows patients to experience flow, which increases access to their higher cognitive processing and working memory. "Co-regulation provides the neural state that supports the establishment of trusting relationships" as Porges describes (2022, p. 12). Feeling safe within the therapeutic alliance and accessing flow states may increase insight, creativity, and a sense of well-being for this reason.

Huotilainen and colleagues (2018), in an article humorously titled, "Why our brains love arts and crafts," write that through accessible art-making practices our embodied cognition allows the body's relaxation response to turn on as art therapy participants co-regulate. Research outside of art therapy has deemed co-regulation to be a precursor to building social and emotional competence which is key for learning to self-regulate (Silkenbeumer et al., 2016; Paley & Hajal, 2022). As we will discuss below, Jones et al. (2018) found military service members in art therapy were able to become more autonomous throughout their art therapy experience, suggesting that further research in the area of intersubjective states of healing is needed to clarify how this transition between co-regulation and self-regulation occurs within the context of art therapy. Therefore, there is a need for art therapy research which takes into account the therapeutic relationship between the patient and the art therapist.

Another variable in art therapy is art media properties, the inherent physical qualities of artistic materials. These can be identified on continuums, such as between resistive and fluid media (Kagin & Lusebrink, 1978; Hinz, 2009). Generally, the patient's choice of art materials is supported by their art therapist, who has specific training and expertise in the selection and use of art materials and therefore can guide material and media choice to support therapeutic goals (Rubin, 2011). Key aspects of art therapy graduate training involve the exploration of *why* an art therapist may support a patient in the use of any particular art material, such as oil pastels which could be considered more fluid, versus another such as wood carving, which could be considered more resistive. Art therapists also consider other factors regarding art media such as the structure, sensorial qualities, symbolic and metaphorical potential, and other critical and practical considerations (Haaga, & Schwartz, 2022; Moon, 2011; Seiden, 2001).

Studies have explored the ways in which the patient's art-making experience is related to their own personal skills and history of artistic accomplishment as well as the qualities of the art materials and the therapeutic alliance (Ball, 2002; Snir & Regev, 2013). A pilot study by Haiblum-Itskovitch, Czamanski-Cohen and Galili (2018) measured emotional response in healthy participants by looking at the association between an emotion self-assessment and changes in (HRV). More variability in heart rate has been theorized to be an indicator of good health. The researchers explored HRV following art-making with three different two-dimensional (2D) art materials ranging in fluidity: pencil (low fluidity), oil-pastels (medium fluidity), and gouache (a bright paint similar to watercolors; high fluidity). They hypothesized that art making with more fluid materials would result in an increase in emotional response, while predicting that gouache would have the most emotional response and pencil would have the least emotional response. They found that during art making, regardless, of material, there were significant differences in HRV indicative of an emotional response to stimuli. However, they found that HRV was not significantly different between materials of different fluidity. Instead, the authors found that the use of oil pastels and gouache paint, but not pencil, improved the participants' emotional valance (positive mood) but found no changes in emotional arousal as measured by an emotion self-assessment. They suggest that the lack of material-related differences in HRV and the emotional arousal subscale could be attributed to the nature of the task not focusing on a particular emotion but instead asking participants to draw freely. They conclude that the tactile experience paired with the fluidity of oil pastels triggers an emotional response during art making in healthy participants. Given the sample limitations, however, additional research is needed to explore the clinical impact of art media properties, as different art media may lead to different HRV responses in different clinical populations.

In addition to 2D drawings and paintings, a commonly used material in art therapy is clay. Both natural earthen clay and air-dry plastic modeling compound have soft, malleable textures which can be manipulated, and over time dry to develop a hard surface. Use of clay involves touch and movement to create three-dimensional (3D) art objects. As touch, movement, and associated sensations are a primary mode of human existence, communication, and expression, creating in 3D may aid in concretization and symbolization (Henley, 2002). Sholt and Gavron (2006) theorized 3D clay art could "function as a central window to ... unconscious, nonverbal representations and may be especially helpful with people who find it hard to express themselves verbally" (p. 67). As this may be a cultural issue with this population (see Text Box: Military Cultural Considerations for Art Therapists) 3D work is of particular interest.

In a mixed methods study with children, Kim (2014) found that 3D use of clay improved locus of control more than 2D drawings. A subsequent randomized control trial with adults experiencing depression found that art therapy that utilized clay was more effective than recreational classes in reducing depression levels, improving daily functioning, general mental health, and well-being (Nan & Ho, 2017). This result was theorized to occur because 3D artwork is created through bodily-based kinesthetic and affective information which enhances the regulatory functions of the autonomic nervous system (ANS) through psychophysiological attunement (Schore, 2009; Hinz, 2009). Thus, 3D artmaking stimulates both motor and somatosensory areas of the brain.

So, let us loop back to our discussion of mask-making. We wonder if part of mask-making's appeal could be due to the 3-D nature of the art form, as well as the ease the patient has in personifying the mask as a version of themselves. Giving an object a human trait has been shown to increase sympathy for the object, something that can promote healing and connection for those that have difficulties identifying and sympathizing with their own emotions (Rosenthal-von der Pütten et al., 2013; White & Remington, 2019). Certainly, we have seen how mask making seems to resonate in military and veteran art therapy settings (Mims, 2021; Walker et al., 2017). Creative Forces has used mask-making in the past (see Table 8.1), in that a 3D paper-mache mask is offered by the art therapist to the service member, with suggestions for use of multiple kinds of art media which can include both fluid media such as paint and clay and more resistive media such as found object assemblage. Often multiple steps are required in the construction of the masks, indicating a moderate level of complexity of the task (Hinz, 2009). Further studies could explore integrating objective tools to directly measure the impact the use of different art therapy materials and processes may have in facilitating the brain health of military-connected populations.

8.7 ART THERAPY INTERVENTIONS USED BY CREATIVE FORCES ART THERAPISTS

With the eventual goal of facilitating multi-site research, Creative Forces is working toward the standardization of art therapy interventions across network sites. As a first step, Creative Forces identified interventions that were theoretically, culturally and trauma informed, and could be protocolized and replicated. Table 8.1 describes clinical art therapy interventions that art therapists working in the Creative Forces network have anecdotally found to be especially helpful for military-connected populations (Table 8.1). The needs and goals are listed as well as a brief description of six typical interventions, followed by the art media properties.

TABLE 8.1 Needs, goals, and art media dimension variables for six typical art therapy interventions used across Creative Forces sites.

Art therapy intervention	Needs & goals:	Art media dimension variables
Population: Active-Duty Military & Veterans with mTBI and associated Psychological Health Conditions		
Mask-making: Service members are provided with a brief orientation to mask-making and paper-mache masks and invited alter their masks using any materials they would like including acrylic paints, modeling clay, and additional sculptural assemblage materials (Walker et al., 2016)	• Regulate emotions • Repair sense of self • Express identity and sense of self • Strengthen cohesion of intersecting identities • Improve cognition and planning • Foster externalization of conflicted inner states	• 3-D • Resistive (inherent structure) • Boundary-determined (solid composition) • Representational
Box Project: Service members are invited to select and alter a box using any materials they would like to, including paint and the assemblage of miscellaneous objects to represent aspects of career and self on the outside of the box and represent private aspects of self, including losses, inside the box (Jones et al., 2018).	• Process complicated grief • Contain obtrusive emotions • Set boundaries with self and others • Express identity and sense of self • Strengthen identity cohesion • Improve cognition and planning • Process specific traumatic events and losses	• 3-D • Resistive (inherent structure) • Boundary-determined (solid composition) • Representational (generally)

(Continued)

TABLE 8.1 (Continued)

Art therapy intervention	Needs & goals:	Art media dimension variables
Montage Painting: Mixed media collage and painting which encourages a layering of materials and images on a contained surface to depict a personal theme related to combat and recovery (Walker et al., 2017).	• Examine identity, stressors, and life transitions after combat injury (Walker et al., 2017). • Integrate past, present, and future experiences (Walker et al., 2017) • Access new meanings via juxtaposition and integration of formerly disconnected visual images (Scotti & Chilton, 2017)	• 2-D • Fluid (paint) and/or resistive (cut collage images) • Boundary-determined (via canvas size) • Representational (generally)
Bridge with Path Drawing: Service members are provided 12x18 drawing paper and drawing materials including pencils, makers, oil and chalk pastels and asked to "Draw a bridge from someplace to someplace. The bridge connects to a path. Draw the path and write where the path leads you to" (Darewych 2014; Hays & Lyons, 1981).	• Bring to consciousness formerly unconscious thoughts through symbols and/or metaphors • Invoke new insights and motivation for change • Explore individuals' experiences of transitions, perceptions of their environments, goals, and possible barriers to goals, future orientation, problem-solving abilities • Assess the presence of and sources of life meaning and purpose	• 2-D • Resistive (pencils) and/or more fluid (chalk pastels) • Boundary-determined (via paper size) • Multiple steps are required, indicating moderate level of complexity and task structure • Representational
Pour Painting: Service members are instructed in a marbling technique achieved by diluting acrylic paint colors and pouring the paint onto a canvas or other substrate, then maneuvering the canvas to create ripples and swirls. Subsequent verbal processing is used to free associate words and images from the abstract designs that emerge (Stamper, n.d.)	• Elicit affect • Communicate emotional expression • Raise emotional self-awareness • Alleviate anxiety • Circumvent immobilizing inhibitions • Access unconscious process • Foster positive emotions • Promote mindfulness	• 2-D • Fluid (easily manipulated or altered) • Quantity-determined (paint amount provides the limit) • Abstract

(*Continued*)

TABLE 8.1 (Continued)

Art therapy intervention	Needs & goals:	Art media dimension variables
Population: Military Families		
Animal Strengths and Family Landscape: Families draw animals symbolic of themselves, then jointly create a landscape where all can live safely together, exploring familial roles, strengths, safety, and needs (Herman & Chilton, 2022)	• Repair attachment bonds disrupted due to family separations • Build communication skills • Provide an intervention developmentally appropriate for children and adolescents	• 2-D (with 3-D optional) • Resistive (inherent structure) • Boundary-determined (paper boundaries) • Multiple steps are required, indicating moderate level of complexity and task structure (Hinz, 2009). • Representational

8.8 CREATIVE FORCES ART THERAPY RESEARCH AND PROGRAM EVALUATION FINDINGS

As noted earlier, Creative Forces' partnership with the DoD first began at the NICoE which included an established art therapy program poised to be replicated across the other Intrepid Spirit Center sites as they were being built. Due to this partnership, much of the Creative Forces' research to date focuses on art therapy for military service members with TBI and associated psychological health conditions. Below are summaries of Creative Forces art therapy research studies and program evaluations; published articles describing them in depth are all accessible through the Creative Forces National Resource Center (www.creativeforcesnrc.arts.gov/). For the purposes of this chapter, we excluded publications that discuss veteran-related research and program evaluations, or that discuss the impact of combined creative arts therapies, and focused exclusively on art therapy research and program evaluation for active-duty service members.

The first Creative Forces publication focused on the impact of the incorporation of art therapy into the interdisciplinary team at the NICoE. Walker et al. (2016) followed the case of a senior ranking military service member with a history of moderate TBI and chronic PTSD who was enrolled in the four-week IOP. He was offered a comprehensive treatment plan which included primary care, neuropsychology, neurology, neuroimaging, and integrative treatments such as acupuncture, mind-body medicine, art therapy, and music therapy. While initially wary of art therapy, after creating artwork of a mask and containing it in a box, he found he could externalize an intrusive image which had been haunting him for seven years. He reported that the image no longer caused him anxiety, and flashbacks of the image were minimal.

His experience in art therapy encouraged him to seek long-term outpatient art therapy sessions at NICoE after completing the IOP. Through art therapy, he was able to externalize intrusive traumatic memories of his lived experiences. The service member's magnetoencephalography (MEG) scan reflected reduced power in the alpha band frequency, compared to other TBI patients, that was localized to Broca's area, or speech–language area of the brain. This finding provided the first neuroimaging evidence supporting why the visual depiction of the service member's "speechless terrors" aided the service member in his treatment when words were not enough (Walker et al., 2016).

In 2017, Walker et al. explored the meaning of approximately 400 masks made in art therapy by service members during the four-week NICoE IOP program (Walker et al., 2017). Mask-making in art therapy is hypothesized to present a visual way for service members to express their sense of self: who they are, who they have become, and who they will be, due to their lived experiences. The researchers categorized visual imagery by analyzing symbols, themes, and formal art elements seen in images captured of the completed masks, as well as the service members' descriptions of what they were trying to convey in the masks as described in clinician notes. The analysis identified patterns and recurring themes in the masks that ultimately contributed to an overarching construct related to their identities. One important limitation of this study was that the assessment of the service members' masks could not be made without the notes that provided the service members' own interpretations of their masks. This limitation further supports the need for art therapists to be included on the interdisciplinary team, as they can help increase the understanding of the service members' injury and recovery experiences to other providers to support specialized treatment planning.

On a broader level, Jones et al. (2018) focused on the overall art therapy treatment dose at an Intrepid Spirit Center in Virginia. Researchers wanted to understand the complexities of short- and long-term group and individual art therapy treatment and to describe the theoretical bases of the art therapy directives implemented for this patient population. They note that group art therapy is used to address relationship building, increase communication, and reduce isolation through the process of creating and talking together about the artwork. In contrast, individual art therapy is used to focus on personal grief and trauma processing. Additionally, they found that short-term art therapy was more of a therapist-led intervention. This could be due to the art therapist's focus on increasing the stabilization of symptoms, increasing the service member's understanding about their symptoms, and establishing safety. Long-term art therapy treatment differed in that it became increasingly patient-led over time. This longer-term journey was reported to help service members to solidify their psychosocial growth and re-establish their agency in creating their lives. In the long-term program, about 30% of service members ended art therapy due to having met their goals, moving, or retiring but about 70% continued art therapy to focus on individual processing of complicated grief and specific traumatic events (Jones et al., 2018). One strength of the study was that the programs investigated had either mixed group and individual sessions or progressed from individual to group open studio sessions and, regardless of the format, the service members also became more autonomous in the open studio group sessions. Therefore, further evaluation of patient autonomy in the short-term vs. long-term individual and group sessions is warranted to understand the impacts of art therapy treatment in these different settings.

Kaimal et al. (2018) took a more clinician-focused approach by looking at the association between clinical symptoms and visual imagery created during art therapy. To do this, they used the mask themes previously identified in Walker et al. (2017) and studied their associations with standardized measures of clinical symptoms of depression, anxiety, and PTS obtained at the start of NICoE's four-week IOP. They found that patients with masks depicting themes of psychological injury reported higher PTS symptoms, and that those with mask themes of fragmented representations of military symbols reported increased anxiety. On the other hand, those with masks depicting themes with metaphors had reduced anxiety symptoms, and those with cohesive (no fragmentation) representations of their military unit identity reported reduced PTS and depression symptoms. Lastly, those with masks containing cultural/historical characters and cultural/societal symbols had reduced anxiety and depression symptoms. The authors concluded that the use of mask-making could potentially help clinicians to identify risk and resilience factors for service members with PTS and TBI (Kaimal et al., 2018). It is important to note that this study does not support evidence of a causal relationship between self-reported symptoms and mask themes. Further research is needed to determine why the metaphorical interpretations by the service members can represent the presence of psychological risk and resilience.

Walker et al. (2018) followed by looking at potential neuroimaging associations with the masks made in art therapy during the NICoE IOP. In this case series, Walker and colleagues focused on the resting state condition to understand how the resting brain innately behaves. Thus, this group studied resting state functional connectivity measures from within the default mode network and the thalamus in a group of ten service members divided into two groups based on themes represented within their masks (Walker et al., 2018). Readers may recall that the default mode network is a network of interacting brain regions involved in memories of self while at rest, transitioning between rest and task performance, and mind-wandering (Raichle et al., 2001; Greicius et al., 2003; Buckner et al., 2008) and has been noted to be disrupted in service members with PTSD and TBI (Spielberg et al., 2015; Dretsch et al, 2019; DiGangi et al., 2016; Nathan et al., 2017; Miller et al., 2017; Sheynin et al., 2020). Additionally, they theorized that the thalamus, a brain region crucial for sensory and motor relay of signals to the rest of the brain, may demonstrate differences in connectivity between groups. Group 1 (n=5) depicted injured/traumatic themes in their masks and researchers found this group to have high PTSD scores, low entropy between thalamic brain regions, and low default mode network functional connectivity. Group 2 (n=5) depicted patriotic themes in their masks and researchers found this group to have low PTSD scores, high entropy between thalamic brain regions, and high default mode network functional connectivity. Although providing preliminary evidence of the associations between mask themes, symptom severity, and neuroimaging metrics, this study had a few limitations. This study included a small sample size without sufficient statistical power and only presented potential associations; no causal relationships could be identified. The researchers pointed to the need to investigate neuroimaging changes pre- and post-art therapy treatment. Additionally, the authors theorized that data may be confounded by career timelines with service members at the end of their military careers feeling more comfortable opening up when processing traumatic content due to less anxiety surrounding removal from duty, while service members still planning to return to duty could be more inclined to focus on patriotic themes surrounding the military experience. Future art therapy research should consider potential implications of career timeline in analyses as well as other miliary cultural concerns (see text box below, Military Cultural Considerations for Art Therapists).

In addition to associations with mask themes, researchers have also studied the use of the mixed media technique of montage painting during group art therapy treatment at NICoE. Montage paintings are created by combining collage and painting materials to create a multilayered image. Berberian, Walker, and Kaimal (2019) examined 240 montage paintings that expressed themes such as trauma narratives and a range of posttraumatic symptoms visually. The authors explained that montage paintings serve as visual reflections of the service members' experiences of TBI and/or psychological health conditions. Additionally, they proposed that the gratification experienced through art therapy increased socialization, pleasure, and enabled service members to become more open to the recovery process. They found art therapy imagery allows the art therapist to engage patients in describing their physical and psychological symptoms related to military experiences, and wondered if other healthcare providers might benefit from collaborating with art therapists to provide integrative care that allows for visual exploration of traumatic experiences which cannot be communicated otherwise (Berberian et al., 2019). As with many retrospective analyses, this study is limited by interpretations based on photographs and brief clinical notes created during group art therapy. However, this limitation continues to highlight the need for the integration of master's level art therapists into interdisciplinary programs as they have the clinical training to facilitate art making while providing the psychological and physical safety needed to explore challenging clinical symptoms in group settings. The service members' ability to explore their military experience through montage painting also highlights the need for informed mixed methods art therapy research.

In 2020, a case study by Maltz et al. sought to understand the impact of art therapy as part of an interdisciplinary clinical team at the Intrepid Spirit Center in Washington state. The study outlined a six-week treatment program focused on cognitive processing therapy (CPT) for PTSD with art therapy being integrated into one branch of the treatment. The team analyzed a mask created by a military service member in art therapy as well as his journal writing throughout the six-week PTSD treatment. Maltz et al. (2020) suggested that art therapy can be a useful assessment tool for capturing improvements in PTSD symptoms not explicitly captured by traditional measures, further supporting the use of art therapy in interdisciplinary clinical programs. However, they were limited by the lack of standardized clinical outcome measures which were inconsistent across the six weeks and suggest that future studies that seek to recruit a larger cohort focuses on the collection of systematic outcomes to better capture potential treatment effectiveness of art therapy.

In 2021, Kaimal et al. built upon the long-term art therapy treatment model described in the Jones et al. (2018) article by conducting a program evaluation using surveys to understand how to improve the quality of its art therapy interventions. A program evaluation is a systematic method for collecting and analyzing information to explore the effectiveness and efficiency of programs (Kaimal & Blank, 2015). Program evaluation data from art therapy programs can help art therapists implement evidence-based practice and advocate for improved art therapy services (Kaimal et al., 2019; Jones et al., 2018). Kaimal et al. (2021) reported that, on average, participants completed about two years of art therapy treatment; however, there was considerable drop-off on completion of survey feedback across that time. Kaimal et al. (2021) found that, at two years, the survey feedback from patients who completed the long-term art therapy treatment (using the last survey as a long-term measure) reflected improved perceived outcomes, an improved ability to communicate with others, and increased awareness of their symptoms, when compared to the start of their treatment (using the second survey as short-term measure). Demographic features such as time of service were associated with most positive impact in survey measures. Kaimal et al. (2019) found similar findings in an earlier program evaluation conducted at the same site, and the authors suggested that art therapy could be most helpful for service members with longer deployments or with chronic symptoms not effectively addressed elsewhere. However, a main limitation to this program evaluation is that the service members' feedback surveys were not validated and did not incorporate validated measures of clinical symptoms, therefore more validated symptom measures are warranted. Other demographic features such as gender were also associated with differences in survey measures. For example, survey feedback from women focused more on positive and future-oriented subject matters, whereas the men's survey feedback focused most on processing negative emotions and past memories; however, the sample of women was too small (n=14) to make any generalizations (Kaimal, et al., 2021). As a large majority of military-related studies have focused only on male service members, this program evaluation reflects the need for the inclusion of women in military-related art therapy studies.

In 2022, additional work investigating the progression of behavioral outcomes associated with the montage painting directive of art therapy at the four-week IOP at NICoE was conducted. Kaimal et al. (2022) examined depression and PTS behavioral measures of 240 service members at the admission and discharge of the four-week IOP. Within the montage paintings, researchers noted that the theme of color symbolism was associated with higher depression and PTS scores at admission but lower scores at discharge. In contrast, the themes of physical injury, psychological injury, and memories of deployment were associated with no change in depression and PTS scores over the four weeks. However, this study was also limited in that it only followed patients through a short 4-week period with the complexities of all other complementary and medical treatment modalities concurrently offered to patients in the NICoE IOP. Therefore, any changes in depression and PTSD scores cannot be attributed to art therapy sessions alone. Thus, this study provided more evidence for the need for pre- and post-art therapy studies to investigate direct relationships between symptom measures and art therapy themes.

An unpublished neuroimaging study, presented at the 2022 Military Health System Research Symposium (MHSRS) by Payano Sosa et al. (2022), analyzed the resting state functional connectivity in 104 service members who participated in the 4-week IOP at NICoE. Researchers assessed functional connectivity with the default mode network, dorsal attention network, amygdala, and hippocampus to further understand how the brain regions, associated with autobiographical memory, attentional focus, emotional processing, and memory respectively, differed between service members who represented the theme of closure and healing within their art therapy masks and those that did not have this represented in their masks. This retrospective study noted that service members who depicted themes of healing and closure within their art therapy masks demonstrated greater connectivity between regions associated with attention (dorsal attention network), memory (hippocampus), and processing of painful stimuli (insula, thalamus, postcentral gyrus). This study also notes the limitations of retrospective work and the inability to make causal interpretations of the data; however, these preliminary results again highlight the need to collect both neuroimaging and behavioral outcomes pre- and post-art therapy treatment.

In sum, this review has condensed the findings and limitations of ten studies conducted with military service members supported by Creative Forces art therapists. These projects have utilized a range of research methods such as program evaluations, case studies, case series, thematic analysis, and the use of retrospective neuroimaging metrics. While limited in scope, the studies exemplified the ethical principles of integrity and respect for persons involved whilst describing in depth and beginning to quantify the physical, emotional, and social impacts of art therapy for miliary populations.

8.9   FUTURE CREATIVE FORCES ENDEAVORS TO ADVANCE ART THERAPY RESEARCH

Creative Forces is continuing to pursue research to provide scientific evidence in support of the use of art therapy to improve outcomes for service members. In 2021, Creative Forces released a call for proposals for clinical research studies addressing the question: How and to what extent does art therapy affect emotional processing and self-regulation for service members and veterans? Funding for two projects was awarded and a collaboration between the University of Pennsylvania and NICoE is currently investigating art therapy and emotional well-being in military populations with PTS using fMRI and behavioral measures pre- and post-art therapy. A second collaboration between the University of Florida, Drexel University, and the Malcom Randall VA is studying the extent to which art therapy decreases PTSD symptoms after TBI, and how it improves self-regulation and affects related indicators of neurophysiological response also using fMRI pre- and post-art therapy. Additional funding opportunities to pursue randomized clinical trials are anticipated to further this line of research.

8.10   CONCLUSION

Many important concepts have been summarized briefly in this chapter, and we encourage further collaboration and exchange of ideas moving forward in advancing the neuroscience of art therapy. As we have discussed, Creative Forces has championed research endeavors for understanding trauma resolution through art therapy treatment with service members. We theorize that repeated exposure to art therapy potentially promotes neuroplasticity in brain circuitry regions possibly associated with TBI/PTS symptom reduction. Current funding is supporting the use of objective and standardized clinical and neurobiological outcome measures pre- and post-art therapy, which will pave the way for further understanding of the mechanisms of action in art therapy. To close, we affirm art therapy is a brain-based profession (King, 2015) that provides a treatment for trauma that may uniquely address the neurobiological, emotional, and cultural needs of the military. Current world events drive the urgent need for effective and accessible brain health and trauma treatments (Kolappa et al., 2022), therefore it is of global significance to advance art therapy clinical practice and research.

Military Cultural Considerations for Art Therapists

The U.S Department of Defense (DoD) provides military forces needed to deter war and ensure our nation's security (www.defense.gov). As most art therapists have not served in the armed forces, it is necessary to study military culture to provide culturally informed treatment (Howie, 2019). Art therapists should become aware of the differences between service branches (Army, Navy, Air Force, Marine Core, Space Force, and Coast Guard) and between enlisted service members and commissioned officers. Of course, each individual person has a complex and nuanced identity which is always a blend of sub-cultural and personal attributes. The following provides a brief summary of some aspects of military culture.

Authority/Chain of Command: Military norms include discipline, acting within the chain of command and respecting authority. Service members give up many areas of personal autonomy when in the military. On the flip side, those in positions of authority often feel great pressure regarding their responsibility for others. Art therapy may be a place to learn to manage stress as well as increase self-knowledge regarding one's individual values and interests though personal creative choices.

Teamwork & Sense of Community: Service members often work in teams, units, platoons, battalions, etc., where there is an emphasis of group cohesion and collective effort. They often develop deep friendships and experience a sense of comradery. During transition out of the military and into civilian life, it is important to build community bonds to decrease the risk of isolation. Group art therapy sessions and local arts engagement programs may provide places to re-build this sense of community.

The Warrior Ethos: Service members often feel a commitment to the values of honor, courage, and selfless service to protect and defend national sovereignty, which can include the intentional use of force (Pressfield, 2011). Warriors will endure adversity and sacrifice their personal good to enact this moral responsibility. They may experience pain without complaint and be willing to sacrifice their lives for the team members standing beside them.

Mission Mindset: "Mission first, People always!" The military mindset is about winning the mission through a call to arms but emphasizes care of its people (Chilton, 2022).

Lifelong Learning: As the military emphasizes practical lifelong training, willingness to "do the work" in therapy to learn new coping skills can be surprisingly congruent with the military mindset, as long as there is a clear goal or "end state" that can be achieved.

Trust: Service members may take effort to enter care, build trust, and engage in a therapeutic alliance. As service members see their role to serve and defend, it can be a challenge to be served and receive help. Any self-disclosure and emotional expression can be seen as counter to the stoicism of the Warrior Ethos, leading to a culture of silence and secrets. Furthermore, combat trauma or other difficult-to-discuss events may be classified or closely held due to national security and/or to protect vulnerable others. Service members and veterans may not be willing to open up, even years after the fact, for any or all of these reasons. When trust is gained, art therapists have an advantage, as art can be a way to safely disclose trauma and moral injury without breaking confidentiality.

Symbols of Identity: Service members and their families may experience immense pride and commitment related to their service branch, which can be a unique core identity – Soldier, Airman, Ranger, Marine, and so forth – felt as strongly as one's race or gender. For this reason, art materials and supplies on which specific markers of identity can be depicted are useful for this work (Jones et al., 2018).

Rituals: Special ceremonies are associated with promotions, deployments, retirement, and receiving service awards. Gratitude and appreciation are offered through formal events, awards and other symbolic means, such as small gift-giving. Funerals are of particular importance to attend. Art therapy can support formal rituals and informal therapeutic performances to mark special moments and ease transitions (Vaudreuil et al., 2019).

Deployments, Temporary Duty Stations (TDY), and Moves: These transitions can impact stability and attachment to family, friends, and communities but can be understood and coped with, sometimes with great pride, as a special part of military culture. Art therapy to address grief, loss, and adjustment during these times of transition may be useful for any member of the family.

Motivations to Join the Service: Individuals join the military for different reasons, such as to support the nation, fight in combat, make a living, support their families, or find one's purpose. Do not assume you know a person's motivation, instead ask to learn their experience.

Military Terms, Acronyms, and Slang: There are many military specific terms used to communicate as well as unique terms to branches and military occupational specialties. Art therapists should make the effort to learn the terms frequently used by the specific populations that they treat, asking for clarification when appropriate.

Media Portrayals: Due to the portrayals of the military in the media many civilians may have stereotypes of service members as having an aggressive disposition, and/or see veterans as heroes, charity cases, or victims (Parrott et al., 2019). Art therapy can help express service members' sense of self and individuality to counter these limiting narratives.

Ethical Complexity: In the military, the nation's needs and interests often take precedent and can sometimes outweigh the needs of the individual. Art therapists may face ethical challenges related to this (Howie, 2019). We advise all therapists to approach this work with cultural humility and explore one's own counter-transference, possible cultural prejudices, and potential ethical questions related to work with the military in order to best treat this population (Jackson, 2020; Mims et al., 2021).

Discussion Questions

- Why is trust vital in the military community?
- How might the art therapy process circumvent the culture of silence in military settings?
- What aspects of the neuroscience of art therapy most intrigues you and why?

ACKNOWLEDGMENTS

We would like to acknowledge those in the United States Armed Forces for their service and sacrifice, and the families who serve alongside them. The authors would also like to recognize the leadership, providers, and staff at the NICoE, Intrepid Spirit Centers, military treatment facilities, and VA hospitals who work diligently to provide treatment to military personnel. Appreciation is extended to Creative Forces®: NEA Military Healing Arts Network, an initiative of the National Endowment for the Arts in partnership with the U.S. Departments of Defense and Veterans Affairs. The initiative seeks to improve the health, well-being, and quality of life for military and veteran populations exposed to trauma, as well as their families and caregivers. Creative Forces is managed in partnership with Americans for the Arts, the Henry M. Jackson Foundation for the Advancement of Military Medicine, and Mid-America Arts Alliance.

REFERENCES

Alexander, C. (2015). Behind the mask: Revealing the trauma of war. *National Geographic, 227*(2), 30–51.

Andrews, R. J., Fonda, J. R., Levin, L. K., McGlinchey, R. E., & Milberg, W. P. (2018). Comprehensive analysis of the predictors of neurobehavioral symptom reporting in veterans. *Neurology, 91*(8), e732–e745. https://doi.org/10.1212/WNL.0000000000006034

Badura-Brack, A., McDermott, T. J., Heinrichs-Graham, E., Ryan, T. J., Khanna, M. M., Pine, D. S., Bar-Haim, Y., & Wilson, T. W. (2018). Veterans with PTSD demonstrate amygdala hyperactivity while viewing threatening faces: A MEG study. *Biological Psychology, 132*, 228–232. https://doi.org/10.1016/j.biopsycho.2018.01.005

Ball, B. (2002). Moments of change in the art therapy process. *The Arts in Psychotherapy, 29*(2), 79–92.

Banaag, A., Korona-Bailey, J., & Koehlmoos, T. P. (2022). Intrepid spirit centers: Considerations for active duty, national guard, reserves, and retirees. *Military Medicine*, usac051. https://doi.org/10.1093/milmed/usac051

Berberian, M., Walker, M. S., & Kaimal, G. (2019). "Master My Demons": Art therapy montage paintings by active-duty military service members with traumatic brain injury and post-traumatic stress. *Medical Humanities*, *45*(4), 353–360. https://doi.org/10.1136/medhum-2018-011493

Bryant, R. A., Kemp, A. H., Felmingham, K. L., Liddell, B., Olivieri, G., Peduto, A., Gordon, E., & Williams, L. M. (2008). Enhanced amygdala and medial prefrontal activation during nonconscious processing of fear in posttraumatic stress disorder: an fMRI study. *Hum Brain Mapp*, *29*(5), 517–523. https://doi.org/10.1002/hbm.20415

Buckner, R. L., Andrews-Hanna, J. R., & Schacter, D. L. (2008). The brain's default network: anatomy, function, and relevance to disease. *Annals of the New York Academy of Sciences*, *1124*, 1–38. https://doi.org/10.1196/annals.1440.011

Campbell, M., Decker, K. P., Kruk, K., & Deaver, S. P. (2016). Art therapy and cognitive processing therapy for combat-related PTSD: A randomized controlled trial. *Art Therapy*, *33*(4), 169–177. https://doi.org/10.1080/07421656.2016.1226643

Chen, J. E., & Glover, G. H. (2015). Functional magnetic resonance imaging methods. *Neuropsychology Review*, 25(3), 289–313. https://doi.org/10.1007/s11065-015-9294-9

Chilton, G. (2007) Altered books in art therapy with adolescents, *Art Therapy*, *24*(2), 59–63, https://doi.org/10.1080/07421656.2007.10129588

Chilton, G. (2013). Art therapy and flow: A review of the literature and applications. *Art Therapy*, *30*(2), 64–70. https://doi.org/10.1080/07421656.2013.787211

Chilton, G., Vaudreuil, R., Freeman, E. K., McLaughlan, N., Herman, J., & Cozza, S. J. (2021). Creative Forces programming with military families: Art therapy, dance/movement therapy, and music therapy brief vignettes. *Journal of Military, Veteran and Family Health*, *7*(3), 104–113.

Chilton, IV, F. S. (2022). *Reflections on Military Culture*. (Unpublished Manuscript).

Cicerone, K. D., & Kalmar, K. (1995). Persistent postconcussion syndrome: The structure of subjective complaints after mild traumatic brain injury. *The Journal of Head Trauma Rehabilitation*, *10*(3), 1–17. https://doi.org/10.1097/00001199-199510030-00002

Combat Exposure. (2022). U.S. Department of Veterans Affairs. www.ptsd.va.gov/understand/types/combat_exposure.asp

Cooper-White, P. (2014). Intersubjectivity. In D. A. Leeming (Ed.), *Encyclopedia of psychology and religion* (pp. 882–886). Springer U.S. https://doi.org/10.1007/978-1-4614-6086-2_9182

Creative Forces National Resource Center (n.d.) National Endowment for the Arts Creative Forces. Retrieved October 2022 from www.creativeforcesnrc.arts.gov/

Creative Forces: NEA Military Healing Arts Network (2022). National Endowment for the Arts. www.arts.gov/initiatives/creative-forces

Crocq, M.-A., & Crocq, L. (2000). From shell shock and war neurosis to posttraumatic stress disorder: A history of psychotraumatology. *Dialogues in Clinical Neuroscience*, *2*(1), 47–55. https://doi.org/10.31887/dcns.2000.2.1/macrocq

Crum-Cianflone, N. F., Powell, T. M., LeardMann, C. A.,Russell, D. W., & Boyko, E. J. (2016). Mental health and comorbidities in U.S. military members. *Military Medicine*, *181* (6), 537–545. https://doi.org/10.7205/MILMED-D-15-00187

Csíkszentmihályi, M. (1996). *Creativity: Flow and the psychology of discovery and invention*. HarperCollins.

Csíkszentmihályi, M. (2004). Flow, the secret to happiness. [Video]. TED Conferences. www.ted.com/talks/mihaly_csikszentmihalyi_flow_the_secret_to_happiness

Damoiseaux, J. S., Rombouts, S. A., Barkhof, F., Scheltens, P., Stam, C. J., Smith, S. M., & Beckmann, C. F. (2006). Consistent resting-state networks across healthy subjects. *Proceedings of the National Academy of Science USA*, *103*(37), 13848–13853. https://doi.org/10.1073/pnas.0601417103

Darewych, O. H. (2014). *The bridge drawing with path art-based assessment: Measuring meaningful life pathways in higher education students*. (Unpublished doctoral dissertation). Lesley University, Cambridge, MA.

Decker, K. P., Deaver, S. P., Abbey, V., Campbell, M., & Turpin, C. (2018). Quantitatively improved treatment outcomes for combat-associated PTSD with adjunctive art therapy: Randomized controlled trial. *Art Therapy*, *35*(4), 184–194. https://doi.org/10.1080/07421656.2018.1540822

DeGraba, T. J., Williams, K., Koffman, R., Bell, J. L., Pettit, W., Kelly, J. P., Dittmer, T. A., Nussbaum, G., Grammer, G., Bleiberg, J., French, L. M., & Pickett, T. C. (2021). Efficacy of an interdisciplinary intensive outpatient program in treating combat-related traumatic brain injury and psychological health conditions [Original Research]. *Frontiers in Neurology, 11.* https://doi.org/10.3389/fneur.2020.580182

DeLucia, J., & Kennedy, B. (2021) A veteran-focused art therapy program: Co-research to strengthen art therapy effectiveness, *International Journal of Art Therapy, 26*(1–2), 8–16. https://doi.org/10.1080/17454832.2021.1889007

Dietrich, A. (2004). Neurocognitive mechanisms underlying the experience of flow. *Consciousness and Cognition, 13,* 746–761.

DiGangi, J. A., Tadayyon, A., Fitzgerald, D. A., Rabinak, C. A., Kennedy, A., Klumpp, H., Rauch, S. A., & Phan, K. L. (2016). Reduced default mode network connectivity following combat trauma. *Neuroscience Letters, 615,* 37–43. https://doi.org/10.1016/j.neulet.2016.01.010

Dretsch, M. N., Rangaprakash, D., Katz, J. S., Daniel, T. A., Goodman, A. M., Denney, T. S., & Deshpande, G. (2019). Strength and temporal variance of the default mode network to investigate chronic mild traumatic brain injury in service members with psychological trauma. *Journal of Experimental Neuroscience, 13,* 1179069519833966. https://doi.org/10.1177/1179069519833966

Dunkley, B. T., Doesburg, S. M., Sedge, P. A., Grodecki, R. J., Shek, P. N., Pang, E. W., & Taylor, M. J. (2014). Resting-state hippocampal connectivity correlates with symptom severity in post-traumatic stress disorder. *NeuroImage: Clinical, 5,* 377–384. https://doi.org/10.1016/j.nicl.2014.07.017

Dunn-Snow, P., & Joy-Smellie, S. (2000). Teaching art therapy techniques: Mask-making, a case in point. *Art Therapy, 17*(2), 125–131.

Focus on Traumatic Brain Injury Research (2022). National Institute of Neurological Disorders and Stroke. www.ninds.nih.gov/current-research/focus-disorders/focus-traumatic-brain-injury-research

Forster, G. L, Simons, R. M., & Baugh, L. A. (2017). Revisiting the role of the amygdala in posttraumatic stress disorder. In (Ed.), *The amygdala – where emotions shape perception, learning and memories.* IntechOpen. https://doi.org/10.5772/67585

Gold, J., & Ciorciari, J. (2020). A review on the role of the neuroscience of flow states in the modern world. *Behavioral Sciences* (Basel, Switzerland), *10*(9), 137. https://doi.org/10.3390/bs10090137

Greicius, M. D., Krasnow, B., Reiss, A. L., & Menon, V. (2003). Functional connectivity in the resting brain: A network analysis of the default mode hypothesis. *Proceedings of the National Academy of Sciences of the United States of America, 100*(1), 253–258. https://doi.org/10.1073/pnas.0135058100

Haaga, M. O., & Schwartz, J. (2022). Understanding media: Laying the groundwork for art-making. In M. Rastogi, R. P. Feldwisch, M. Pate, & J. Scarce (Eds.), *Foundations of art therapy* (pp. 31–80). Academic Press. doi.org/10.1016/B978-0-12-824308-4.00013-2

Haiblum-Itskovitch, S., Czamanski-Cohen, J. and Galili, G. (2018). Emotional response and changes in heart rate variability following art-making with three different art materials. *Frontiers of Psychology, 9,* 968. https://doi.org/10.3389/fpsyg.2018.00968

Hall, N. A., Everson, A. T., Billingsley, M. R., & Miller, M. B. (2022). Moral injury, mental health and behavioural health outcomes: A systematic review of the literature. *Clinical Psychology & Psychotherapy, 29*(1), 92–110. https://doi.org/10.1002/cpp.2607

Hayes, J. P., LaBar, K. S., McCarthy, G., Selgrade, E., Nasser, J., Dolcos, F., VISN 6 Mid-Atlantic MIRECC workgroup, & Morey, R. A. (2011). Reduced hippocampal and amygdala activity predicts memory distortions for trauma reminders in combat-related PTSD. *Journal of Psychiatric Research, 45*(5), 660–669. https://doi.org/10.1016/j.jpsychires.2010.10.007

Hays, R., & Lyons, S. (1981). The bridge drawing: A projective technique for assessment in art therapy, *The Arts in Psychotherapy, 8,* 3–4, 207–217. https://doi.org/10.1016/0197-4556(81)90033-2

Henley, D. (2002). *Clayworks in art therapy: Plying the sacred circle.* Jessica Kingsley.

Herman, J., & Chilton, G. (2022). *Animal Strengths and Family Environment Directive in Family Art Therapy with Military Families.* [Manuscript submitted for publication.] Creative Forces®: NEA Military Healing Arts Network; Intrepid Spirit Center, Fort Belvoir, VA.

Hinz, L. (2009). *The Expressive Therapies Continuum.* Routledge. https://doi.org/10.4324/9780203893883

Hoover, P. J., Nix, C. A., Llop, J. Z., Lu, L. H., Bowles, A. O., & Caban, J. J. (2022). Correlations between the neurobehavioral symptom inventory and other commonly used questionnaires for traumatic brain injury. *Military Medicine*, usab559. Advance online publication. https://doi.org/10.1093/milmed/usab559

Howie, P. (2019). A part of, yet separate: Ethical issues arising in art therapy with combat service members and their families. In A. Di Maria (Ed.), *Exploring ethical dilemmas in art therapy: 50 clinicians from 20 countries share their stories* (pp. 91–96). Routledge.

Howie, P. (Ed.). (2017). *Art therapy with military populations: History, innovation, and applications.* Routledge.

Howie, P., & Sobol, B. (2013). Cultural considerations in family art therapy. In P. Howie, S. Prasad, & J. Kristel (Eds.), *Using art therapy with diverse populations: Crossing cultures and abilities* (pp. 245–225). Jessica Kingsley.

Hughes, K. C., & Shin, L. M. (2011). Functional neuroimaging studies of post-traumatic stress disorder. *Expert Review of Neurotherapeutics, 11*(2), 275–285. https://doi.org/10.1586/ern.10.198

Huotilainen, M., Rankanen, M., Groth, C., Seitamaa-Hakkarainen, P., & Mäkelä, M. (2018). Why our brains love arts and crafts: Implications of creative practices on psychophysical well-being. *Form Akademisk, 11*(2), 1–18. https://doi.org/10.7577/formakademisk.1908

Huskey, R., Craighead, B., Miller, M. B., & Weber, R. (2018). Does intrinsic reward motivate cognitive control? A naturalistic-fMRI study based on the synchronization theory of flow. *Cognitive, affective & behavioral neuroscience, 18*(5), 902–924. https://doi.org/10.3758/s13415-018-0612-6

Jackson, L. (2020). *Cultural humility in art therapy: Applications for practice, research, social justice, self-care, and pedagogy.* Jessica Kingsley.

Jones, J. P. (2017). Complicated grief: Considerations for treatment of military populations. In P. Howie (Ed.), *Art therapy with military populations* (pp. 98–110). Routledge.

Jones, J. P., Walker, M. S., Drass, J. M., & Kaimal, G. (2018). Art therapy interventions for active duty military service members with post-traumatic stress disorder and traumatic brain injury. *International Journal of Art Therapy, 23*(2), 70–85. https://doi.org/10.1080/17454832.2017.1388263

Joseph, K., Bader, K., Wilson, S., Walker, M., Stephens, M., & Varpio, L. (2017). Unmasking identity dissonance: Exploring medical students' professional identity formation through mask making. *Perspectives on Medical Education, 6*(2), 99–107.

Judkins, J. L., Moore, B. A., Collette, T. L., Hale, W. J., Peterson, A. L., & Morissette, S. B. (2020). Incidence rates of posttraumatic stress disorder over a 17-year period in active duty military service members. *Journal of Trauma Stress, 33*(6), 994–1006. https://doi.org/10.1002/jts.22558

Kagin, S. L., & Lusebrink, V. B. (1978). The expressive therapies continuum. *Art Psychotherapy, 5*(4), 171–180. https://doi.org/10.1016/0090-9092(78)90031-5

Kaimal, G., & Blank, C. A. L. (2015). Program evaluation: A doorway to research in the creative arts therapies. *Art Therapy, 32*(2), 89–92. https://doi.org/10.1080/07421656.2015.1028310

Kaimal, G., Jones, J. P., Dieterich-Hartwell, R., & Wang, X. (2021). Long-term art therapy clinical interventions with military service members with traumatic brain injury and post-traumatic stress: Findings from a mixed methods program evaluation study. *Military Psychology, 33*(1), 29–40. https://doi.org/10.1080/08995605.2020.1842639

Kaimal, G., Jones, J. P., Dieterich-Hartwell, R., Acharya, B., & Wang, X. (2019). Evaluation of long- and short-term art therapy interventions in an integrative care setting for military service members with post-traumatic stress and traumatic brain injury. *The Arts in Psychotherapy, 62*, 28–36. https://doi.org/10.1016/j.aip.2018.10.003

Kaimal, G., Walker, M. S., Herres, J., French, L. M., & DeGraba, T. J. (2018). Observational study of associations between visual imagery and measures of depression, anxiety and post-traumatic stress among active-duty military service members with traumatic brain injury at the Walter Reed National Military Medical Center. *BMJ Open, 8*(6), e021448. https://doi.org/10.1136/bmjopen-2017-021448

Kaimal, G., Walker, M. S., Herres, J., Berberian, M., & DeGraba, T. J. (2022). Examining associations between montage painting imagery and symptoms of depression and posttraumatic stress among active-duty military service members. *Psychology of Aesthetics, Creativity, and the Arts*, *16*, 16–29. https://doi.org/10.1037/aca0000316

Khatri, N., Sumadhura, B., Kumar, S., Kaundal, R. K., Sharma, S., & Datusalia, A. K. (2021). The complexity of secondary cascade consequent to traumatic brain injury: Pathobiology and potential treatments. *Current Neuropharmacology*, *19*(11), 1984–2011. https://doi.org/10.2174/1570159X19666210215123914

Kim, J. (2014). *The impact of two-dimensional versus three-dimensional art therapy on locus of control in special needs children in South Korea* (Doctoral dissertation, The Florida State University).

King, J. L. (2016). *Art therapy, trauma, and neuroscience*. New York, NY: Routledge.

King, J. L. (2015). Art Therapy: A Brain-based Profession. In D. Gussak & M. Rosal (Eds.), *The Wiley handbook of art therapy* (pp. 77–89). Wiley-Blackwell.

Kolappa, K., Seeher, K., & Dua, T. (2022). Brain health as a global priority. *Journal of the Neurological Sciences*, *439*(15), 120326. https://doi.org/10.1016/j.jns.2022.120326

Kong, L. Z., Zhang, R. L., Hu, S. H., & Lai, J.-B. (2022). Military traumatic brain injury: a challenge straddling neurology and psychiatry. *Military Medical Research*, *9*(2). https://doi.org/10.1186/s40779-021-00363-y

Lee, K. M., Greenhalgh, W. M., Sargent, P., Chae, H., Klimp, S., Engel, S., Merritt, B. P., Kretzmer, T., Bajor, L., Scott, S., & Pyne, S. (2019). Unique features of the U.S. Department of Defense Multidisciplinary Concussion Clinics. *Journal of Head Trauma Rehabilitation*. *34*(6), 402–408. https://doi.org/10.1097/HTR.0000000000000526

Leite, L., Esper, N. B., Junior, J. R. M. L., Lara, D. R., & Buchweitz, A. (2022). An exploratory study of resting-state functional connectivity of amygdala subregions in posttraumatic stress disorder following trauma in adulthood. *Scientific Reports*, *12*(1). https://doi.org/10.1038/s41598-022-13395-8

Litz, B. T., Stein, N., Delaney, E., Lebowitz, L., Nash, W.P., Silva, C., & Maguen, S. (2009). Moral Injury and Moral Repair in War Veterans: A Preliminary Model and Intervention Strategy. *Clinical Psychology Review*, *29*(8), 695–706

Lobban, J., & Murphy, D. (2019). Understanding the role art therapy can take in treating veterans with chronic post-traumatic stress disorder. *The Arts in Psychotherapy*, *62*, 37–44. https://doi.org/10.1016/j.aip.2018.11.011

Maltz, B., Hoyt, T., Uomoto, J., & Herodes, M. (2020). A case analysis of service-member trauma processing related to art therapy within a military-intensive outpatient program. *Journal of Clinical Psychology*, *76*(9), 1575–1590. https://doi.org/10.1002/jclp.22929

Mancini M. A. (2020). Trauma-Informed Behavioral Health Practice. *Integrated Behavioral Health Practice*, 191–236. https://doi.org/10.1007/978-3-030-59659-0_7

Military Health System (2022). Brain injury awareness to improve readiness. Military Health System. www.health.mil/Military-Health-Topics/MHS-Toolkits/Brain-Injury-Awareness

Miller, D. R., Hayes, S. M., Hayes, J. P., Spielberg, J. M., Lafleche, G., & Verfaellie, M. (2017). Default Mode Network Subsystems are Differentially Disrupted in Posttraumatic Stress Disorder. *Biological psychiatry. Cognitive Neuroscience and Neuroimaging*, *2*(4), 363–371. https://doi.org/10.1016/j.bpsc.2016.12.006

Mims, R. (2021). *Art therapy with veterans*. Jessica Kingsley.

Mims, R., Mcmackin, M., Chilton, G., Buotte, P., & D'Augustine, K. (2021). Countertransference when working with military service members and veterans. In R. Mims, (Ed.), *Art Therapy with Veterans* (p. 185). Jessica Kingsley.

Molendijk, T., Kramer, E. H., & Verweij, D. (2018). Moral aspects of "moral injury": Analyzing conceptualizations on the role of morality in military trauma. *Journal of Military Ethics*, *17*(1), 36–53.

Moon, C. H. (2011). *Materials & media in art therapy: Critical understandings of diverse artistic vocabularies*. Routledge.

Nan, J. K. M., and Ho, R. T. H. (2017). Effects of clay art therapy on adults outpatients with major depressive disorder: A randomized controlled trial. *Journal of Affective Disorders*, *217*, 237–245. https://doi.org/10.1016/j.jad.2017.04.013

Nancarrow, S. A., Booth, A., Ariss, S., Smith, T., Enderby, P., & Roots, A. (2013). Ten principles of good interdisciplinary team work. *Human Resources for Health*, *11*(1), 19. https://doi.org/10.1186/1478-4491-11-19

Nathan, D. E., Bellgowan, J. A. F., French, L. M., Wolf, J., Oakes, T. R., Mielke, J., Sham, E. B., Liu, W., & Riedy, G. (2017). Assessing the impact of post-traumatic stress symptoms on the resting-state default mode network in a military chronic mild traumatic brain injury sample. *Brain Connectivity*, *7*(4), 236–249. https://doi.org/10.1089/brain.2016.0433

NEA and DOD Launch Creative Forces: NEA Military Healing Arts Network. (2016). Americans for the Arts. www.americansforthearts.org/news-room/americans-for-the-arts-news/nea-and-dod-launch-creative-forces-nea-military-healing-arts-network

Ng, S. Y., & Lee, A. Y. W. (2019). Traumatic brain injuries: Pathophysiology and potential therapeutic targets. *Frontiers in Cellular Neuroscience*, *13*, 528. https://doi.org/10.3389/fncel.2019.00528

Nicholson, A. A., Rabellino, D., Densmore, M., Frewen, P. A., Paret, C., Kluetsch, R., Schmahl, C., Théberge, J., Ros, T., Neufeld, R., McKinnon, M. C., Reiss, J. P., Jetly, R., & Lanius, R. A. (2018). Intrinsic connectivity network dynamics in PTSD during amygdala downregulation using real-time fMRI neurofeedback: A preliminary analysis. *Human Brain Mapping*, *39*(11), 4258–4275. https://doi.org/10.1002/hbm.24244

Operation Homecoming: Writing the Wartime Experience. (n.d.). National Endowment for the Arts. Retrieved October, 2022 from www.arts.gov/initiatives/creative-forces/operation-homecoming

Our Impact. National Endowment for the Arts Creative Forces (2022). www.creativeforcesnrc.arts.gov/

Paley, B., & Hajal, N. J. (2022). Conceptualizing emotion regulation and coregulation as family-level phenomena. *Clinical Child and Family Psychology Review*, *25*(1), 19–43. https://doi.org/10.1007/s10567-022-00378-4

Parrott, S., Albright, D. L., Dyche, C., & Steele, H. G. (2019). Hero, charity case, and victim: How U.S. news media frame military veterans on Twitter. *Armed Forces & Society*, *45*(4), 702–722.

Payano Sosa J., Srikanchana R., Walker M., Stamper A., King, J., Ollinger, J., Bonavia, G., Christensen, A., Darda, K., Chatterjee, A., & Sours Rhodes, C. (2022). *Learning to heal through art therapy: Military service members presenting closure and healing mask themes have higher connectivity between brain regions associated with memory and pain* [Poster]. Military Health System Research Symposium (MHSRS), Kissimmee, FL.

Peterson, A. L., Young-McCaughan, S., Roache, J. D., Mintz, J., Litz, B. T., Williamson, D. E., Resick, P. A., Foa, E. B., McGeary, D. D., Dondanville, K. A., Taylor, D. J., Wachen, J. S., Fox, P. T., Bryan, C. J., McLean, C. P., Pruiksma, K. E., Yarvis, J. S., Niles, B. L., Abdallah, C. G., … the Consortium to Alleviate, P. (2021). STRONG STAR and the Consortium to Alleviate PTSD: Shaping the future of combat PTSD and related conditions in military and veteran populations. *Contemporary Clinical Trials*, *110*, 106583. https://doi.org/10.1016/j.cct.2021.106583

Phillips, M. M. & Wang, S. S. (2014). War veterans try yoga, hiking, horseback riding to treat PTSD. *The Wall Street Journal*. www.wsj.com/articles/war-veterans-try-yoga-hiking-horseback-riding-to-treat-ptsd-1410537293

Porges, S. W. (2022). Polyvagal theory: A science of safety. *Frontiers in Integrative Neuroscience*, *16*. https://doi.org/10.3389/fnint.2022.871227

Pressfield, S. (2011). *The warrior ethos*. Black Irish Entertainment LLC.

Raichle, M. E., MacLeod, A. M., Snyder, A. Z., Powers, W. J., Gusnard, D. A., & Shulman, G. L. (2001). A default mode of brain function. *Proceedings of the National Academy of Sciences of the United States of America*, *98*(2), 676–682. https://doi.org/10.1073/pnas.98.2.676

Ramchand, R., Schell, T. L., Karney, B. R., Osilla, K. C., Burns, R. M., & Caldarone, L. B. (2010). Disparate prevalence estimates of PTSD among service members who served in Iraq and Afghanistan: possible explanations. *Journal of Trauma Stress*, *23*(1), 59–68. https://doi.org/10.1002/jts.20486

Ramirez, J., Erlyana, E., & Guilliaum, M. (2016). A review of art therapy among military service members and veterans with post-traumatic stress disorder. *Journal of Military and Veterans Health, 24*(2), 40–51.

Rasmussen, T. E., Reilly, P. A., & Baer, D. G. (2014). Why military medical research? *Military Medicine, 179*(suppl_8), 1–2.

Ray, S. K., Dixon, C. E., & Banik, N. L. (2002). Molecular mechanisms in the pathogenesis of traumatic brain injury. *Histology and Histopathology, 17*(4), 1137–1152. https://doi.org/10.14670/HH-17.1137

Robb, R. (2012). The history of art therapy at the National Institutes of Health. *Art Therapy, Journal of the American Art Therapy Association, 29*(1), 33–37. https://doi.org/10.1080/07421656.2012.648097

Rosenthal-von der Pütten, A.M., Krämer, N.C., Hoffmann, L., Sobieraj, S., & Eimler, S. C. (2013). An experimental study on emotional reactions towards a robot. *International Journal of Social Robotics, 5*, 17–34. https://doi.org/10.1007/s12369-012-0173-8

Ross, M. C., & Cisler, J. M. (2020). Altered large-scale functional brain organization in posttraumatic stress disorder: A comprehensive review of univariate and network-level neurocircuitry models of PTSD. *NeuroImage: Clinical, 27*, 102319. https://doi.org/10.1016/j.nicl.2020.102319

Rubin, J. A. (2011). *The art of art therapy: What every art therapist needs to know.* Routledge.

Rubinov, M., & Sporns, O. (2010). Complex network measures of brain connectivity: uses and interpretations. *NeuroImage, 52*(3), 1059–1069. https://doi.org/10.1016/j.neuroimage.2009.10.003

Schore, A. N. (2009). Relational trauma and the developing right brain: An interface of psychoanalytic self psychology and neuroscience. *Annals of the New York Academy of Sciences, 1159*(1), 189–203.

Scotti, V., & Chilton, G. (2017). Collage as arts-based research. In P. Leavy (Ed.), *Handbook of arts-based research* (pp. 355–376). Guilford Press.

Seiden, D. (2001). *Mind over matter: The uses of materials in art, education and therapy.* Magnolia Street Publishers.

Shay, J. (1994). *Achilles in Vietnam: Combat trauma and the undoing of character.* New York: Scribner.

Shear, M. K. (2015). Complicated grief. *New England Journal of Medicine, 372*(2), 153–160. https://doi.org/10.1056/NEJMcp1315618

Sheynin, J., Duval, E. R., King, A. P., Angstadt, M., Phan, K. L., Simon, N. M., Rauch, S., & Liberzon, I. (2020). Associations between resting-state functional connectivity and treatment response in a randomized clinical trial for posttraumatic stress disorder. *Depression and Anxiety, 37*(10), 1037–1046. https://doi.org/10.1002/da.23075

Shin, L. M., Wright, C. I., Cannistraro, P. A., Wedig, M. M., McMullin, K., Martis, B., Macklin, M. L., Lasko, N. B., Cavanagh, S. R., Krangel, T. S., Orr, S. P., Pitman, R. K., Whalen, P. J., & Rauch, S. L. (2005). A functional magnetic resonance imaging study of amygdala and medial prefrontal cortex responses to overtly presented fearful faces in posttraumatic stress disorder. *Archives of General Psychiatry, 62*(3), 273–281. https://doi.org/10.1001/archpsyc.62.3.273

Sholt, M., & Gavron, T. (2006). Therapeutic qualities of clay-work in art therapy and psychotherapy: A review. *Art Therapy, 23*(2), 66–72. https://doi.org/10.1080/07421656.2006.10129647

Silkenbeumer, J., Schiller, E. M., Holodynski, M., & Kärtner, J. (2016). The role of co-regulation for the development of social-emotional competence. *Journal of Self-regulation and Regulation, 2*, 17–32. https://doi.org/10.11588/josar.2016.2.34351

Snir, S., & Regev, D. (2013). A dialog with five art materials: Creators share their art making experiences. *The Arts in Psychotherapy, 40*(1), 94–100. https://doi.org/10.1016/j.aip.2012.11.004

Spielberg, J. M., McGlinchey, R. E., Milberg, W. P., & Salat, D. H. (2015). Brain network disturbance related to posttraumatic stress and traumatic brain injury in veterans. *Biological Psychiatry, 78*(3), 210–216. https://doi.org/10.1016/j.biopsych.2015.02.013

Spooner, H., Lee, J. B., Langston, D. G., Sonke, J., Myers, K. J., & Levy, C. E. (2019). Using distance technology to deliver the creative arts therapies to veterans: Case studies in art, dance/movement and music therapy. *The Arts in Psychotherapy, 62*, 12–18.

Sripada, R. K., King, A. P., Garfinkel, S. N., Wang, X., Sripada, C. S., Welsh, R. C., & Liberzon, I. (2012). Altered resting-state amygdala functional connectivity in men with posttraumatic stress disorder. *Journal of Psychiatry & Neuroscience: JPN, 37*(4), 241–249. https://doi.org/10.1503/jpn.110069

Stamper, A. (n.d.). *Pour painting directives and justification.* Unpublished manuscript, Creative Forces®: NEA Military Healing Arts Network.

Tanielian, T. & Jaycox, L. (Eds.). (2008). *Invisible wounds of war: Psychological and cognitive injuries, their consequences, and services to assist recover.* RAND Corporation.

Ulrich, M., Keller, J., Hoenig, K., Waller, C., & Grön, G. (2014). Neural correlates of experimentally induced flow experiences. *NeuroImage, 86,* 194–202. https://doi.org/10.1016/j.neuroimage.2013.08.019

Vaudreuil, R., Bronson, H. and Bradt, J. (2019). Bridging the clinic to community: Music performance as social transformation for military service members. *Frontiers of Psychology, 10*(119). https://doi.org/10.3389/fpsyg.2019.00119

Walker, M. S. (2017). Integrative approaches to treating PTSD and TBI: Art therapy approaches within the National Intrepid Center of Excellence at Walter Reed National Military Medical Center. In P. Howie, Ed., *Art therapy with military populations* (pp. 111–123). Routledge.

Walker, M. S. (2019). Outcomes of art therapy treatment for military service members with traumatic brain injury and post-traumatic stress at the National Intrepid Center of Excellence. In J. L. Contreras-Vidal, D. Roblemann, J. G. Cruz-Garza, J. M. Azorín, & C. S. Nam (Eds.), *Mobile brain-body imaging and the neuroscience of art, innovation and creativity* (pp. 115–124). Springer.

Walker, M. S., Kaimal, G., Koffman, R., & DeGraba, T. J. (2016). Art therapy for PTSD and TBI: A senior active duty military service member's therapeutic journey. *The Arts in Psychotherapy, 49,* 10–18. https://doi.org/10.1016/j.aip.2016.05.015

Walker, M. S., Kaimal, G., Gonzaga, A. M. L., Myers-Coffman, K. A., & Degraba, T. J. (2017). Active-duty military service members' visual representations of PTSD and TBI in masks. *International Journal of Qualitative Studies on Health and Well-being, 12*(1), 1267317. https://doi.org/10.1080/17482631.2016.1267317

Walker, M. S., Stamper, A. M., Nathan, D. E., & Riedy, G. (2018). Art therapy and underlying fMRI brain patterns in military TBI: A case series. *International Journal of Art Therapy, 23*(4), 180–187. https://doi.org/10.1080/17454832.2018.1473453

Weber, R., Tamborini, R., Westcott-Baker, A., & Kantor, B. (2009). Theorizing flow and media enjoyment as cognitive synchronization of attentional and reward networks. *Communication Theory, 19*(4), 397–422. https://doi.org/10.1111/j.1468-2885.2009.01352.x

White, R. C., & Remington, A. (2019). Object personification in autism: This paper will be very sad if you don't read it. *Autism: The International Journal of Research and Practice, 23*(4), 1042–1045. https://doi.org/10.1177/1362361318793408

Wix, L. (2000). Looking for what's lost: The artistic roots of art therapy: Mary Huntoon. *Art Therapy, 17*(3), 168–176. https://doi.org/10.1080/07421656.2000.10129699

World Health Organization. (2015). *International statistical classification of diseases and related health problems* (10th revision, 5th ed., 2016 ed.). WHO. https://apps.who.int/iris/handle/10665/246208

CHAPTER 9

THE INTERPOSITIONAL ROLE OF ART THERAPY IN MUSEUM SETTINGS

Denise Wolf, Kathryn Snyder, and Raquel Farrell-Kirk

9.1 INTRODUCTION

This chapter reflects the diverse work facilitated and researched by these authors across many museums. Collectively, we identify and seek to continue the dialogue surrounding the role of art therapists in art education, museum spaces, and the community, predicated on the notion that a museum is a place of community engagement and learning and art is a powerful mechanism for self-reflection, identification, understanding, and personal and collective healing.

The authors explore how artwork within a museum's collection functions as a resource for utilizing art in a therapeutic context (de Botton & Armstrong, 2013) by supporting emotional integration and resilience, and providing a place to reflect on injustice, as well as to address and ameliorate the impact of trauma and oppression as it has been represented historically and contemporaneously. As de Botton and Armstrong (2013) reflect, there are seven functions of art: remembering our whole humanity, encouraging hope, dignifying sorrow, rebalancing towards what is good and right, guiding us into self-understanding, extending us into growth, and fostering appreciation which sensitizes us to the world all around.

We explore a framework, developed by Snyder (2022), for understanding the opportunity for art therapists to work within museums. This framework is built upon the public nature of the institution, the objects within the institution, and the call for collaboration between museum professionals (educators, curators, directors) and art therapists in the provision of ethical care that benefits from a shared endeavor of human progress, transformation, and learning through arts experiences (Snyder, 2022). Contemporary neuroscience offers the theory of embodied cognition (Galetzka, 2017) to understand the mechanisms of change at work while King's (2016) three tenets of art therapy serve as a means to connect the application of museum-based art therapy to our understanding of neuroplasticity and the amelioration of the sequelae of trauma.

There is increasing interest in expanding the therapeutic capacity of museums (Chatterjee & Noble, 2013; Cowan et al., 2020; Watson et al., 2021). Perhaps, beginning with Silverman's (2010) appeal to museums to become places of "social work," to more contemporary efforts endorsing "social prescribing" – having medical professionals prescribe their patients visits to museums or participation in other cultural activities and experiences. In September of 2021, doctors in Brussels began to recommend museum visits to their patients being treated for stress, which they could attend free of cost (Boffey, 2021). The Massachusetts Cultural Council launched the CultureRx Initiative in 2021, a social prescription pilot program

DOI: 10.4324/9781003348207-9

with the intent to provide access to culture and arts experiences to promote well-ness through the positive therapeutic effect of arts engagements (Swaback, 2021). There is an effort to utilize the benefits of museum visits to ameliorate the intensi-fying stress of the crises of recent years that have resulted in growing mental health concerns: extreme political division, police brutality, and the COVID-19 pandemic. This nexus point between medical prescription practices and art and culture can provide an optimal entry point for art therapists to focus on for legitimizing a museum-based practice while simultaneously advocating for mental health and community care.

We assert that there is increasing evidence to support museum-based art therapy practices with a specific emphasis on the value of community-based service provision for the work of healing both individual and collective trauma. The expertise of art therapists combined with museums' public accessibility and rich collections of art and artifacts can transform museum spaces into highly potent venues for a wide array of art therapy services. These designations can range from consultation with museum staff, to supporting accessibility programming and art education, and/or the provision of direct services through clinical art therapy programming.

9.2   MUSEUM HISTORY AND THE IDEA OF RELEVANCE

Historical and contemporary goals of museums align in the common mission of fos-tering a space that compels visitors to engage in a social process of discovery and rediscovery (Watson et al., 2021). For some time, museum professionals in the United States have been calling for a rethinking of museum mission statements, shifting away from embedded colonial histories implicit in many museum artifacts acquired through theft, exploiting cultural, spiritual, and religious beliefs vis-à-vis relics dis-played as "exotic" (Anderson, 2019, p. 4). An essential function of a museum mission statement, according to Anderson (2019) should be to offer a guide in providing access and interaction with the community. It must also consider how to align its statement with contemporary issues and realities in confluence with a socially just focus (Coleman, 2016; Raicovich, 2021; Simon, 2016). New mission statements and their enactment must engage the public, diverging from abstract or academic con-structs to encompass real-world, real-time experiences and needs in conjunction with interpretive strategies (Anderson, 2019; Decter et al., 2022).

International communities have been debating the definition of "museum" for several years, resulting in the International Council of Museums (ICOM) formula-tion of a new definition in August of 2022. This new definition includes an empha-sis on the participation of the community, inclusivity, accessibility, and sustainability with the statement, "They [museums] operate and communicate ethically and pro-fessionally with the participation of communities, offering varied experiences for education, enjoyment, and reflection and knowledge sharing" (The Extraordinary General Assembly of International Council of Museums, 2022). As part of this re-thinking, museum professionals are pushing for more dialogue about how muse-ums are and can be part of larger initiatives of contemporary importance.

Varutti (2022) asks that we consider an "empathic museum" that acknowl-edges how attending to viewers' experience of museum spaces can foster social change and enhance connection to the community. Museums have the capability and even perhaps responsibility to consider how an affective response can be harnessed within exhibits to impact empathy, foster emotions such as awe, and support people when viewing challenging and upsetting works related to war, genocide, and other atrocities (Varutti, 2022). Similarly, curation goals have shifted from the acquisition of a publicly accessible collection of artifacts to include artifacts that illuminate the community about culture, history, and science; a shift from "authoritative knowledge" to a co-created influence of human experience (Annechini et al., 2020).

According to the model, espoused by many museum professionals, where a museum is a place for social work, inclusivity, and relevance, museums exist only with consideration to the audience that comes to view the collection, making this an enterprise that is dependent on reciprocity and dialogue, associating "object" with learning (Anderson, 2019; Coleman, 2016; Simon, 2016; Raicovich, 2021). Full consideration of the audience through awareness of relevant social needs creates fertile grounds for direct art therapy practice as well as the use of art therapists as consultants to help the museum truly function as a living institution.

9.3   FRAMEWORK AND NEUROLOGICAL MECHANISMS OF ART THERAPY

A framework for understanding a museum as a place for art therapy practice is based on three primary factors: (1) the public nature of the space affords an opportunity for the greater public good in the form of activities and engagements that promote health, well-being, and deep social connection, (2) the objects within the space of the museum offer opportunities for individuals and groups to connect with ideas, experiences, and feelings expressed within these artifacts which supports deeper personal meaning-making, and (3) collaboration must take place between highly trained museum professionals and credentialled art therapists who can fully support the mental health and rehabilitation needs of the participants and create programs that are considerate of therapy and the unique goals of the individuals while utilizing and respecting the artwork, collection, and space of the museum.

This framework supports the new definition and defined purpose of museums which runs analogous to the definition and purpose of art therapy. Art therapy is an integrative mental health profession that includes the use of art and art making to support the emotional, mental health, and rehabilitation needs of people of all ages and stages of life and to foster self-awareness and growth and includes an emphasis on community well-being (AATA, 2022; BAAT, 2022). Similarly, museums are redefining themselves with a focus on supporting wellness, meeting important needs in their communities, and serving as a resource for a wide cross-section of community members (Simon, 2016; Snyder, 2022). While not named explicitly, a space that can enable a creative process is implicit to the work of art therapy. Museums offer powerful images and evocative objects in a public space that can be supportive in containing affect and emotional response, personal and interpersonal dialogue, and meaning-making (Coles, 2020; Ioannides, 2016).

Borrowing from contemporary neuroscience, we can utilize the lens of embodied cognition and its appreciation for the role of the body's interaction with the environment to help us consider, understand, and explain the therapeutic potential of art therapy in a museum space (Coles et al., 2019; Timm-Bottos & Reilly, 2015). In this construct, semantic meaning is made when an object is perceived and linked to experiences, memories, and emotions. These may in turn evoke bodily responses and activate sensorimotor areas of the brain (Galetzka, 2017). Repeated experiences build upon themselves, creating complex neurological patterns and personal meaning. King's (2016) three tenets of art therapy serve as means to connect the application of museum-based art therapy practices to our understanding of neuroplasticity and the amelioration of the sequelae of trauma through art therapy practices; the artwork itself embodies an essential component to treatment within a therapeutic relationship, creative expression is restorative and enriching unto itself, and the materials and methods promote self-expression and emotion regulation when applied in specialized ways. "The fundamental power of art therapy [within a museum setting] rests in the three-way process between the client, the therapist, and the image or artifact" (Ioannides, 2016, p. 99).

The very structure of the museum can be experienced as an enchanting entity, not just the objects within (Annechini et al., 2020). The aesthetics of the exterior structure of museums may arouse feelings of comfort and nurturance, and fuel a creative urge for expression (Hutchison, 2015). "The architectural boundaries—including size, scale, lighting, temperature, circulation, display and layout—along with the appraisals visitors make of these elements, delineate the museum and the outside world" (Ioannides, 2016, p.104). The use of a beautifully appointed space, the connection to art, and a social network of shared viewers within the context of working with an art therapist has profound implications for museum art therapy practice.

Art and artifacts in the collection of a museum are also important opportunities for people to engage in a direct experience with objects that spark connections, associations, histories, and projective meanings. Direct engagement sparks sensory awareness and immersion while narrative and further meaning-making can be explored. These objects may be historic connections to cultures and heritages with inherent significance for an individual who is from that culture as well as for a wider array of people as we make sense of our diverse world and the deep history that we are all a part of. Empathy is built when we make such connections, which results in greater respect and understanding of others in our communities. A neuroaesthetic perspective may support our understanding that there is a profound and deep impact on viewing art and dialoguing with others, professionals and otherwise, to enhance the emotional connections, sensory and motor activation, and the way that meaning emerges (Chatterjee & Vartanian, 2014).

An experienced clinician with an intuitive sense of how our brains engage in emotional processing can incorporate core concepts of aesthetic space, symbolic content, and responses to aesthetic experiences into (museum-based) clinical practice (King et al., 2019). A novice understanding of our neurological relationship to art, aesthetics, and healing practices supports our notion that work within museums has the potential to impact the neural circuitry of the brain (Koban et al., 2021; Lusebrink & Hinz, 2020), connecting experiences with art to mechanisms of change that we might harness for therapy, healing, and overall health.

9.4   ART THERAPY PRACTICES IN MUSEUMS

Art therapy sits at the intersection of the changing museum philosophy – towards relevance and meeting the social needs of their communities – and the Arts in Health movement (Aspen Institute, 2021) where social prescribing of arts and culture experiences is being explored as robust health supports. Writing about the potential for art therapy programs in art museums, Watson, Coles, and Jury (2021) capitalize on the notion of accessible space and social inclusion within museums. Utilizing a philosophy of placed-based learning and service provision (Vander Ark et al., 2020), art therapists have been working in museums in attenuated and prescribed ways (Watson et al., 2021) as well as in full-time and integrative ways such as the full-time position at The Montreal Museum of Fine Arts where Stephan Legari was hired to develop partnerships and programming around art therapy (Vartanian, 2019).

Consideration of space, collections, art education practices, docent-led public tours, and de-stigmatization of mental health care all work to support the opportunity for art therapy to be considered in museum practices. The study done by Watson et al. (2021) suggests that the museum setting itself is a therapeutic factor. They report that their art therapy client participants attributed feelings of value due to the setting because of their perception of the way society values a museum itself, its contents, and the education about artwork that is offered. Other therapeutic aspects of consideration noted were the participants' experiences of personal identification and inspiration from viewing artworks and objects, enhanced creative and therapeutic processes, and their ability to move within the museum space as well as within the public domain. Importantly, the idea of reducing power dynamics and hierarchical relationships between client participants and therapists and museum professionals was also valued by participants in reflecting on their experiences. Finally, the relaxed nature of viewing artwork in a museum allowed for the process of therapy to slow down and for participants to find ease and comfort in relating (Watson et al., 2021).

With an explicit mission to care for their community, The Studio Museum of Harlem New York encompasses the community in every stage of development. Chloe Hayward at The Studio Museum sees her role as an art therapist and art educator as one of supporting the health and well-being of every visitor by utilizing her skills in art, education, and therapy to create opportunities for safety, reflection, and personal aesthetic integration within exhibits, in programming, and with the staff (Snyder, 2022a). This integrated approach to art therapy/art education in a museum offers a model where trauma-informed care and emotion-centered exhibits merge with the broadest perspective of art therapy.

Similarly, an initiative at the Cincinnati Art Museum in Ohio brought in art therapists to educate docents on the potential needs of visitors to the museum (A. Palamara, personal communication, August 20, 2020). This trauma-aware lens of consultation by art therapists is another opportunity to consider the integration of professional knowledge into museums, holding the premise of emotions as a catalyst and fulcrum for enhancing the goals of the museum experience. Andrew Palamara, the docent coordinator who initiated this program, went on to form a small working group of allied professionals during the COVID-19 pandemic who are dialoguing about trauma-aware practices in museums, specifically focused on education divisions within museums (Palamara et al., 2020).

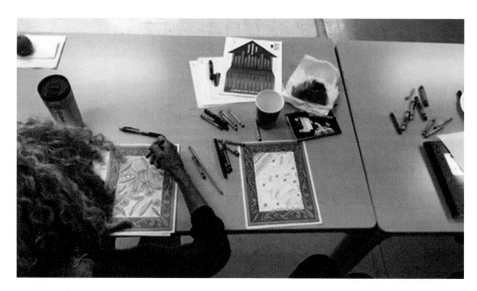

FIGURE 9.1 Art museum educators learn to use "framing" as a tool for supporting regulation and containment in art experiences

Wolf and Snyder were invited into the Philadelphia Museum of Art in Philadelphia, Pennsylvania, to provide professional development to museum educators in 2016 and 2017. Educators were interested in learning more about trauma-informed education, noting that many of their students, young and old, come into the museum carrying the burdens of their past traumas, which will show up in a wide variety of ways when engaging with art in the collection and during art making in the museum's classrooms. Wolf and Snyder presented participants with a theoretical overview of the neurobiological impact of trauma and the potential positive impact of arts experiences followed by engaging in interactive, participatory art making (Figure 9.1) and dialogue prompting personal exploration of their own neurodiverse experiences, responses to art, and needs for safety, support, and experiential integration.

The art therapy perspective provided educators invaluable insight into verbal and non-verbal cues that may indicate emotion dysregulation. Educators also learned verbal and non-verbal means of supporting individuals while they are in a dysregulated state. Educators learned how use of materials, media, and art prompts that enhance museum experiences can help create positive boundaries and allow for personal exploration around challenging experiences without delving into the realm of psychotherapy.

An additional workshop was offered at the Philadelphia Museum of Art to provide support for museum educators when they confront difficult or challenging subject matter in the museum (Synder & Wolf, 2018) (Figure 9.2). The educators identified these images as well as several other paintings, objects, and collections as catalysts for visible emotional responses from museum goers. Themes of provocative imagery, race, oppression, and representation were brought up as specific areas of concern. Facilitators and educators engaged in dialogue around the ways that

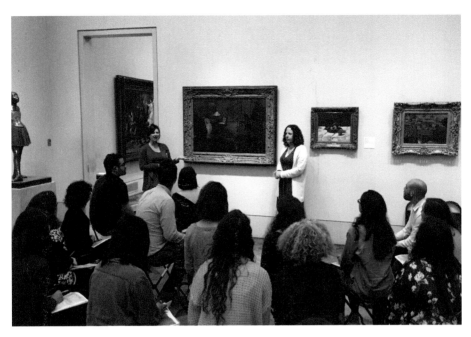

FIGURE 9.2 Wolf and Snyder at Philadelphia Museum of Art Educator Workshop. Note: Photo of Snyder (left) and Wolf (right) discussing the museum goers experience of Degas' *Interior* with museum educators

museum goers have expressed concern, distress, overwhelm, and a need to process their experience when visiting the museum as well as when engaging in programming with the educational staff.

A specific painting identified was *Mrs. Peale Lamenting the Death of Her Child/Rachel Weeping* (Figure 9.3). At the initial display of this painting in 1782, the artist Charles Wilson Peale, screened the painting behind a curtain which held a warning pinned to it, "Before you draw this curtain Consider whether you will afflict a Mother or Father who has lost a Child" (*Mrs. Peale Lamenting the Death of Her Child*, n.d. https://philamuseum.org/collection/object/71982). It is still reported to "afflict" viewers over 200 years later. *Interior* (Figure 9.4) has been said to emanate "sexual menace" (Interior, n.d., https://philamuseum.org/collection/object/82556). Museum educators had observed that this painting prompted strong emotional responses from patrons such as tears, anxiety, and/the unprompted disclosure of their own personal experience with sexual violence. Subsequently, Wolf and Snyder led participants through the museum collection to bear witness to identified objects in the collection. In the gallery space, they engaged in discussion with the educators, and identified ways to utilize the space of the museum, the viewing of additional objects, and ways to facilitate boundary settings to safely contain dysregulation while providing exceptional gallery experiences.

The Coral Springs Museum of Art (Coral Springs, FL) launched a community-wide open studio art therapy event mere days after the school shooting at Marjorie Stoneman Douglas, just minutes away in Parkland, Florida. At the time of publication,

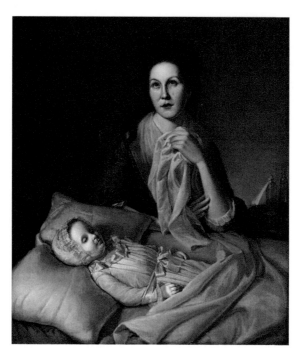

FIGURE 9.3 Peale, C. (1772; enlarged 1776; retouched 1818). *Mrs. Peale Lamenting the Death of Her Child/Rachel Weeping* [painting]. Retrieved from https://philamuseum.org/collection/object/71982

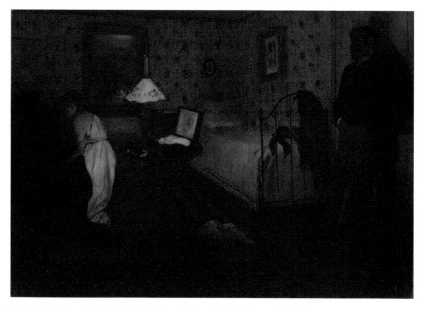

FIGURE 9.4 Degas, E. (1868–69). *Interior* [painting]. https://philamuseum.org/collection/object/82556

this remains the deadliest high school shooting in United States history and grief and disbelief rippled through the quiet suburban town. The speed with which this much needed and well received response was mounted was due, in part, to a pre-existing relationship with art therapists and an understanding of the mechanisms for establishing a program. This partnership was a direct result of local art therapy advocacy and public awareness aimed at museum professionals and galleries that had occurred over the preceding years. "An open, drop-in art therapy studio accommodated people with a broad range of trauma impacts and offered a stigma-free, accessible place for initial support or referrals to more intensive services" (Farrell-Kirk, 2021, p. 214).

The museum leveraged the inherent benefits of the museum space by housing the multi-day event not in its classrooms but in the spacious main gallery. With its open floor plan, floor to ceiling windows flooding the room with natural light, and walls of art on display, the space provided participants with a serene environment intended to bolster the emotional regulation being facilitated by the art making and therapeutic support being offered. The physical location of the space itself allowed community members to attend a therapeutic program without having to enter a traditional treatment setting, thereby removing some of the stigma that may have served as a barrier to seeking help. Farrell-Kirk and the team of art therapists utilized a trauma-sensitive approach to provide services to those impacted by the shooting, including students, faculty, and community members. Participants were supported to create art to memorialize friends lost and received referrals to long-term support if indicated. What began as a response to the crisis flourished into the development and funding of ongoing art therapy groups at the museum that continued for over two years. Additionally, the program served as the inspiration for Power of Art, a series of public art and art therapy offerings that was awarded a highly competitive $1M grant from Bloomberg Philanthropies. This grant furthered the program's impact, extending beyond the museum walls into wide-reaching, community-based art making.

Although having an established partnership is useful in mounting a quick response to unexpected trauma, it is not required. Art therapist Farrell-Kirk was part of a team from the Florida Art Therapy Association (FATA) who quickly and skillfully implemented a community trauma response after the unexpected collapse of a 12-story beachfront condominium in Surfside, Florida that took 98 lives, despite no art therapy and museum partnerships in the area. They formulated a response based on Farrell-Kirk's previous experience in Parkland and approached the Bass Museum (Miami Beach, FL) who agreed to work alongside the art therapy team to coordinate a community-wide event that provided access to art therapy for a wide cross-section of the community. Though initially envisioned as an event-specific response, it spurred the museum to hire one of the team members, a local art therapist, to create and facilitate consistent art therapy programming. In both Parkland and Surfside, museums stood in the midst of community traumas with resources at their disposal and staff eager and motivated to help, while art therapists stood in possession of the skills, knowledge, and specialized training to help provide healing, but without large-scale spaces and access to the community. Through collaboration, they realized the potential positive impact on the community members exceeded what they could have accomplished alone.

Research conducted by Snyder (2022b) as part of her doctoral research fellowship and practicum at Drexel University focuses on the perspective of a variety of museum professionals on the potentials and challenges of providing art therapy in museums. Results suggest considerable interest in museum communities and stakeholders in having art therapy programming within museums. Museum professionals indicated previously having utilized art therapists for consultation on highly provocative shows such as the recent show at the Philadelphia Museum of Art, "Elegy: Lament in the 20th Century." Additionally, the professionals interviewed were increasingly aware of the mental health and social concerns rising in their communities and unmistakably evident in audiences within their museums. Many were engaged in robust dialogues within their cities around how to be of service during the pandemic and were extending their roles in novel ways to meet these needs, such as situating the museum as a hub for food distribution and other social services while their communities were in the shut-down.

The Fitchburg Museum in Massachusetts has been instrumental in revitalizing their small, post-industrial city, meeting regularly with city officials toward that end. Beyond considering a creative economy, they see their mission as a museum as one of service to the community. During the pandemic they offered relief in the form of food aid packages through their Fitchburg Families First program (FAM, 2022) among other initiatives. They have hosted art therapy programming to provide services for specific mental health and substance abuse needs, expressing a strong desire to make this a regular part of their offerings, along with highly supportive educational programming for school children. Like many of the participants, finding qualified art therapists in the community has been a significant challenge.

Additional findings from Snyder's (2022b) research show that museum professionals are involved in working with local medical centers to provide support for patients, justice systems to engage youth and others in re-entry and skill development, creating experiences to support participants with dementia and Alzheimer's and their caregivers, along with many other peripheral wellness programs such as mindfulness, meditation, and yoga that involve viewing artwork and being in gallery spaces. In considering the way that their museum engages ideas of wellness in robust and supportive ways, one participant stated, "Our bread and butter is really what we do with the things that are on view. It's interpretation, it's having conversations, it's training individuals to look and think and be more aware of people." In all these cases, the professionals identified that coordination with an art therapist would significantly enhance these programs.

An additional reflection on art therapy and professional development or support from a participant offered:

> I think using the tools you have at your disposal; on your gallery walls to just better reflect on the social welfare of your own staff could be a first step into really understanding … maybe it could work for the community down the street. And just making time for that kind of self-reflection.

From consideration of the use of art and art therapy techniques for staff support and development, to implementing care groups for other health and education professionals and providing consultation on museum spaces and shows, to developing mental health art therapy groups, museum professionals are asking for art therapy to support their innovative work.

9.5   SCOPE OF PRACTICE AND TRAUMA

Several models of art therapy work in a museum include consultant on shows, docent programs, and education programs; part-time facilitator of specific therapeutic or therapy groups; partner with mental health organizations to bring sub-groups in for specific programming; work within education department with dual degree; work full time within museum to create programming and partnerships.

There are many ways that art therapy is being imagined (and can be imagined) in terms of work within museums. Art therapists may serve as expert consultants, provide specific art therapy groups or therapeutic experiences in response to an event, a population, or a show, or be employed by the museum itself as a full-time art therapist. Stephan Legari is a credentialed art therapist working at Montreal Museum of Fine Arts, often proclaimed to be the first full-time, museum-based, art therapist (Meistere, 2021; Vartanian, 2019). For museum-based art therapy practice to become well established, art therapists are best served with a framework to rely on (Coles & Harrison, 2018). When considering their work and dialogue across professional sectors, a foundational framework that identifies guidelines for urgent response to community needs, consideration of professional ethics in public or semi-public spaces, identification of emotional and physical boundaries, funding, and development of employment contracts would help to strengthen and expand museum-based art therapy practice.

While docents and educators can receive supplemental training to support trauma-sensitive and therapeutic practices, art therapists possess a comprehensive set of specific skills well suited to providing a deeper/broader/more specialized range of outreach within the museum. They are proficient in direct provision of therapy, assessment of client needs, and planning of art experiences to respond to those needs. They also have the knowledge and skills needed to do this while managing risks and upholding their ethics as a mental health practitioner (Coles & Harrison, 2018). Ioannides (2016) states that various cross-sections of the community access art therapy in museum settings, including those with mental health diagnosis, people experiencing job-related stress, students undergoing medical training, youth with academic challenges, individuals with visual impairments, those managing responses to medical illnesses such as cancer, Alzheimer's, addiction and substance use disorders, as well as people who have experienced trauma, amongst a plethora of other reasons people may seek support, connection, and validation (Ghadim & Daugherty, 2021). Credentialed art therapists are guided in their responses to this multiplicity of participant identities and resultant museum-based practices by their ethical principles (AATA, 2017).

9.6   WHAT CAN BE DONE? RECOMMENDATIONS FOR BEST PRACTICE

Cowan, Laird, and McKeown (2020) have written about the potential for mental health programs and services to be hosted within museums. While they expound upon the potential benefits, they also caution that museums are not inherently spaces where clinical therapy takes place. This is a necessary caution that we should heed.

A lack of privacy and confidentiality is certainly a primary concern, though careful planning and consideration can mitigate this. And while the reduction of stigmatization and isolation may also be a benefit of the use of museum spaces, therapists and museum staff must carefully assess the needs of each individual as well as the group (when this is the format), in order to meet therapy goals and create enough safety for the individual to attend to their specific needs, concerns, and unpredictable emotional states.

It is important to also recognize potential barriers related to attending therapy in a museum setting. While housing art therapy at a museum can remove the stigma often associated with seeking mental health care and resources, some attendees may hold negative associations to museums as places that are stiff, unwelcoming, boring, or reserved for elite members with knowledge, affluence, or familiarity that they perceive themselves as lacking (Toolis, 2018). Returning to our framework, the use of public spaces (even when brought into private rooms or cordoned off) is an important consideration. The social justice-minded aspects of this setting allows therapy to be accessed in greater ways and brings the public dialogue about mental health and social services into a public realm. Museums have an implicit mandate to be as inclusive as possible and work in a trauma-informed, trauma-aware, and/or sensory and developmentally aware ways, which are critical in expanding the community that a museum serves, including anyone with mental health and developmental needs. Museums offer "third spaces" where place-based learning and psychological development can occur, "where shared authority, inclusion, and social action are at the heart of … doing work in the neighborhood or community" (Rowson-Love & Szymanski, 2017, p. 196).

Even in the absence of a specific traumatic event, art therapists can lend valuable support to museums through the provision of trauma-sensitive services, outlooks, and specific programming. Support for staff in handling their daily stressors in addition to the ongoing stress of the pandemic and world affairs, as well mounting a response when a specific traumatic event in the community happens are all areas that art therapy can address within museums. Additionally, museum-based art therapy practices can engage in prevention through fostering resilience and connection amongst community members. At the Miami Children's Museum in Miami, Florida, Farrell-Kirk assisted staff and visiting artists in the planning and execution of a series of interactive art-making workshops for children and their families. Consultations with museum leadership, artists, and docents helped ensure the media, directives and overall program was inclusive and accessible.

Exhibits like *A New Kind of House* (Figure 9.5) at Drexel University seeks to engage in "creative placemaking and art for social justice" by hanging photography of contemporary students and neighbors alongside the university's permanent collection featuring colonial imagery in an effort to begin a "rich dialogue" (*A New Kind of House*, 2022). Wilson (2022) interviewed a university student who commented, "Having local high school students work next to a traditional oil painting is a way to say, 'We're here. This is what Drexel looks like now'."

Collaboration between museum staff and art therapy professionals is a critical link to successfully develop and implement museum-based services. The expertise of the museum professional provides context of the object/s as well as the collection and artist or socio-cultural location. This information can further the multiplicity

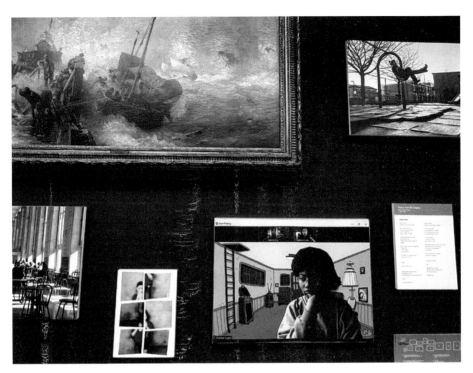

FIGURE 9.5 *A New Kind of House* (2022, October 7). Drexel University exhibitions & events from https://guides.himmelfarb.gwu.edu/APA/web-page-no-author

of meaning that is explored in the therapeutic context, in that they possess an intimate knowledge of the museum and how to navigate its physical space as well as the administrative components. Working with a qualified art therapist ensures that consideration has been made for psychological safety and meeting individual treatment goals and objectives.

While there seems to be a growing investment in health, wellness, and social/ emotional services within museums, many barriers and challenges exist to promote the work of art therapy within museum settings. As mentioned, finding qualified art therapists is a challenge. Many communities do not have access to art therapists within their community and states vary regarding licensure and qualifications. This fact not only leads to confusion about who is and is not qualified but also questions about payment for services. Rightfully, all involved are concerned with providing ethical care with fully qualified art therapists, trained staff, and adequate boundaries relative to privacy, confidentiality, space, treatment goals, and expectations of all involved. Finally, through interprofessional collaboration, experiences and positive outcomes for participants are enhanced. Opportunities exist to act as a bridge between the museum and medical and health-care systems; art therapists can help museum staff have a better understanding of mental health and in turn mental and medical health providers can become more aware of museums and galleries as a resource for treatment (Coles & Harrison, 2018).

9.7   SUMMARY AND CONCLUSION

The mission of a museum is currently undergoing metamorphosis, moving away from "serving people" (Plumley, 2020), towards providing a guide for access and interaction with the community (Coleman, 2016; Raicovich, 2021; Simon, 2016) that interconnects these disciplines in new ways that promote healing (Gruenwald, 2021). Art therapists can offer insight and perspective within museums on the ways that varied intersectional identities may interact with the art and how viewing art may impact their psychological self, especially when the art itself is experienced as provocative or disturbing. Art therapists can also support deepening conversations elicited from art and artifacts for personal growth and psychological transformation. This combination of space, which offers a place along with containment of aroused affect and behavior, the artwork, which is provocative and evocative, and the professional collaboration between museums professionals and art therapists presents a unique and robust opportunity for widespread community mental health care, social support, and socially active and engaged community dialogue and healing.

REFERENCES

American Art Therapy Association. (2022). About Art Therapy. https://arttherapy.org/about-art-therapy/

American Art Therapy Association. (2017). Ethical principles for art therapists. Retrieved December 2, 2022, from https://arttherapy.org/wp-content/uploads/2017/06/Ethical-Principles-for-Art-Therapists.pdf

A New Kind of House (2022, October 7). *Drexel University exhibitions & events.* https://guides.himmelfarb.gwu.edu/APA/web-page-no-author

Anderson, G. (2019). *Mission matters: Relevance and museums in the 21st century.* Rowman & Littlefield.

Annechini, C., Menardo, E., Hall, R., & Pasini, M. (2020). Aesthetic attributes of museum environmental experience: A pilot study with children as visitors. *Frontiers in Psychology, 11*, 300. https://doi.org/10.3389/fpsyg.2020.508300

Aspen Institute. (2021). *NeuroArts Blueprint* (Executive Summary). Johns Hopkins University.

BAAT (British Art Therapy Association) (2022). *Definition of art therapy.* https://baat.org/art-therapy/

Boffey, D. (2021, September 2). Brussels doctors to prescribe museum visits for Covid stress. *The Guardian.* www.theguardian.com/world/2021/sep/02/brussels-doctors-to-prescribe-museum-visits-for-covid-stress

Chatterjee, H., & Noble, G. (2013). *Museums, health and well-being.* Ashgate Publishing.

Chatterjee, A., & Vartanian, O. (2014). Neuroaesthetics. *Trends in Cognitive Sciences, 18*(7), https://doi.org/10.1016/j.tics.2014.03.003

Coleman, L. E. (2016). The socially inclusive museum: A typology re-imagined. *The International Journal of the Inclusive Museum, 9*(2). https://doi.org10.1080/09647779800401704

Coles, A., & Harrison, F. (2018). Tapping into museums for art psychotherapy: An evaluation of a pilot group for young adults. *International Journal of Art Therapy, 23*(3), 115–124. https://doi.org/10.1080/17454832.2017.1380056

Coles, A., Harrison, F., & Todd, S. (2019) Flexing the frame: Therapist experiences of museum-based group art psychotherapy for adults with complex mental health difficulties. *International Journal of Art Therapy, 24*(2), 56–67. https://doi.org/10.1080/17454832.2018.1564346

Coles, A. (Ed.). (2020). *Art therapy in museums and galleries: Reframing practices.* Jessica Kingsley.

Cowan, B., Laird, R., & McKeown, J. (2020). *Museum objects, health and healing.* Routledge de Botton, A., & Armstrong, J. (2013). *Art as therapy*. Phaidon Press.

Decter, A. Y., Semmel, M. L., & Yellis, K. (Eds.). (2022). *Change is required: Preparing for the post-pandemic museum*. Rowman & Littlefield.

Degas, E. (1868–69). *Interior* [Painting]. The Philadelphia Museum of Art, Philadelphia, PA, United States. https://philamuseum.org/collection/object/82556

Farrell-Kirk, R. (2021). Art therapy after the Stoneman Douglas High School shooting. In J. Scarce (Ed.), *Art therapy in response to natural disasters, mass violence, and crises* (pp. 212–225). Jessica Kingsley. ProQuest Ebook Central. http://ebookcentral.proquest.com/lib/drexel-ebooks/detail.action?docID=6825639

Fitchburg Art Museum (FAM). (2022). *2021 Annual Report*. Author.

Galetzka, C. (2017). The story so far: How embodied cognition advances our understanding of meaning-making. *Frontiers in Psychology*. https://doi:10.3389/fpsych.2017.01315

Ghadim, M. R., & Daugherty, L. (2021). *Preface*. In M. R. Ghadim & L. Daugherty (Eds.), *Museum-based art therapy* (p. xv). Routledge.

Gruenewald, T. (2021). *Curating America's painful past: Memory, museums, and the national imagination*. University Press of Kansas.

Hutchinson, S. (2015). Working with foster carers in the role of therapist at a local gallery. *British Art Therapy Association Newsbriefing*. www.atmag.org/wp-content/uploads/2013/12/Pages-from-News-briefing-December-2015-1.pdf

Ioannides, E. (2016) Museums as therapeutic environments and the contribution of art therapy. *Museum International*, *68*(3 –4), 98–109. https://doi.org/10.1111/muse.12125

King, J. L. (Ed.). (2016). *Art therapy, trauma, and neuroscience: Theoretical and practical perspectives*. Routledge.

King, J.L., Kaimal, G., Konopka, L., Belkofer, C., & Strang, E. (2019) Practical applications of neuroscience-informed art therapy. *Journal of the American Art Therapy Association*, *36*(3), 149–156. https://doi.org/10.1080/07421656.2019.1649549

Koban, L., Gianaros, P. J., Kober, H., & Wager, T. D. (2021). The self in context: Brain systems linking mental and physical health. Nature reviews. *Neuroscience*, *22*(5), 309–322. https://doi.org/10.1038/s41583-021-00446-8

Lusebrink, V. B., & Hinz, L. D. (2020). Cognitive and symbolic aspects of art therapy and similarities with large scale brain networks. *Art Therapy*, *37*(3), 113–122. https://doi.org/10.1080/07421656.2019.1691869

Meistere, U. (2021, September 1). *Museotherapy – the museum as a prescription*. Arterritory. https://arterritory.com/en/visual_arts/interviews/25738-museotherapy_-_the_museum_as_a_prescription/

Palamara, A., Ostheimer, R.T., Legari, S., Wiskera, E., & Evans, L. (2020, June 29). Trauma-aware art museum education: Principles & practices. *Art Museum Teaching*. https://artmuseumteaching.com/2020/06/29/trauma-aware-art-museum-education-principles-practices/

Peal, C. (1772; 1776; 1818). *Mrs. Peale Lamenting the Death of Her Child/Rachel Weeping* [Painting]. The Philadelphia Museum of Art, Philadelphia PA, United States. https://philamuseum.org/collection/object/71982

Plumley, A. (2020, Apr 2). *Museums and equity in times of crisis*. American Alliance of Museums. www.aam-us.org/2020/04/02/museums-and-equity-in-times-of-crisis/

Raicovich, L. (2021). *Culture strike: Art and museums in an age of protest*. Verso.

Rowson Love, A., & Szymanski, M. (2017). A third eye or a third space? Systems thinking and rethinking physical museum spaces. In Y. Jung & A. Rowson Love (Eds.), *Systems thinking in museums: Theory and practice* (pp. 195–204). Rowman & Littlefield

Simon, N. (2016). *The art of relevance*. Santa Cruz, CA: Museum 2.0.

Silverman, L.H. (2010). *The social work of museums*. Routledge.

Snyder, K. (2022). *Museum-based art therapy: Exploring possibilities and barriers with museum professionals*. [Manuscript submitted for publication]. Department of Creative Arts Therapies, Drexel University.

Snyder, K. (2022a). A museum's centering on healing through community care and social responsibility: A dialogue with Chloe Hayward of The Studio Museum of Harlem (USA). *Museological Review, 26*, 127–133. www.le.ac.uk/museological-review

Snyder, K. (2022b, June 2). An offering of hope and connection: The potential for art therapy in museum and cultural spaces [Poster]. Creative Interdisciplinary Research in Graduate Education (CIRGE) Creativity Salon, Drexel University, College of Arts and Sciences. https://drexel.edu/soe/research/research-initiatives/Creative-Interdisciplinary-Research-in-Graduate-Education/

Snyder, K., & Wolf, D. (2018, June 13). *Teaching tough topics: Trauma informed education, regulation and expression.* [Workshop Presentation. Philadelphia Museum of Art, Visual Arts Sources for Teaching Summer Workshop, Philadelphia, PA.

Swaback, K. (2021, Dec. 8). *Social Prescription Pilot explores positive health impacts of cultural experiences for people and communities.* Mass Cultural Council. https://massculturalcouncil.org/blog/social-prescription-pilot-explores-positive-health-impacts-of-cultural-experiences-for-people-communities/

The Extraordinary General Assembly of International Council of Museums. (2022, August 24). *Museum definition.* International Council of Museums. https://icom.museum/en/resources/standards-guidelines/museum-definition/

Timm-Bottos, J., & Reilly, R. C. (2015). Learning in third spaces: Community art studio as storefront university classroom. *American journal of community psychology, 55*(1), 102–114.

Toolis, E. (2018). *Museums as sites of social change: Exploring processes of placemaking and barriers to access and participation for underrepresented communities.* University of California, Santa Cruz.

Vander Ark, T., Liebtag, E., & McClennen, N. (2020). *The power of place: Authentic learning through place-based education.* ASCD.

Vartanian, H. (2019, March 22). *A museum hires a full-time therapist.* Hyperallergic. https://hyperallergic.com/491210/a-museum-hires-a-full-time-therapist/

Varutti, M. (2022, September 14). *The "emotional turn" in museum practice.* International Council of Museums (ICOM). https://icom.museum/en/news/the-emotional-turn-in-museum-practice/

Watson, E., Coles, A., & Jury, H. (2021). "A space that worked for them": Museum-based art psychotherapy, power dynamics, social inclusion and autonomy. *International Journal of Art Therapy.* https://doi.org/10.1080/17454832.2020.1866046

Wilson, L. (2022, Summer). More than writing, it's community. *Cross Roads.* https://drexelmagazine.org/2022/crossroads-more-than-writing-its-community/

CHAPTER 10

VOICES

Addressing Parkinson's Disease Symptomatology with Clay Manipulation

Morgan Gaydos and Deborah Elkis-Abuhoff

Parkinson's disease (PD) is a progressive, movement disorder that affects a large number of individuals on a global scale, with an estimated 10 million identified as living with PD worldwide (Parkinson's Foundation, 2022a). PD occurs when there is a loss of dopamine producing cells with the substantia nigra region of the midbrain; this area is primarily responsible for the body's ability to execute and coordinate movement. Although symptoms are unique to each individual, common motor symptoms include resting tremors in limbs, muscle stiffness, slowness of movement (bradykinesia), and loss of balance/freezing gait (Parkinson's Foundation, 2022b). The rise of PD awareness and research has also identified the presence of non-motor symptoms, which can include depression, anxiety, apathy, and changes in cognition (Parkinson's Foundation, 2022c). Alongside medication to treat symptoms, supportive therapies have been shown to not only support both motor and non-motor symptoms, but also to help individuals adjust to PD changes in lifestyle and improve quality of life (Michael J. Fox Foundation, 2022).

Art therapy has been found effective in treating individuals diagnosed with PD (Cucca et al., 2021; Elkis-Abuhoff & Gaydos, 2018; Junakovic & Telarovic, 2021), which starts with the understanding of the three tenets of art therapy: therapeutic relationship, creative process, and materials/methods (King, 2016). In the work of Elkis-Abuhoff and colleagues (2008; 2013; 2018; Goldblatt et al., 2010; Table 10.1), the material/method of clay manipulation largely played a role in observing improved physiological/motor symptoms and reported a decrease in areas of depression, anxiety, phobia, and obsessive-compulsive thinking.

With the clay manipulation directive, participants were invited to gently squeeze a ball of clay with each hand, warming up their hands while also becoming engaged with the material. Once ready, participants were instructed to break the material up into as many pieces as desired before integrating the clay back into a shape other than a ball. Through this hands-on approach, individuals diagnosed with PD demonstrated creative engagement, as the art material and process provided an integrative experience for verbal and visual responses, notable changes in affect, and improved flow/content of speech. This creative process also allowed for individuals to reflect on past memories and meaningful family relationships that brought them a sense of purpose and helped re-establish parts of their identity within a progressive diagnosis. The tactile material, flexible and adaptive in nature, provided an intimate sensory experience which contributed to the therapeutic relationship, as individuals opened up to share their appreciation for the safe space and verbalize meaning within their art. Rapport was created through this immersive experience and participants expressed wanting to continue the art therapy sessions as the therapeutic space

DOI: 10.4324/9781003348207-10

TABLE 10.1 Published work of Elkis-Abuhoff and colleagues

Authors	n =	Assessments/ Materials	Outcomes
Elkis-Abuhoff, D. L., Goldblatt, R. B., Gaydos, M., & Corrato, S. (2008). Effects of clay manipulation on somatic dysfunction and emotional distress in patients with Parkinson's disease. *Art Therapy: Journal of the American Art Therapy Association,* 25(3), 122–128.	n = 41	Brief Symptom Inventory (BSI) Clay manipulation One-time session	– A decrease in symptom severity for all 9 BSI domains for the PD group – Greater decrease in somatic symptoms and emotional distress in the PD group vs non-PD group
Goldblatt, R., Elkis-Abuhoff, D., Gaydos, M., & Napoli, A. (2010). Understanding clinical benefits of modeling clay exploration with patients diagnosed with Parkinson's disease. *Arts & Health,* 2(2), 140–148.	n = 22	Brief Symptom Inventory (BSI) Clay manipulation One-time session	– Three measures emerged as indicators for PD individuals' psychological adjustment: depression, obsessive- compulsive behaviors, and phobic anxiety – Significant decrease in all three indicators with scored closer to the adult norm after clay manipulation
Elkis-Abuhoff, D. L., Goldblatt, R. B., Gaydos, M., & Convery, C. (2013). A pilot study to determine the psychological effects of manipulation of therapeutic art forms among patients with Parkinson's disease. *International Journal of Art Therapy,* 18(3), 113–121.	n = 7	Brief Symptom Inventory (BSI) and Perceived Stress Scale 4 (PSS-4) Various types of clay medium 6-week group program, pre/post assessments at Week 1, 3, and 6	– The three BSI subscales of depression, obsessive-compulsive behaviors, and phobic anxiety all demonstrated a decrease pre/post – PSS-4 showed an increase at Week 1, but a decrease for Week 3 and Week 6 – Qualitative findings supported the group process, as comradeship and trust emerged from the process

Source: Published work of Elkis-Abuhoff and colleagues.

held trust, emotional expression, and self-exploration (Elkis-Abuhoff et al., 2013). In addition, notable results were found to support the use of clay manipulation within art therapy from a more scientific standpoint. Neurological responses were inferred by observing positive changes in participant behavior and improvements on a self-report symptom inventory (Table 10.1). When considering the results of these studies, the team began to examine the neurological effects of clay manipulation and how art therapy can improve symptomology by targeting areas of the brain.

Neuroplasticity, the brain's ability to physiologically rewire itself when one is engaged in a desired activity and/or learning something new, is a natural component within the art therapy process (Hass-Cohen & Findlay, 2015). This can be attributed to the notion that the act of creating art allows for the mind and body to work in tandem; art making requires physical movement, which leads the way to emotional processing and internal exploration (Elkis-Abuhoff & Gaydos, 2018). When engaged in a tactile/kinesthetic material, that relies on physical touch, stimulation from the area of the body engaged provides kinesthetic feedback to the brain. Sensory input from the art material appeared to result in improved motor output, where participants were observed with less rigidity in their hands and more physical control directly after engagement with clay (Elkis-Abuhoff et al., 2008). The final result is an immersive, creative experience that can lead to changes in affect/mood, improved cognition, and relief from PD symptoms within the moment (Elkis-Abuhoff & Gaydos, 2018).

Reestablishing connections within the brain through art making also plays a role in establishing feelings of resiliency within a diagnosis (Hass-Cohen & Findlay, 2015). In the work of Elkis-Abuhoff and colleagues, clay manipulation was able to accommodate a wide range of palm grips and levels of rigidity. Providing an art material that can be successfully used at many levels of symptomatology can allow participants to experience a sense of mastery after engagement as they were observed taking their time to work through motor symptoms, specifically hand tremors/rigidity; participants reported feeling a sense of relief when clay manipulation led to increased physical flexibility (Elkis-Abuhoff & Gaydos, 2018). The immersion and symbolism behind the clay manipulation translated into overcoming their limitations within the moment and adapting to changes cause by the PD diagnosis. Results from the work of Elkis-Abuhoff and colleagues, including improved motor ability and an emotional shift in the areas of depression, anxiety, and phobia, are highlighted in Table 10.1.

As the field of art therapy continues to acknowledge the natural, neuroscience component underscored when an individual engages in active art making, there is a need for future research and collaboration across disciplines, such as working alongside neurologists and occupational therapists. As PD continues to progress and increase on a global level, a reliance on allied care professions, such as art therapy, can help individuals learn to manage their symptoms and move forward within their diagnosis (Michael J. Fox Foundation, 2022). Clinicians within the art therapy and neuroscience fields can come together to broaden the effectiveness of treatment by addressing the whole person and their range of symptoms, while simultaneously utilizing the creative capacities of each individual.

Applied Educational Neuroscience©

Lori Desautels and Ashlee Harmon

The framework of AEN© addresses brain and nervous system development through an educator's lens as we explore the four pillars that support physiological, emotional, social, and cognitive well-being (Figure 10.1). The pillars lean into one another and include educator brain and body state, touch points, co-regulation, and teaching students and staff about their neuroanatomy and nervous systems (Desautels, 2020). The four pillars reinforce a relational, preventative, and nervous system-aligned discipline lens that addresses the sensations, feelings, thoughts, and

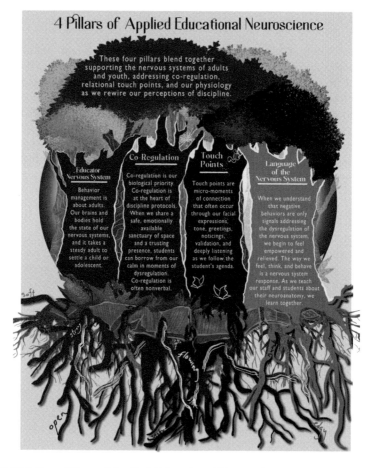

FIGURE 10.1 Four Pillars of Applied Educational Neuroscience

behaviors of students and staff. This relational and preventative perception of discipline is a conceptual approach cultivating co-regulatory practices which strengthen connections in the classroom, integrated through educator procedures, routines, and transitions throughout the day to build a nurturing and inclusive environment. The foundation of this framework begins with adult nervous system awareness and regulation. When adults are attending to their autonomic state functioning, there is more capacity to co-regulate a difficult experience, condition, or event with students. The AEN© framework supports relational nervous system-aligned and preventative trauma-sensitive discipline protocols by addressing the sensory systems that lie beneath misunderstood behaviors (Desautels, 2020). When we activate the regions of the brain we want to develop, we are providing practices that can lead to changes in brain function and structure, enhancing emotional and social well-being and improved academic performance (Perry & Winfrey, 2021).

10.1   FOCUSED ATTENTION PRACTICES

We are implementing Focused Attention Practices in the schools for all ages. Focused Attention Practices can calm or energize the nervous system and support self-regulation. Approaching students and staff in ways that align with their brain and nervous system states is critical for our emotional, mental, and physiological well-being. These practices can generate energy for sleepy, tired, or immobilized nervous systems or they can calm the nervous system for learning, addressing our sensory and nervous systems, accessing the frontal cortex where executive functions are activated. We integrate these practices at the beginning of class or class period, throughout the day as needed, and closing the school day or class period. When our autonomic states find a balance of steadiness, we can think clearly, problem-solve, and hold stronger memory with increased attention (Desautels, 2020).

Ashlee Harmon, sixth-grade teacher and former graduate student of Dr. Lori Desautels in the *Applied Educational Neuroscience* certification program at Butler University, founded *Mindful Artists Club* to bridge creation with artistic mediums and neuroanatomy education for students. Since 2019, *Mindful Artists Club* functions as a community of regulation, neuroscience innovation, and artistic creativity for fifth- and sixth-grade students at Avon Intermediate School West in Avon, Indiana. Students meet monthly to create artistic representations of how they are experiencing their nervous systems throughout the day, paired with learning critical processes of the brain.

At the start of each *Mindful Artists Club* meeting, students engage in a focused attention practice designed specifically for the theme of our meeting to prime their nervous system for accessing regulation. Color-oriented focused attention practices are most commonly used in our meetings as students explore the value and power of connecting colors to brain state illustrations. *Colors of My Heart* is a focused attention practice where students use colored pencils to first draw a heart and then fill the heart with shapes and colors that identify their current brain state. Students similarly engage with colors in *Color Palette Breathing*. In this focused attention practice, students begin by viewing a color palette, then choosing one color from the palette that represents a positive emotion students want to feel. Students close their eyes, if they feel comfortable, and take mindful, slow breaths while visualizing that color entering their nervous system. Both of these color-oriented focused attention practices also yield invaluable conversation and discovery of each student's unique perspective on colors and the sensations they bring to our meetings.

10.2   TEACHING NEUROANATOMY

While exploring the merging of art with awareness of brain state, students in *Mindful Artists Club* engage in hands-on learning of neuroanatomy concepts appropriate for upper-elementary learners. This is a critical first step for *Mindful Artists Club* students before they begin to create their artistic representations of neuroscience. At our first meeting of the year, students are introduced to three-dimensional brain models of the six major structures of the brain (frontal lobe, parietal lobe, occipital lobe, temporal lobe, cerebellum, and brain stem). As students physically hold the brain models and analyze their different parts, *Artistic Neuroscience Mentors* (previous student members who receive training by Ashlee on how to instruct their peers on neuroanatomy) lead lessons on the functions of each region of the brain. Sparking connections and interests in neuroanatomy creates excitement, joy, and curiosity as our students see first-hand the wonderment of our neurological workings and the possibilities of accessing moments of emotional regulation.

In the artistic application of our neuroanatomy lessons, *Mindful Artists Club* students create a variety of colorful representations of neuroanatomy through the lens of achieving regulation and awareness of brain state. For example, in *My Brain Model*, students use the medium of clay to craft models of their brain. As a precursor to this project, students use three-dimensional brain models to touch and manipulate the lobes of the brain to feel and see the neuroanatomy they will be replicating. To connect with color association practices, students paint each lobe with a color they associate with each function.

10.3   NEUROPLASTICITY

As *Mindful Artists Club* students engage in additional sessions on brain anatomy, we begin to transition to experiences with neuron models. In efforts to merge art making with theories of neuroplasticity, it is imperative that *Mindful Artists Club* students first engage in neuroanatomy lessons to visualize the processes behind neuron functions and the importance of repetition in neural thoughts and actions. During our beginning stages of learning about neurons, students interact with an enlarged neuron model in conjunction with lessons about the sensations and miracles of our nervous system that lead to our greatest superpower: neuroplasticity. From these hands-on interactions with the nervous system, students view media (e.g., three-dimensional renderings of synaptic transmission) to see neuroplasticity in action.

Artistic representations of neuroplasticity are a focal point in our latter sessions of the year as students engage in applying knowledge from their nervous system lessons. *Neuroplasticity is My Superpower* is one project students create through the artistic medium of either colored pencils or markers. Students begin this project by jotting down a few words that represent dysregulating emotions and/or sensations they are experiencing (e.g., shaky, cold, confined, etc.). With the mentorship of our *Artistic Neuroscience Mentors*, students are taught to add reframing words to the emotions and/or sensations they listed (e.g., shaky to stable, cold to warm, confined to free, etc.). This reframing process is taught through the lens of neuroplasticity, and students begin to create their *Neuroplasticity is My Superpower* project. Students first draw themselves as a superhero with a cape. On the cape, students include their reframing words as a visual reminder of their neuroplasticity superpower. This illustration is encouraged to be kept in a place where students can regularly see it.

10.4 TOUCHPOINTS

Bridging the natural rhythms, motions, and other sensory experiences of art with educational neuroscience knowledge guides many art projects in *Mindful Artists Club*. The variety of artistic mediums that are accessible for learners of all ages yields opportunities for students to use the colors and textures of their world for tier-one practices that support a calmer nervous system. One of *Mindful Artists Club*'s first meetings involves creating *Sensory Cubes* where students choose from a variety of fabric textures to create sensory cubes that promote regulation, creating a touch point for accessing their frontal lobe. Students are given a blank wooden cube, glue, and a variety of fabrics, from leather to sequins to plush. The process of students choosing their preferred textures creates calm as they fire up their neural signals of touch and sight to identify what feels calm and safe.

The natural artistry of light and darkness also connects with regulation as students study their "upstairs brain" (prefrontal cortex) and "downstairs brain" (brain stem) (Real Happy Endings, 2021). In our *Upstairs Brain vs. Downstairs Brain Illustrations* project, students use the framework of the sun (bright spots of calmness) and the moon (dark spots of dysregulation) to create illustrations of what makes them feel regulated vs. dysregulated using the medium of markers. This project removes the stigma of dysregulation as students are taught that our natural world has a day and night just like our natural bodies have regulation and dysregulation.

The framework of Applied Educational Neuroscience cultivates co-regulatory and sensory practices that move children and youth from autonomic states of protection to autonomic states of growth. When we meet our youth in their emotional and sensory states, integrating art, rhythm, breath, and movement, we help them to access the cortical regions of the brain where sustained attention, working memory, problem-solving and creativity can be activated.

Neuro-informed Art Therapy, Trauma, and Supervision Training Approach, Guided by the Principles of Adlerian Psychology

Erin Rafferty-Bugher

As the mental health field expands and develops in-depth understanding of neuroscience-informed psychotherapy and trauma frameworks (Cozolino, 2017), art therapy master's degree programs have a responsibility to integrate neuroscience-informed trauma approaches into training and supervision curricula. Neurocounseling (Miller, 2016; Miller & Beeson, 2020) is the inclusion of neuroscience-informed approaches in counseling education and has been introduced within counselor educator supervision training. Neurocounseling provides practitioners with a rationale to integrate neuroeducation into training, naming externalization, empathy, universality, regulation, and engagement as key therapeutic factors used to support the developing professional. Three concepts are highlighted in neurocounseling to incorporate into professional training: (1) neuroeducation; psychoeducation on brain functions and structures including an emphasis on neuroplasticity; (2) neurofeedback; supports awareness of a person's innate ability to be aware of, regulate, and monitor their biological internal systems and functions; and (3) metaphor-based approaches in teaching neuroscience principles using experiential and creative methods for integration of learning and knowledge acquisition (Duenyas & Luke, 2019). Similar to counselor training, art therapy training and supervision may consider incorporating these three neuroscience concepts for the emerging art therapy professional.

Art therapy research continues to expand and confirms the significant connection of art therapy and neuroscience (Kaimal et al., 2016; King, 2016; King et al., 2019). These researchers specifically highlight the impact of neurobiological processes involved in art therapy when engaging with art materials and the impact on various structures and mechanisms involved within brain systems (Lusebrink, 2010). The Expressive Therapies Continuum® (ETC) framework advances application practices and further developed neuroscience-informed therapeutic applications and engagement with art materials and media (Hinz, 2009). The ETC proposes that optimal, well-functioning brain activity includes healthy neuronal networking towards holistic brain integration (Lusebrink & Hinz, 2016). Art therapy applications informed by the ETC framework is foundational in developing neuro-informed art therapy and trauma prepared professionals, and placement should be considered in the beginning of art therapy programs when considering a neuro-informed curriculum.

Integrating and centering a culturally responsive approach in neuro-informed art therapy education training and supervision is a professional ethical responsibility (Awais & Blausey, 2021; Jackson, 2020; Kuri, 2017; Menakem, 2017; Potash, 2018;). Adlerian psychology offers a comprehensive theoretical approach as a foundational framework for connecting overarching neuroscience concepts to anchor in training (Miller et al., 2016). Adlerian theory links neuroscience concepts based on the tenets of "belonging, socially embedded connections, holism, and considers the individual's unique cognitive worldview or lifestyle" (p. 125). Adlerian theory grounds postmodern, collectivist, social–relational approaches for emerging art therapy professionals (Aslinia et.al, 2011; Irvine et.al, 2021). This integrated framework posits an ethically responsible neuro-informed art therapy and trauma model in training and supervision for professional preparation, practice, and application of skills and knowledge.

Models for teaching within this context incorporate neuro-informed trauma concepts within course content and deliver opportunities for those concepts to be reinforced and applied in internship supervision for professional preparedness. The courses would be best served to provide foundational teaching on neuroanatomy in a developmental progression, designed to prepare students to integrate and synthesize neuro-informed concepts learned, practiced and eventually applied into client case conceptualization. Examples of student art-based assignments aligning the three neurocounseling concepts within teaching this model are presented to highlight potential neuro-informed considerations for inclusion in training and supervision. An example of neuroeducation represents a student's synthesis and understanding of general brain functionality, processes, and mechanisms in an assignment to create a model of the brain (Figure 10.2). Figure 10.3 reflects

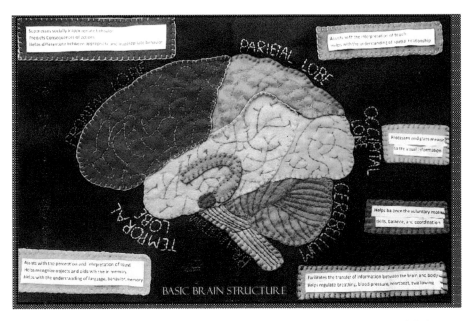

FIGURE 10.2 Neuroeducation example; neuroanatomy of the brain. A model demonstrating synthesis of general brain functionality, processes, and mechanisms. Felt stitching by Maria Siddiqui

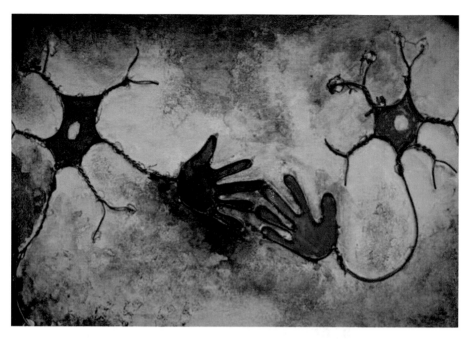

FIGURE 10.3 Neuroeducation emphasizing neuroplasticity example; includes cellular representation of neurotransmitter and dendrite synaptic connection within a trusting therapeutic relationship. Paint and wire by Maria Siddiqui

another example of neuroeducation with specific emphasis on neuroplasticity, a key concept in neuro-informed trauma training. This image represents cellular structures and includes dendrite connectivity that highlights, through metaphor and symbol, the significance of a trusting therapeutic relationship or perception of safety in therapy neuroception; all suggested key concepts in neuro-informed trauma training. Figure 10.4 is an image that reflects a metaphor-based synthesis of a student's understanding of the autonomic nervous system and its biological response to trauma and adversity. The image reflects the polyvagal theory; a conceptual framework in therapy to provide understanding of autonomic reactivity (Dana, 2018). This image is also an example of neurofeedback, as a metaphor highlights the significance of biological-based opportunities to engage in regulatory experiences. There are numerous neuro-and trauma-informed considerations to include within art therapy graduate training and supervision preparation that creatively integrate the increasing developmental complexity and relevance for the emerging professional art therapist.

Art therapy education has historically incorporated experiential, art-based creative approaches (Leigh, 2021) emphasizing insight and the development of self-awareness as integral key components in training and supervision. The process of connecting sensations, feelings, and perceptions into cognitive awareness is a crucial factor in training for the development of an ethical, culturally responsible, emerging professional art therapist; encouraging the radical consciousness of the self as a culturally responsive professional (Talwar, 2019). Figure 10.5 highlights an

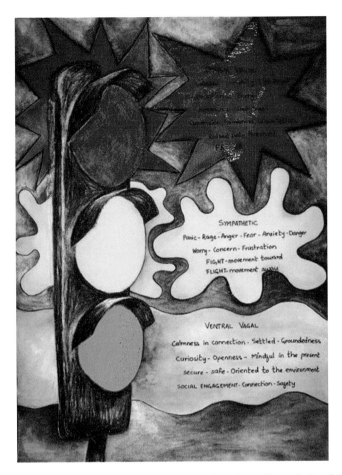

FIGURE 10.4 Neurofeedback; example of a metaphor for self-regulation based on the polyvagal theory in therapy and the autonomic nervous systems role in biological responses to trauma. Colored pencil and pen by Maria Siddiqui

example of a metaphor-based approach using response art in internship supervision as a self-reflective and insight-oriented practice (Fish, 2019). The assignment includes prompts that further engage exploration and investigation of a tree as a metaphor for the self, centering cultural identity as an emerging professional as integral to the assignment. Art-based reflection and inquiry, using the ETC framework within a neuro-informed context, provides a method and approach to directly access implicit perceptions, thoughts, and feelings using media and materials as the bridge or conduit connecting conscious cognitive awareness (King et al., 2019, p. 151). This approach links key neuroscience concepts for consideration in art therapy education, training, and supervision.

Arts-based metaphor and experiential teaching methods informed by the tenets of neurocounseling, ETC framework and Adlerian principles, provide a neuro-informed trauma training approach that includes an emphasis on self-reflective and conscious awareness practice, bringing implicit and unconscious material into

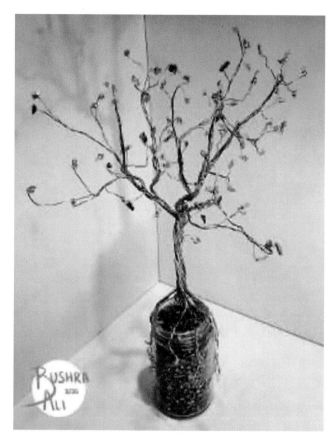

FIGURE 10.5 Metaphor-based approach example of resiliency. Art response assign-
          ment as a self-reflective practice within internship supervision course.
          Wire, glass and beads by Bushra Ali

conscious awareness (Figure 10.5). The model may offer a theoretical structure to
guide neuro-informed art therapy and trauma training and supervision. This framework provides a holistic training method promoting the opportunity for healthy integrated individuals and a more resilient and thriving community.

Storycloths

Lisa Garlock

On the placard next to the soft looking, cream-colored quilt at the Smithsonian Renwick Gallery, I read,

Comforter …
Paul Villinski began making this comforter while recovering from drug and alcohol addiction. He recalls, "I needed a way to sit still, especially at night, so I spent multiple hours hand-stitching most evenings for about six months. I was coming to understand that I had been taking the comfort needed to survive from drugs and booze, but I was learning in sobriety to find that comfort in other human beings." The artist often held hands with others during recovery meetings. He stitched together these work gloves—turned inside out to reveal the soft interior—to suggest the warmth and stability of a community wrapping its arms around him. Each stitch reflects the journey of his mind and hands and his restoration and connectedness.
(Smithsonian Art Museum, This Present Moment:
Crafting a Better World exhibit, 2022–23) (Figure 10.6)

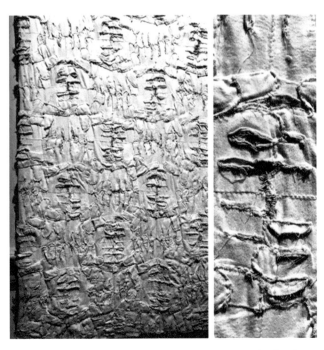

FIGURE 10.6 Hand stitched, inside-out work glove quilt by Paul Villinski. Smithsonian Art Museum, This Present Moment: Crafting a Better World exhibit, 2022–23

This short description of an artwork reveals multiple layers of complexity inherent in healing using hand stitching. This piece falls within the realm of storycloths, which are also known as story quilts, arpilleras, memory cloths, and narrative textiles (Garlock, 2021). A story cloth is a narrative that is told visually, using fabric; often the fabrics have meaningful histories – remnants of favorite clothing, cloth from a grandparent, ritual fabric, handwoven or hand dyed cloth. Using these types of fabric in narrative textiles adds to the idea of "making special" (Dissanayake, 1988, p. 92), which is also an important concept in art therapy. Images are created using a wide variety of techniques, depending on culture, skills, and materials. The quilt described above is metaphorical, symbolic and abstract, rather than narrative, yet each stitch may represent a memory, feeling, thought, or hope. The artist used this project in order to "sit still," and it most likely became a meditative and calming way to reflect, while creating and exploring comfort, connection, and sobriety.

In art therapy, textiles are considered a non-traditional art material; the art therapy founders were specific in choosing fine art materials with which to work (Moon, 2010). However, using a needle and thread is as traditional as charcoal on a cave wall; the needle as technology is basically the same as it was 40,000 years ago (Pagano, 2019). According to Robson and Kaplan (2003, in Huotilainen, et al., 2018),

> Arts and crafts were a crucial ingredient in the lives of hunter-gatherer groups and were passed on from one generation to the next. The link between our bodily activities, such as use of the hands, and our cognitive abilities, such as perception, memory, attention or creativity, can be understood in the light of this link in hunter-gatherer life.
>
> (p. 12)

Cutting, placing, and sewing, plus texture, pattern, color, and organizing the details of the story with textiles connects the here and now with deep roots of our ancestors.

In many cultures, traditionally people sewed in community. They gathered to work on individual projects, on collective pieces, or on projects that benefited the entire community. This idea reflects the above artist's recognition of connecting with others as a path to "comfort." In Common Threads Project, an integrative trauma recovery program, sewing circles are key to being able to heal from the trauma of sexual violence. In a sewing circle, participants can focus on their hands and sewing, while also listening and talking as stories unfold. From feminist, multicultural, and narrative perspectives, people stitching and sewing in community can create an egalitarian environment where power differentials are leveled. Cooperation, collaboration, and lifting each other up become the norm as people share fabrics, trade threads and techniques, appreciate each other's work, and realize that they all have stories to which others can relate. Additionally, textile work has also been shown to reduce depression, anxiety, and trauma-related symptoms (Cohen, n.d.; Collier et al., 2016; Reynolds, 2000). Reducing depression implies an increase in the ability to experience pleasure, which many people cited as a reason to make with textiles (Collier, 2012). Reduction in anxiety can mean fewer activating thoughts, a calming of the autonomic nervous system, and a lower heart rate. Fewer trauma-related symptoms may reflect being in the here and now, with tactile and kinesthetic materials, and experiencing repetitive, rhythmic, and rewarding movements of hands as the images take shape (Perry, 2006).

In Common Threads Project, the goal is to evolve from therapist facilitated circles, to independent, peer support circles. Advocacy also plays a role in healing from trauma, and each group can decide if they want to exhibit their storycloths, tell their stories in public, and work on educating, reducing stigma and empowering others (Cohen & Butterly, 2020). Likewise, by making art, exhibiting it, and discussing his own struggles with addiction, Villinski ("Comforter" creator) advocates for others who may be in similar situations.

Hand stitching a narrative also taps strongly into neurological underpinnings. Research has found that engaging in complex creative tasks, such as quilting, is important for developing new neural pathways, activating various parts of the brain, and increasing learning and memory (McDonough et al., 2015). Lusebrink's Expressive Therapies Continuum (ETC) constructs a theory of how the brain develops and works in relation to art-making and materials. Using the ETC, art therapists understand how art materials help children with their development on multiple levels (Hinz, 2020). Hinz discusses the idea of large-scale brain networks, where multiple areas of the brain interact in order to facilitate learning, memory, attention, and other complex elements of perception and behavior (Koziol et al., 2014, in Hinz, 2020). McDonough et al. (2015) saw more brain area activation in older people engaged in challenging activities (quilting), and very little activation when engaging in low challenge activities.

Throughout the process of creating a story cloth, all levels of the ETC are engaged – kinesthetic/sensory, affective/perceptual, cognitive/symbolic, and creative (Figure 10.7). Storycloth making requires creativity in the inception of the idea

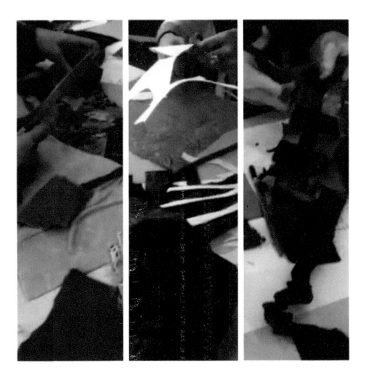

FIGURE 10.7 Images showing aspects of designing, laying out, and choosing materials

and throughout the process as the maker continually contemplates the design and layout and moves pieces around as the storycloth develops. Cognitive skills are used in planning the design, decision making, storytelling and story writing, organization and figuring out the steps, measuring, and conferring with others about techniques. Emotional content varies depending on the story and what the maker chooses to show, yet emotions elicited while working may be deep, surprising, and enlightening. Fabric color, texture, pattern, and image, along with types of stitches, can all work together for affective impact. As with most art media, the storycloth process is very kinesthetic, activating most of the senses: vision, the sense of smell, touch, hearing, and movement. Occasionally, certain fibers can cause sneezing or mild allergies if participants are sensitive.

Storycloth making is a multistep, slow process that lends itself well to working through traumatic experiences. Both hands are being used simultaneously when hand sewing (Figure 10.8), and the eyes are moving slightly to the left and right as stitches are being made; the sewer can also focus on their breathing to match the rhythm of their stitching, as in a mindfulness practice which is associated with increased mental wellness and decreased negative feelings (Huotilainen et al., 2018). Storycloth making in community encourages relationship building; research

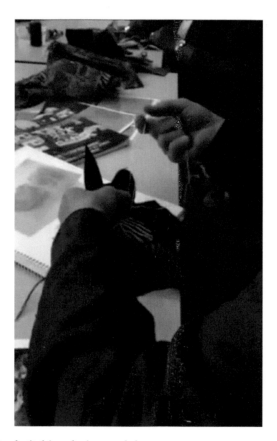

FIGURE 10.8 Hand stitching during workshop

is showing that in groups, brains can become synchronized, creating "similarity in brain responses" depending in part on "the common ground created by having a conversation" (Leong, in Hughes, 2022). Relating personal and universal stories serves to connect people, create bonds and friendships, and strengthen community. Making storycloths works well for processing trauma, elevating mood, mastering challenging materials, and using multiple areas of the brain in order to learn, grow, and heal.

Connecting Neuroscience to Caribbean Art Therapy Trauma Practice

Sarah Soo Hon and Karina Donald

Caribbean nations are categorized as a group of small island developing states (United Nations, 2020). As a multicultural region, nations share histories from indigenous groups of Taino and Kalinago peoples to colonization by Western Europe until the 20th Century. As former colonies, nations also share similar cultures (Burton, 2009) steeped in centuries of slavery and indentureship. Over time, these nations are known to use the arts in performances to process trauma and music to articulate social and cultural identities (Mahabir, 2015). These developing states still have much to understand about art therapy practices because of limited resources for mental health practice and research (Walker et al., 2022). In addition, there is urgency for art therapy interventions to redress cross-cultural issues (Hocoy, 2002) and develop a decolonizing approach to cultural competence (Potash et al., 2017). In view of this, the following vignettes illustrate the importance of culturally informed practice and how art is used to process traumatic experiences in two nations: Grenada and Trinidad and Tobago. Here, we consider the potential for a theoretical underpinning of neuroscience to inform a broadened understanding of resilience within a contextualized practice of communal and individualized art therapy.

The spontaneous use of movement, music, and singing are aspects of Caribbean culture (Allen, 2019) that are integrated into art therapy trauma treatment. Acknowledging that the body holds memories of trauma (Van der Kolk, 2014) facilitated trauma processing for a 6-year old Grenadian female. The client was referred for trauma processing of sexual abuse. In the first three sessions, the client was inconsolable by her family members and the therapist. She was preoccupied with being in a closed room and seemed tense because she assumed that she must talk about her trauma. The client was resistant to art-based trauma protocols, which did not integrate music and movement – common practices in the Caribbean context. Drawing on the strengths of her Caribbean value for artistic expressions through music and dance, the client's level of arousal decreased. By using the kinesthetic–sensory approach to treatment (Hinz, 2020), 18 by 24 and 24 by 30-inch sheets of paper were taped to the walls and floors of the therapy room, which created reflective distance and anxiety management (Hass-Cohen et al., 2014). The gradual exploration of her favorite songs with spontaneous singing and large arm and leg movements aided in differentiating current and past emotions related to trauma. The client's engagement in rhythmic movements created a state of flow by using a well-timed intervention (Wilkinson & Chilton, 2013) that encouraged her cultural strength (Csíkszentmihályi, 1991) of music and movement.

After those sessions, other novel art materials were gradually introduced that increased interest in the creative process while also moderating cortisol, noradrenaline, and dopamine levels (Hass-Cohen et al., 2014). The client added her art to pre-drawn outlines of figures aligned with the expressive culture of boundaries (Mahabir, 2015). She used markers and oil pastels first to relate happy feelings, and at the midpoint of treatment showed a reduction of anxiety (Eaton & Tieber, 2017). In later sessions, she requested sheets of paper taped to walls to allow for spontaneous dancing, and hand movement to process trauma. Opportunities for kinesthetic art engagement grounded in Caribbean culture supported cognitive processing of trauma and release of physical tension in ways that would not have been possible with the use of protocols that were not culturally informed.

The integration of performance, music, and visual art into the communal response to trauma is also observed in Trinidad and Tobago (Soo Hon, 2021). Community violence has a documented impact on the psychosocial well-being of adolescents in Trinidad and Tobago (Rollocks et al., 2013; Soo Hon, 2021), with homicide considered to be the leading cause of death for adolescent boys (UNICEF, 2014). The Office of the Special Representative of the Secretary-General (SRSG) on Violence against Children (2016) points out that community violence can have a cumulative negative effect on children, leading to death, injury, life-long mental and emotional harm, lowered academic performance, risk of becoming violent, and undesired societal and cultural effects. In exploring how adolescents may use culturally relevant arts practices to support their own psychosocial well-being, expressions of loss following the sudden death of an adolescent boy illustrated the potential for group art to support the processing of a traumatic experience.

During data collection for a wider research project at a high school situated in Laventille, a community in Trinidad where there is a high incidence of gang-related activity and violence (Adams et al., 2018; Seepersad, 2016), news reports confirmed that a student was killed outside of his home in a drive-by shooting. While the range of staff and student responses to this experience of loss included musical tributes, public demonstrations, and media appeals for a safer community, one particular response that is highlighted in this vignette is the emergence of graffiti on the walls and ceiling of the student's classroom. According to Hass-Cohen et al. (2014), "traumatic memories present as strongly nonverbal, situational, emotional, and sensory experiences along with relatively weak verbal representations of those experiences" (p. 69). The graffiti observed in the classroom was a spontaneous tribute to the deceased student and was initiated by his peers. This body of work preceded group discussions and appeared to express a sense of loss not readily verbalized by students in discussion or informal conversations.

Key elements of this body of work included multiple contributors, the repetition of phrases such as "RIP" (Rest in Peace) and "SIP" (Sleep in Peace) and its large scale when viewed as a whole, encompassing four walls, the ceiling and outer wall of the classroom. More detailed elements included posters made of bristol paper with a pasted image of the deceased boy and personal messages of love. This mural-like graffiti evidences both sensorimotor (Hass-Cohen et al., 2014) and communal (Kapitan et al., 2011) experiences toward neurobiological processing, healing, and reconciliation. The sensorimotor process described by Hass-Cohen et al. (2014) suggests that expressive activities stimulate coping, mastery, and control, as well as support feelings of safety, and cognitive and emotional flexibility that enable neurobiological processing of traumatic narratives. The communal process articulated by Kapitan et al. (2011) involves critical inquiry using the creative arts to develop the capacity to reflect and respond to adverse situations. As the graffiti covered a large area of the classroom, kinesthetic (Hinz, 2020) and sensorimotor experiences (Hass-Cohen et al., 2014) can be inferred from the resulting imagery. Additionally, the graffiti, as a student-led initiative, reflects the potential for communities to use the arts to help its members transform personal tragedy into shared experiences that restore collective identity (Kapitan et al., 2011).

Although there is still much to be explored within the intersections of neuroscience, art therapy, and culture, these vignettes illustrate the potential for neuroscience to deepen understanding of how culturally relevant arts practices can be integrated into trauma treatment to support individual and community resilience.

Connecting the Words of Healing through Amorphous Art

Laura Gruce

This vignette is from an art therapist, working with a combat veteran during his treatment in a residential program at a Veteran's Hospital in South Florida. The veteran is referred to as "Paul" to protect his identity. Paul was experiencing symptoms from post-traumatic stress disorder (PTSD), isolation, and anxiety. Paul had withdrawn significantly from peers and loved ones.

During the beginning weeks of the art therapy group, Paul presented with much resistance to this treatment. He did not believe art was the correct modality for him and could not understand how it could help. Paul would not talk or emote much during his initial art therapy sessions.

In the art therapy group, we worked together to establish a safe place with the reiteration of boundaries, confidentiality, and respect for others. A multisensory approach was used, combining a visual and tactile process to the materials. Art materials ranged from abstract paints to more tactile, grounding materials. Breathing exercises, guided imagery, and relaxing music helped ease feelings of resistance. These exercises seemed to help stabilize Paul's nervous system and connected him with the present moment in preparation for the art directives.

WEEK 1

The initial group session began with a theme of identity, starting with self-portraits. I established a therapeutic relationship with the group while working to establish an individual connection with each group member. Topics focused on identity, self-esteem, and those times where there may be self-doubt or feelings of their loss of self. During this group, the other members were able to create their self-portraits. Paul responded as having difficulty with this exercise and just observed the group, interacting socially.

WEEK 2

Group members were encouraged to draw their "opposite" self by creating a portrait that represented the opposite way they were identifying or feeling at the time. Various art materials were introduced and modified as necessary. Paul was not too engaged in this group. He talked to the art therapist and shared a photo of his favorite place during this session. Paul shared that he did not feel like an artist. He shared that his "opposite self" would be that one day he would be able to draw this favorite photo. It was a photo of a lounge chair, in ocean water, in a tropical setting.

WEEK 3

The group created their "future-self" and what that might look like. Paul identified feelings on the inside that did not align with what he created in the artwork, which could indicate isolation of affect, and could mean that it was necessary for Paul to compartmentalize his feelings. Paul was still not openly sharing or making evident connections to his art, compared to the other group members that were.

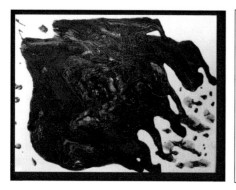

Journal (Week 4) "I picked up my first colors sort of bright ... sprayed the canvas knew this wasn't for me. The colors looked like happiness and I was not happy. I have to show some frustration. I look at some other colors and all bright colors things started to mesh, okay so this is how I feel; angry, mad, depressed, anxious, hate, hopeless, helpless, so many negative feelings on this canvas. "I drew what I feel – all the hate and frustration I have inside – even though on the outside I look happy – I am not."

FIGURE 10.9 Journal Week 4. Cara, V., David, D., & Gruce, L., (2019). *There and Back Again, Art as a Journey Through One's Hell – Case Report ID 449*

WEEK 4

The intervention transitioned to abstract art by working with acrylic pouring. This fluid medium is hard to control, as it lacks in defined shapes or forms. This type of amorphous art can help with patience, and the challenges of frustration tolerance. The kinetic process of the moving and mixing of the paints seemed to evoke a regression in Paul; he appeared to rely on primitive defenses to help tolerate his anxiety. Paul had difficulty finding words. Using the art materials, I encouraged Paul to find those pathways to his true self. Paul was very focused and engaged when working with the abstract art materials. Paul's first reaction to his painting (Figure 10.9) were that the colors were too bright and happy. He insightfully understood how he had presented this way to others, superficially as "bright and happy"; however, on the inside he was feeling anger and isolation. This was a great exercise for Paul to practice letting go of his attachment to outcomes, and past ideologies. From his journal notes, Paul had begun to make a therapeutic shift as he recognized that the brighter colors were meshing with the darker colors, and his real feelings began to emerge. This experience seemed to bring him more peace, and less frustration. He began connecting to his authentic self.

WEEKS 5–6

We continued with abstract directives that encouraged self-expression. During week 6, the art therapy group was asked to think about patterns in their lives. Members were encouraged to create a visual interpretation of those behavioral patterns.

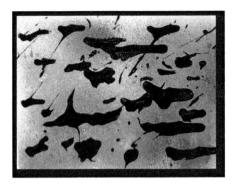

Journal (Week 6) **"I did not realize how there is life and positive things for me. I just kept closing and isolating from help. I believed I was doing the right thing, becoming so selfish. I was hurting one and loved ones."**

FIGURE 10.10 Journal Week 6. Cara, V., David, D., & Gruce, L., (2019). *There and Back Again, Art as a Journey Through One's Hell – Case Report ID 449*

I offered examples to the group, such as spirals, grids, or waves, that may replicate internal feelings. Paul created a spotted, amorphic pattern, continuing with his primal spontaneous expression without any attachment to symbols. Paul continued to resist vocalizing his true feelings. At this time, he started with bright pink and blue paint colors and then added the darker red amoebic forms in the foreground. He did not share much verbally (Figure 10.10). In his journal quote, Paul recognized how his past behavioral patterns were hurting himself and his loved ones. Here we are working within that safe realm between verbal and non-verbal expression, while maintaining the therapeutic relationship (King, 2016).

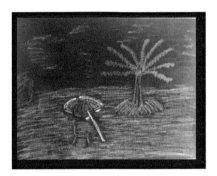

Journal (Week 7) **"The more I expressed my feelings (in the other classes and group activities) the more I would relate it to my art therapy. I felt everything was falling back into place. I was being more creative and actually drawing where I would like to be in the future. Every subject, staff, material that I was taught in the other therapeutic modalities, I would practice in art therapy. By expressing art, I was expressing my feelings. I went from anger and dark colors to bright and feeling happy. I'm starting to see that I can change and have a positive life."**

FIGURE 10.11 Journal Week 7. Cara, V., David, D., & Gruce, L., (2019). *There and Back Again, Art as a Journey Through One's Hell – Case Report ID 449*

WEEK 7

As a grounding exercise, I asked the group to create their safest place, to show where they would like to exist in the future. This supported a "Bottom-up approach" (Shnider, 2018) that encouraged sensory engagement of and a reflected change for Paul from his older restricted ideas. Paul was becoming more invested in the art process. He drew a picture of his favorite place, using oil pastels on black construction paper. His bright colors and lines were striking and appeared brighter than his past work. This mirrored his affect, and he was improving his ability to share and socialize with confidence. Paul created a drawing of his perfect, desired outcome. Paul's art became more representational, as he became more verbally insightful (Figure 10.11).

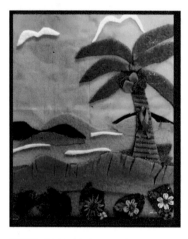

Journal (Weeks 9 & 10) **"She gave me back my faith and hope. I realized that art therapy is not about a famous person, but that I am the famous painter, its my work, and I understand my work. In the time I was here, I noticed my progress in many ways, but in my art, I can demonstrate my feelings more."**

FIGURE 10.12 Journal Week 9 and 10. Cara, V., David, D., & Gruce, L., (2019). *There and Back Again, Art as a Journey Through One's Hell – Case Report ID 449*

WEEKS 9–10

For the final project, the group members were encouraged to re-create their favorite image using sensory materials. Paul was eager to work on this with much focus and enthusiasm. This exercise seemed to elicit increased self-awareness and insight from Paul. He wanted to make sure he had enough time to create this image. He spent extra time, during his last two group sessions to make certain his art was completed. His finished piece was a tropical scene that depicted Paul's home; with a palm tree, and seagulls, big ocean waves, flowers, and bright green grass with lots of texture and detail (Figure 10.12).

The intentional material choice seemed to elicit creative expression from Paul within the therapeutic relationship. By incorporating the three tenets therapeutic bond, creative process, materials, and methods (King, 2016), I observed positive improvements in Paul. He had engaged in both verbal and non-verbal explorations that yielded visible, observed changes with improved affect, confidence, awareness, and self-reflection. "The veteran experienced improvement with his overall affect, his insight and awareness. He showed a significant reduction in his symptomatology" (Cara et al., 2020). Paul's self-doubt, anxiety, and strong resistance to me and his artwork had diminished. He adopted a positive outlook on his life and connections to others.

Short Perspective: Neurobiologically Informed Art Therapy Work Within the Context of Complex Socio-Political Realities

Einat Metzl

Reflecting on my art therapy experiences in the Middle East (in particular, in Israel), Latin America (in particular, in Mexico and Chile), and the U.S. (mainly in Los Angeles and New Orleans) over the last decade and a half, I realize that much of my clinical and creative intuition, research, and teaching could well be framed within the growing understanding of what we do from a neurobiological and interpersonal perspective.

Art therapy offers an additional relationship between the person and their creation, and between the creator and materials with which they work. A resonance/empathy occurs through the engagement of the client during the process of creating, which allows for an active body–mind connection beyond the person to person relationship in talk therapy. In addition, the therapeutic relationship with one's artistic creation can continue to form, promote internal dialogue and mentalization between face-to face therapy sessions, as the creator contemplates the art made in session or continues to add to it.

To provide an example: I was working with a young man who identifies as Palestinian, gay, and a creative performer, who suffers from extreme social anxiety. Let's call him Ken (pseudonym). Ken was offered asylum in Israel as a political refugee due to severe violence and death threats. He was residing at a friend's house, had no art materials, and was only able to meet me at night via zoom. I'm a middle-aged Israeli woman whom he never met and who works predominantly through art engagements. However, during a session he accepted an invitation to take a pen and three small pieces of paper and created symbols for his past, present, and future, which allowed him to connect the terror he had felt, and the strife he is currently experiencing with the hope he still holds for himself. At the end he was amazed by how profound the art could be "although it was just a brief sketch, and with so little materials or thinking. Ken also commented that it was because of the trust we had been able to build between us, that he was "even able to draw something."

It is incredible how our minds allow us to take audio-visual signals someone generates in an entirely different house (as this was a zoom-mediated art therapy session), and those resonant with an internal experience – a felt sense generated by the engagement with the art and another. Technology allows us to receive those signals from so far apart, but the essence is still, in my mind, that our brains can take these audio-visual inputs and allow those to be received and trigger our own experiences and empathy toward another, that truly creates the difference.

The underpinning of this perspective is based on understanding the centrality of therapeutic relationship to healing, creative process as a force for expression, personal reflection and insight, and our offering of materials and methods as integrative spaces of somatic–cognitive–emotional and spiritual–collective knowing.

1   The centrality of therapeutic relationship to healing – the importance of relational and socio-cultural safety as well as a secure attachment to the developing (or healing) brain (for example in Hass-Cohen & Clyde Findlay, 2019). This concept of sound relationship and structure which is so synonymous with the setting of therapy and the centrality of concepts such as the therapeutic relationship, transference and countertransference, empathy and projections are all directly linked to how we now understand emotional and cognitive empathy. Our understanding of these concepts is now informed by an increased understanding of how the brain uses large-scale networks for processing of emotion, cognition, and consciousness (Han et al., 2021; Koban et al., 2021), thus our perceptions, experiences and interactions are integrative by their nature.

2   The creative process as a force for expression, personal reflection, and insight – we all intuitively know that the creative process offers opportunity to integrate memories with current experiences, fears, and wishes regarding the future. The process of creating reflects trying to make sense of what it is that we are doing, and then continuing to shape and be shaped by our creations. This parallels the notion of neuroplasticity in which connections in the brain form and re-form throughout life and may hold the ability to bounce back (often conceptualized as resilience) after adversity/trauma. In fact, a cornerstone of the art therapy profession might be framed in terms of how creative thinking and creative production propel well-being following adversity. That is the idea that art making and creative expression of an experience forms and strengthens new associations in the brain, creates new neutral pathways linked to perceptual, somatic, emotional, cognitive, and culturally relevant encoded information.

In an exploration of creativity and resilience in New Orleans after Hurricane Katrina (Metzl, 2009) the importance of creative thinking, specifically flexibility and originality, stood out as predictive of resilient adaptation a year after losing one's house due to hurricane Katrina, even after taking socioeconomic standing and other socio-cultural variables into account. Neuroplasticity & resilient adaptation seem to be linked and data suggest that creative thinking and creative production are both the outcome of neuroplasticity and the result of it (Orwig et al., 2021; Schlegel et al., 2015; Sun et al., 2016, 2020). Walker and colleagues (2018) echo the potential I witnessed when working with a wonderful team of art therapy volunteers led by Karla Leopold with displaced survivors of hurricane Katrina (www.nytimes.com/2007/09/17/arts/design/17ther.html). When offered convenient and relevant opportunities to create with others who shared their experiences, relationships emerged, and the environment of the RVs in which they lived seemed more livable. One art piece at a time, one story, one acknowledgment from another – participants were able to express pain and hardship as well as ground themselves in their strength and ability to adapt.

3   Our offering of materials and methods as integrative spaces of somatic–cognitive–emotional and spiritual–collective knowing. Active engagement in

physical and socio-emotional ways with one's surroundings had frequently been linked to well-being, consistent with models of therapy that emphasize having a full, integrative engagement between the body, thoughts, and feelings. According to Nadal and Chatterjee (2019) The aesthetic experience – "being moved" – engaging the salience network, the reward network, engages target-focused behavior and assessment and an embodied simulation. In art therapy, models such as the Expressive Therapies Continuum (ETC) (Lusebrink & Hinz, 2020) explore how engagement with different art materials invites foci on different levels and movement toward creative integration.

Similarly, art offers integration, validation, and connection for elderly adults suffering from Alzheimer's disease. For example, as the disease progresses and verbal and cognitive limitations mark more and more the abilities for one to function and express themselves verbally as in the past, dopamine replacement therapy seems to enhance motivation for creative expression, allowing for alternative self-expression (Demarco, 2021). These findings remind me of work that I had done with either 0–5-year-old children as well as in a dementia treatment center where I offered art therapy groups. In both cases, while insight and verbal narrations were at times important for some clients, the centrality of the work was centered around engagement with the materials on the somatic and perceptual levels first, often through non-verbal play, and then, through cognitive or affective engagement, into a sense of being moved by the aesthetic experience created by oneself or others in the group. I remember once an elderly woman who joined my group with a big smile. She could not remember her name and barely spoke but recognized the sewing materials and immediately engaged in sewing. She was not at all focused on the product but worked with deep contemplation. Memories of her life as a seamstress emerged, coupled with funny and sad recollections of life. All other participants in the group as well as the staff members were all shocked – stating they had never heard her speak so much.

It was clear to me this was not anything I had intentionally done or offered; it was simply the material and the movement linked to years of repetition, procedural/socio-physiological memory that were suddenly accessible when re-engaging in sewing. In some way reminiscent of the engagement of young children with materials they have encountered many times, the emotional ease and skilled sensorimotor execution are linked with an engaged, active yet focused state of mind (flow).

A final note is that we truly still know very, very little about art therapy and the brain. While the models we have developed are lovely and they receive more and more support through research, much of what I have said here is an intuition based on my clinical experience. There are so many variables and mysteries about how our brains work, how and why we are creative, and what causes what when we do so. It is important to remember there are limitations with current research that we must acknowledge (e.g. Walker et al., 2018; King et al., 2019) as we can continue to creatively explore, learn, and remember that there are some mysteries we as humans might never completely understand.

The Integration of Imagery Rehearsal Therapy and Art Therapy (IRT + AT) for Post-traumatic Nightmares (PTN)

Adrienne Stamper

Post-traumatic nightmares (PTN) occur in approximately 90% of individuals with PTSD (Creamer et al., 2018). One study found that patients who cited significant distress from PTN were about ten times more likely to report suicidal ideation, compared to those who did not (Paxton Willing et al., 2021). Imagery Rehearsal Therapy (IRT) is a short, CBT-based treatment targeting the reduction of PTN by reconstructing them into something more benign (Krakow & Zadra, 2006). Though specific protocols may vary, IRT typically entails a written narrative of the nightmare and then a re-scription of the dream in a way that changes the emotional content from negative to positive (Kunze et al., 2016). Art therapy (AT) uses visual imagery to express feelings and experiences that may be difficult to verbalize. Between these two treatments, there is a shared principle of externalizing something painful and then transforming it into something meaningful. A potential integration of IRT+AT invites the patient to create an artistic depiction of a new dream, using an art medium of their choice. The patient is then instructed to rehearse the new dream using the visual support of the artwork to replace the habit of the nightmare. In a sense, IRT translates an imagery-based nightmare into words, and then incorporating AT helps to translate those words back into imagery. The following examples were conducted as part of a treatment program with active-duty military personnel.

In one case example a service member (SM) was suffering from very graphic PTN and constant intrusive thoughts. At the time of his referral for IRT, he had already tried many forms of therapy without success and was very discouraged about his symptoms ever getting better. He stated that he was "tired of the visual images of hurting others or strangling the life out of a faceless shadow ... tired of [his] brain altering combat events in [his sleep] and making them worse." After writing down his nightmare, the SM chose to rescript his dream into a peaceful day at the beach with his children. However, upon trying to visualize his written "new dream," the SM found himself being bombarded with images of his children swept away into the ocean. The SM was then invited to depict his new dream through art in order to help replace these unwanted images. As he painted, the SM began spontaneously adding symbols of protection, to include: a life jacket and two hands clasped in prayer (Figure 10.13). On the back of the canvas, the SM wrote a bible passage which he dedicated to his children ("Behold, I am going to send an angel before you to guard you along the way and to bring you into the place which I have prepared" (Exodus 23:20)). The SM described his process as a "mental barrier to stop [the negative images] which in turn allowed [him] to continue to visualize my new dream the way it was intended." Ultimately, he proudly brought his artwork home, shared it with his children, and displayed it in his house. After completing his treatment, he experienced a cessation of both nightmares and intrusive thoughts. He then expressed

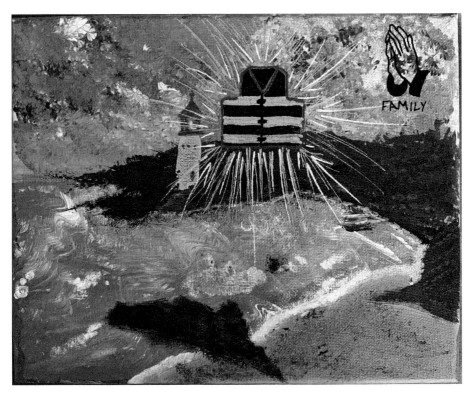

FIGURE 10.13 A painting of the beach created to rescript a service members post-traumatic nightmares

feeling more hopeful and equipped for his life moving forward, stating that IRT + AT offered "great coping mechanisms to bring you back into the present. I was able [to] confront my demons using visual imagery and learn new ways to redirect my focus and pull me away from my negative thoughts."

In a separate case example, a SM used a papier-mâché mask to depict his dream transformation. He wrote "I could feel that the years of traumatic experiences from my deployments were pushing me further and further away from my family. I was suppressing all the rage and pain of what I had seen and been through ... and it was turning me into someone I no longer recognized." In his nightmare, the SM had the face of a monster and his skin was being painfully peeled back. He chose to transform this into his "new dream" by peeling back the face of the "monster" – but this time revealing his "true self" and core values underneath. Behind the monster, the SM collaged a picture of his family with the sun shining down over them, and then added symbols for faith, hope, and love (Figure 10.14). The SM stated: "As I did this, I began to see myself and my life in a new light; finally shedding the 'monster' and leaving it behind me."

Ultimately, IRT can be difficult for some patients to grasp through writing alone. In these cases, writing can feel more like an objective, cognitive exercise, in contrast to the significant sensory and emotional content of a nightmare. One potential

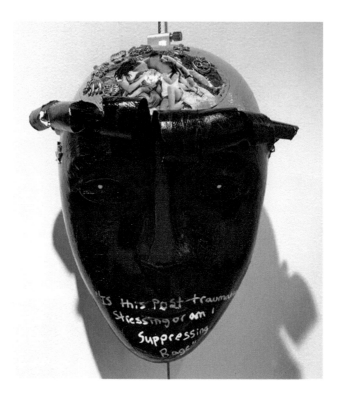

FIGURE 10.14 A papier-mâché mask that depicts a service member's dream transformation

explanation is that art making and trauma are associated with the right hemisphere of the brain; whereas speech and language are housed in the left hemisphere (Van der Kolk, 2014). Thus, the combination of art and writing may promote "neural integration" and communication between the hemispheres of the brain, which is important for the resolution of trauma (Faustino, 2022). Early work suggests IRT+AT may be a viable approach to address the needs of military patients with nightmares that are not adequately addressed with currently available treatments.

Redrawing Value: Gaining New Understanding of Identity through Art Therapy

Barbara van der Vossen

"I'm not really a creative person but my neurologist thinks that art therapy will give me something to do," said R in our first session. At the Indiana University Neuroscience Center where R is a patient, neurologists often refer patients with complex clinical symptoms to the art therapy program to support their healing process and improve their quality of life as a component of comprehensive neurorehabilitation (Kline, 2016). Art making promotes use-dependent plasticity, the ability of the brain to undergo changes when certain areas are activated (Kline, 2016), and the expressive nature of art making provides patients with a powerful avenue for coping with medical traumas (Lusebrink, 2004). R is a 37-year-old 10-year stroke survivor who had just experienced the latest in a series of employment search disappointments. The hiring manager did not call him back, an example of a social interaction that left him feeling invisible and frustrated. R believed that his aphasia led people to view him as unintelligent and unworthy. The eldest son of Hmong refugees from Laos, R's sense of value was culturally and personally tied to a strong work ethic and success in employment.

From my clinical observations, rigid, binary thought patterns are undercurrents in the art therapy process with traumatic brain injury survivors. Initiating an art therapy directive with *I feel, I need, I have, I hope …* often helps to understand a patient's need "to have value." For many survivors, exploring a sense of self becomes a primary therapy goal, as the self before the injury is perceived to have value, the self after the injury is perceived to be a burden. Time becomes a simultaneous ally and enemy; while days feel slower and years longer, there is anxiety around its scarcity and a strong attachment to the past. "*When will I get back to who I was? Do I have enough time?*" In an early session with R, he created a found object mandala that seemed to indicate a desire for symmetry that his body no longer has, and he selected "only perfect leaves, without any cracks," perhaps unconsciously processing the visible scar that runs along the top of his head (Figure 10.15). Gravitating to a person-centered approach in art therapy, I felt that mentioning the observation would be too direct in our young therapeutic relationship. We revisited the piece toward the closing of our work nearly two years later and were able to reflect on how much his perception of himself had shifted.

Art therapy also offered R the opportunity to express and process feelings that he considered unacceptable, such as anger and frustration. When I first suggested expressing anger through art he chuckled, "Oh no, my family doesn't do that, we don't talk about feelings." But, as trust in the therapeutic relationship developed, his personal narratives began to unfold through kinetic drawings of his family. Art offered a safe way for him to externalize experiences that otherwise felt risky to

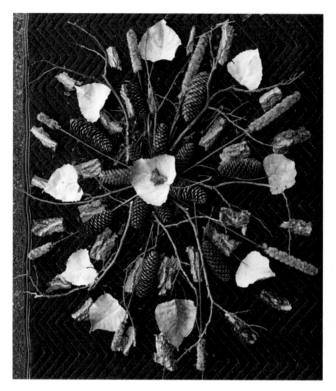

FIGURE 10.15 Found object mandala consisting of twigs, dried leaves, and pinecones. R. Vue (consent for artwork)

define (King et al., 2019). Role confusion seemed apparent in the content choices he made in artwork: he drew a Thanksgiving feast where he is inside the home with the women while his father and brother maintained the fire outside. In a portrait of his family symbolized by animals, he drew each family member as an animal except himself, whom he drew in a closed crate with a question mark. As R processed his personal and family history, conflicts, traumas, and the Third Culture Kid experience (Van Reken et al., 2017) of being the son of Hmong Lutheran refugees, his perspectives began to shift. He noticed a theme of himself as a mediator between family members, offering him a new valued role in his family system. Expressing himself visually and verbally in art therapy helped him practice and model open communication. He began to talk about his grief with his family outside of therapy, and in one particularly meaningful session invited his parents to join him in the culminating activity of an extended directive: together they mourned R's past self in a Hmong-inspired memorial burning of a box that R spent several weeks decorating and filling with past attachments he wanted to release; drawings of his previous career in Information Technology, a romantic relationship that ended, hobbies that no longer felt attainable, and even uncomfortable interactions from his youth that were unrelated to his injury.

Another shift occurred when I noticed that R's drawings of people in motion, gardens, and animals reminded me of a *storycloth*, where personal narratives and

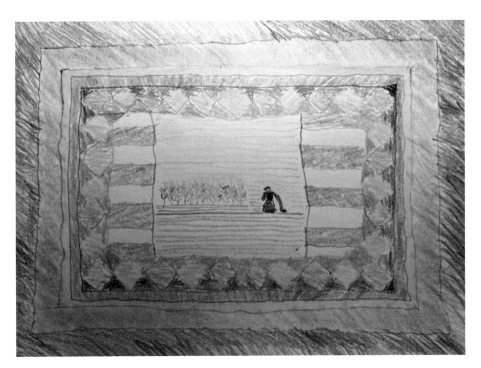

FIGURE 10.16 Drawing of a figure working in a garden, surrounded by a colorful border of geometric shapes

cultural histories are stitched onto fabric. I asked if he was familiar with the concept, which turned out to be a hilarious question! R's mother and late grandmother are acclaimed storycloth artists whose work has been featured in books. Walker et al. (2018) indicated that visual imagery referencing community, purpose, and belonging are associated with improved thalamic activity in brain injury survivors. Indeed, connecting R's drawings to his culture and family was emotional for him; he was contributing to a cultural practice of processing trauma and family lore through narrative art making. He began to intentionally draw storycloth-like pieces, with traditional border edges and color choices (Figure 10.16). For R, the connection to his culture restored a sense of identity and a new understanding of his role in the family. Person-centered, narrative art-making allowed R to re-envision himself in a new, forward oriented manner. Over time, newfound esteem facilitated a return to employment and outspoken art therapy advocacy in brain injury survivor communities.

REFERENCES

Adams, E. B., Morris, P. K. & Maguire, E. R. (2018). The impact of gangs on community life in Trinidad. *Race and Justice*, 1–24. https://doi.org/10.1177/2153368718820577

Allen, R. (2019). Harlem Calypso and Brooklyn Soca: Caribbean carnival music in the diaspora. *Ethnic and Racial Studies: Special Issue: Music, Migration and the City*, 42(6), 865–882. https://doi.org/10.1080/01419870.2019.1544374

Aslinia, S. D., Rasheed, M., & Simpson, C. (2011). Individual psychology (Adlerian) applied to international collectivist cultures: Compatibility, effectiveness, and impact. *Journal for International Counselor Education*, *3*, 1–12. http://digitalcommons.library.unlv.edu/jice

Awais, Y., & Blausey, D. (2021). *Foundations of supervision*. Routledge.

Burton, R. (2009). Globalisation and cultural identity in Caribbean society: The Jamaican case. *Caribbean Journal of Philosophy*, *1*(1). http://ojs.mona.uwi.edu/index.php/cjp/article/viewFile/285/185

Cara,V., David, D., & Gruce, L. (2020, August). *There and back again, art as a journey through one's Hell.* [Poster Presentation] Miami Veterans Medical Center. Miami, Florida. *Caribbean culture*. Ian Randle.

Cohen, R. (n.d.). *Review of pilot studies 2014–2018*. Common Threads Project. https://static1.squarespace.com/static/5b7eeaf2c258b4a04473be79/t/6099c6cafa12a81aef912f2a/1620690642127/Pilot+Review_New_v7+%281%29.pdf

Cohen, R. & Butterly, C. (2020). *The fabric of healing*. EuropeNow. www.europenowjournal.org/2020/10/11/the-fabric-of-healing/

Collier, A., Wayment, H., & Birkett, M., (2016). Impact of making textile handcrafts on mood enhancement and inflammatory immune changes. *Art Therapy*, *33*(4), 178–185.

Cozolino, L. (2017). *The neuroscience of psychotherapy: Healing the social brain* (3rd ed.). W.W. Norton.

Creamer, J. L., Brock, M. S., Matsangas, P., Motamedi, V., & Mysliwiec, V. (2018). Nightmares in United States military personnel with sleep disturbances. *Journal of Clinical Sleep Medicine*, *14*(3), 419–426. https://doi.org/10.5664/jcsm.6990

Csíkszentmihályi, M. (1991). *Flow: The psychology of optimal experience*. Harper Perennial.

Cucca, A., Di Rocco, A., Acosta, I., Beheshti, M., Berberian, M., Bertisch, H. C., … & Ghilardi, M. F. (2021). Art therapy for Parkinson's disease. *Parkinsonism & Related Disorders*, *84*, 148–154.

Dana, D. (2018). *The polyvagal theory in therapy: Engaging the rhythm of regulation*. W.W. Norton.

DeMarco, S. (2021). Prescribing art therapy for Parkinson's disease. *Neuroscience*, *3*, 4.

Desautels, L. L. (2020). *Connections over compliance: Rewiring our perceptions of discipline*. Wyatt-MacKenzie.

Dissanayake, E. (1988). *What is art for?* University of Washington Press.

Duenyas, D., & Luke. C. (2019). Neuroscience for counselors: Recommendations for developing and teaching graduate courses. *The Professional Counselor*, *9*(4), 369–380.

Eaton, J., & Tieber, C. (2017). The effects of coloring on anxiety, mood, and perseverance. *Art Therapy: Journal of the American Art Therapy Association*, *34*(1), 42–46. https://doi.org/10.1080/07421656.2016.1277113

Elkis-Abuhoff, D. L., & Gaydos, M. (2018). Medical art therapy research moves forward: A review of clay manipulation with Parkinson's disease. *Art Therapy: Journal of the American Art Therapy Association*, *35*(2), 68–76.

Elkis-Abuhoff, D. L., Goldblatt, R. B., Gaydos, M., & Convery, C. (2013). A pilot study to determine the psychological effects of manipulation of therapeutic art forms among patients with Parkinson's disease. *International Journal of Art Therapy*, *18*, 113–121. https://doi.org/10.1080/17454832.2013.797481

Elkis-Abuhoff, D. L., Goldblatt, R. B., Gaydos, M., & Corrato, S. (2008). Effects of clay manipulation on somatic dysfunction and emotional distress in patients with Parkinson's disease. *Art Therapy: Journal of the American Art Therapy Association*, *25*, 122–128. https://doi.org/10.1080/07421656.2008.10129596

Faustino, B. (2022). Minding my brain: Fourteen neuroscience-based principles to enhance psychotherapy responsiveness. *Clinical Psychology & Psychotherapy*, 1–22. https://doi.org/10.1002/cpp.2719

Fish, B. (2019) Response art in art therapy: Historical and contemporary overview. *Art Therapy*, *36*(3), 122–132. https://doi.org/10.1080/07421656.2019.1648915

Garlock, L. (2021). Alone in the desert: Making sense of the senseless through story cloths. In L. Leone (Ed.), *Craft in art therapy* (pp. 190–203). Routledge.

Goldblatt, R., Elkis-Abuhoff, D., Gaydos, M., & Napoli, A. (2010). Understanding clinical benefits of modeling clay exploration with patients diagnosed with Parkinson's disease. *Arts & Health*, *2*, 140–148. https://doi.org/10.1080/17533010903495405

Han, M.-E., Park, S.-Y., & Oh, S.-O. (2021). Large-scale functional brain networks for consciousness. *ACB: Anatomy & Cell Biology, 54*(2), 152–164. https://doi.org/10.5115/acb.20.305

Hass-Cohen, N., & Clyde Findlay, J. M. A. (2019). The art therapy relational neuroscience and memory reconsolidation four drawing protocol. *The Arts in Psychotherapy, 63,* 51–59.

Hass-Cohen, N., & Findlay, J. C. (2015). *Art therapy and the neuroscience of relationships, creativity, and resiliency: Skills and practices.* W.W. Norton.

Hass-Cohen, N., Clyde Findlay, J., Carr, R., & Vanderlan, J. (2014). "Check, change what you need to change and/or keep what you want": An art therapy neurobiological-based trauma protocol. *Art Therapy, 31*(2), 69–78. https://doi.org/10.1080/07421656.2014.903825

Hinz, L. D. (2009). *Expressive therapies continuum.* Routledge.

Hinz, L. D. (2020). *Expressive Therapies Continuum: A framework for using art in therapy* (2nd ed.). Routledge.

Hocoy, D. (2002). Cross-cultural issues in art therapy. *Art Therapy: Journal of the American Art Therapy Association, 19*(4), 141–145. www.tandfonline.com/doi/pdf/10.1080/07421656.2002.10129683

Hughes, V. (2022). How to change minds? A study makes the case for talking it out. *The New York Times.* www.nytimes.com/2022/09/16/science/group-consensus-persuasion-brain-alignment.html?smid=nytcore-ios-share&referringSource=articleShare

Huotilainen, M., Rankanen, M., Groth, C., Seitamaa-Hakkarainen, P., and Mäkelä, M. (2018). Why our brains love arts and crafts: Implications of creative practices on psychophysical well-being. *Form Academic,* 11(2), 1–18. https://doi.org/10.7577/formakademisk

McDonough, I., Haber, S., Bischof, G., & Park, D. (2015). The Synapse Project: Engagement in mentally challenging activities enhances neural efficiency. *Restorative Neurology and Neuroscience, 22,* 865–882. https://doi.org/10.3233/RNN-150533

Irvine, T., Labarta, A., Emelianchik-Key, K, (2021). Using a relational-cultural and Adlerian framework to enhance multicultural pedagogy. *The Professional Counselor, 11*(2), 233–247). http://tpcjournal.nbcc.org

Jackson, L. (2020). *Cultural humility in art therapy: Applications for practice, research, social justice self-care, and pedagogy.* Jessica Kingsley.

Junakovic, A., & Telarovic, S. (2021). The effects of art therapy on Parkinson's and Alzheimer's disease. *Medicina Fluminensis, 57*(3), 236–243.

Kaimal, G., Ray, K., & Muniz, J. M. (2016). Reduction of cortisol levels and participants' responses following artmaking. *Art Therapy: Journal of the American Art Therapy Association, 33*(2), 74–80. https://doi.org/10.1080/07421656.2016.1166832

Kapitan, Litell, M., & Torres, A. (2011). Creative art therapy in a community's participatory research and social transformation. *Art Therapy, 28*(2), 64–73. https://doi.org/10.1080/07421656.2011.578238

King, J. L. (Ed.). (2016). *Art therapy, trauma, and neuroscience: Theoretical and practical perspectives.* Routledge.

King, J., Kaimal, G., Konopka, L., Belkofer, C., & Strang, C. (2019) Practical applications of neuroscience-informed art therapy. *Art Therapy: Journal of the American Art Therapy Association, 36*(3), 149–156. https://doi.org/10.1080/07421656.2019.1649549

Kline, T. (2016). Art therapy for individuals with Traumatic Brain Injury: A comprehensive neurorehabilitated-informed approach to treatment. *Art Therapy, 33*(2), 67–73. https://doi.org/10.1080/07421656.2016.1164002

Koban, L., Gianaros, P. J., Kober, H., & Wager, T. D. (2021). The self in context: brain systems linking mental and physical health. *Nature Reviews Neuroscience, 22,* 309–322. https://doi.org/10.1038/s41583-021-00446-8

Krakow, B., & Zadra, A. (2006). Clinical management of chronic nightmares: Imagery rehearsal therapy. *Behavioral Sleep Medicine, 4*(1), 45–70. https://doi.org/10.1207/s15402010bsm0401_4

Kunze, A. E., Lancee, J., Morina, N., Kindt, M., & Arntz, A. (2016). Efficacy and mechanisms of imagery rescripting and imaginal exposure for nightmares: Study protocol for a randomized controlled trial. *Trials, 17*(469). https://doi.org/10.1186/s13063-016-1570-3

Kuri, E. (2017). Toward an ethical application of intersectionality in art therapy. *Art Therapy, 34*(3), 118–122. https://doi.org/10.1080/07421656.2017.1358023

Leigh, H. (2021). Signature pedagogies for art therapy education: A Delphi study. *Art Therapy, 38*(1), 5–12. https://doi.org/10.1080/07421656.2020.1728180

Lusebrink, V. B. (2004). Art therapy and the brain: An attempt to understand the underlying processes of art expression in therapy. *Art Therapy, 21*(3), 125–135. https://doi.org/10.1080/07421 656.2004.10129496

Lusebrink, V. B., & Hinz, L. (2016). The expressive therapies continuum as a framework in the treatment of trauma. In J. L. King (Ed.), *Art Therapy, trauma, and neuroscience: Theoretical and practical perspectives* (pp. 42–66). Routledge.

Lusebrink, V. B., & Hinz, L. D. (2020). Cognitive and symbolic aspects of art therapy and similarities with large scale brain networks. *Art Therapy, 37*(3), 113–122. https://doi.org/10.1080/07421656. 2019.1691869

Lusebrink, V. B. (2010). Assessment and therapeutic application of the Expressive Therapies Continuum: Implications for brain structures and functions. *Art Therapy: Journal of the American Art Therapy Association, 27*(4), 168–177.

Mahabir, K. (2015). Chutney music in carnival: Re-defining national identity in Trinidad and Tobago. In B. Boufoy-Bastick, & S. Chinien (Eds.), *Caribbean dynamics: Re-configuring Caribbean culture.* Ian Randle.

Malik, S. (2021). Using neuroscience to explore creative media in art therapy: A systematic narrative review. *International Journal of Art Therapy, 2,* 1–13.

Menakem, R. (2017). *My grandmother's hands: Racialized trauma and the pathway to mending our hearts and bodies.* Central Recovery Press.

Metzl, E. S. (2009). The role of creative thinking in models of resilience. *Psychology of Aesthetics, Creativity, and the Arts, 3*(2), 112–123.

Michael J. Fox Foundation. (2022). *Allied care.* www.michaeljfox.org/news/allied-care.

Miller, R. (2016). Neuroeducation: Integrating brain-based psychoeducation into clinical practice. *Journal of Mental Health Counseling, 38*(2), 103–115. https://doi.org/10.17744/mehc.38.2.02

Miller, R., Dillman, & Taylor, D. (2016). Does Adlerian theory stand the test of time? Examining individual psychology from a neuroscience perspective. *Journal of Humanistic Counseling, 55,* 111–128.

Miller, R., & E. Beeson (2020). *Neuroeducation toolbox: Practical translations of neuroscience in counseling and psychotherapy.* Cognella.

Moon, C. (2010). A history of materials and media in art therapy. In C. H. Moon (Ed.), *Materials and media in art therapy: Critical understandings of diverse artistic vocabularies.* Routledge.

Nadal, M., & Chatterjee, A. (2019). Neuroaesthetics and art's diversity and universality. *WIREs Cognitive Science, 10*(3), e1487. https://doi.org/10.1002/wcs.1487

Orwig, W., Diez, I., Bueichekú, E., Vannini, P., Beaty, R., & Sepulcre, J. (2021). Cortical networks of creative ability trace gene expression profiles of synaptic plasticity in the human brain. *Frontiers in Human Neuroscience, 15.* https://doi.org/10.3389/fnhum.2021.694274; www.frontiersin.org/article/10.3389/fnhum.2021.694274

Pagano, J. (2019, January 25). *Sewing needles reveal the roots of fashion.* Sapiens. Wenner-GrenFoundation & University of Chicago Press. www.sapiens.org/archeology/fashion-history-sewing-needles/

Parkinson's Foundation. (2022a). *Statistics.* www.parkinson.org/understanding-parkinsons/statistics.

Parkinson'sFoundation. (2022b).*Movementsymptoms.*www.parkinson.org/understanding-parkinsons/movement-symptoms

Parkinson's Foundation. (2022c). *Non-movement symptoms.* www.parkinson.org/understanding-parkinsons/non-movement-symptoms.

Paxton Willing, M. M., Pickett, T. C., Tate, L. L., Sours Rhodes, C., Riggs, D. S., & DeGraba, T. J. (2021). Understanding the role of sleep on suicidal ideation in active duty service members: Implications for clinical practice. *Practice Innovations, 6*(2), 67–76. https://doi.org/10.1037/pri0000146

Perry, B. (2006). Applying principles of neurodevelopment to clinical work with maltreated and traumatized children: The neurosequential model of therapeutics. In N. B. Webb (Ed.), *Working with traumatized youth in child welfare* (pp. 27–52). Guilford Press.

Perry, B. D., & Winfrey, O. (2021). *What happened to you?: Conversations on trauma, resilience, and healing* (1st ed.). Flatiron Books.

Potash, J. (2018) Relational social justice ethics for art therapists. *Art Therapy, 35*(4), 202–210. https://doi.org/10.1080/07421656.2018.1554019

Potash, J. S., Bardot, H., Hyland Moon, C., Napoli, M., Lyonsmith, A., & Hamilton, M. (2017). Ethical implications of cross-cultural international art therapy. *The Arts in Psychotherapy, 56*, 74–82. http://dx.doi.org/10.1016/j.aip.2017.08.005

Real Happy Endings. (2021, February 22). *The Whole Brain Child, by Daniel J. Siegel & Tina Payne Bryson Summary (Part 1 of 2)* [Video]. YouTube. www.youtube.com/watch?v=RcTxHZNLrZQ

Reynolds, F. (2000). Managing depression through needlecraft creative activities: A qualitative study. *The Arts in Psychotherapy, 27*(2), pp.107–114.

Rollocks, S., Dass, N., Hutchinson, G., & Mohammed, L. (2013). The associations observed between experiencing multiple traumatic events and mental health symptoms among adolescents in Trinidad. *Journal of Child and Adolescent Trauma, 6*, 246–259. https://doi.org/10.1080/19361521.2013.836583

Schlegel, A., Alexander, P., Fogelson, S. V., Li, X., Lu, Z., Kohler, P, J., Riley, E., Tse, P. U., & Meng, M. (2015). The artist emerges: Visual art learning alters neural structure and function, *NeuroImage, 105*, 440–451, ISSN 1053-8119, https://doi.org/10.1016/j.neuroimage.2014.11.014

Seepersad, R. (2016). *Crime and violence in Trinidad and Tobago: IDB series on crime and violence in the Caribbean.* https://publications.iadb.org/publications/english/document/Crime-and-Violence-in-Trinidad-and-Tobago-IDB-Series-on-Crime-and-Violence-in-the-Caribbean.pdf

Shnider, D. H. (2018). *Bottom up: An integrated neurological and cognitive behavioral book which addresses the key principles of neuro-psychotherapy. Five important emotional parts of the brain with skills training.* AuthorHouse.

Soo Hon, S. (2021). On using participatory ethnography to explore the relevance of cultural arts practices to the psychosocial well-being of adolescents affected by violence in Trinidad and Tobago. In U. Herrmann, M. Hills de Zarate, & S. Pitruzzella (Eds.), *The mental health of children and young people: International research and contemporary practice in the arts therapies* (Vol. 1). Routledge.

SRSG (Office of the Special Representative of the Secretary-General) on Violence against Children. (2016). *Protecting children affected by armed violence in the community.* https://violenceagainstchildren.un.org/sites/violenceagainstchildren.un.org/files/documents/publications/2._protecting_children_affected_by_armed_violence_in_the_community.pdf

Sun, J., Chen, Q., Zhang, Q., Li, Y., Li, H., Wei, D., Yang, W., & Qiu, J. (2016). Training your brain to be more creative: Brain functional and structural changes induced by divergent thinking training. *Human Brain Mapping, 37*, 3375–3387. https://doi.org/10.1002/hbm.23246

Sun, J., Zhang, Q., Li, Y., Meng, J., Chen, Q., Yang, W., Wei, D., & Qiu, J. (2020) Plasticity of the resting-state brain: static and dynamic functional connectivity change induced by divergent thinking training. *Brain Imaging and Behavior, 14*, 1498–1506. https://doi.org/10.1007/s11682-019-00077-9

Talwar, S. (2019). *Art therapy for social justice: Radical intersections.* Routledge.

UNICEF. (2014). *United Nations Children's Fund: Hidden in plain sight: A statistical analysis of violence against children.* http://files.unicef.org/publications/files/Hidden_in_plain_sight_statistical_analysis_EN_3_Sept_2014.pdf

United Nations. (2020). *Country classification. World Economic Situation and Prospects.* www.un.org/development/desa/dpad/wp-content/uploads/sites/45/WESP2020_Annex.pdf

van der Kolk, B. (2014). *The body keeps the score: Brain, mind, and body in the healing of trauma.* Viking.

Van der Kolk, B. (2014). *The body keeps the score: Brain, mind, and body in the healing of trauma.* Sage.

Van Reken, R. E., Pollock, M. V., & Pollock, D. C. (2017). *Third culture kids 3rd edition: Growing up among worlds.* Nicholas Brealey.

Villinski, P. (1994). Comforter (quilt). Smithsonian Art Museum. This present moment: Crafting a better world exhibit, 2022–2023, Washington, DC

Walker, I. F., Asher, L., Pari, A., Attride-Stirling, J., Oyinloye, A. O., Simmons, C., Potter, I., Rubaine, V., Samuel, J. M., Andrewin, A., Flynn, J., McGill, A. L., Greenaway-Duberry, S., Malcom, A. B., Mann, G., Razavi, A., & Gibson, R. C. (2022) Mental health systems in six Caribbean small island developing states: A comparative situational analysis. *International Journal of Mental Health Systems*, *16*, 39. https://doi.org/10.1186/s13033-022-00552-9

Walker, M. S., Stamper, A. M., Nathan, D. E., & Riedy, G. (2018). Art therapy and underlying fMRI brain patterns in military TBI: A case series. *International Journal of Art Therapy*, *23*(4), 180–187.

Wilkinson, R. A., & Chilton, G. (2013). Positive art therapy: Linking positive psychology to art therapy theory, practice, and research. *Art Therapy*, *30*(1), 4–11. https://doi.org/10.1080/07421656.2013.757513

CHAPTER 11

CONCLUSION

Kerry Kruk-Borisov, Juliet L. King, and Christianne E. Strang

Since the first version of this text was published in 2016, we have seen an expansion of research to practice initiatives that explore how neuroscience evidence and principles influence our understanding of the therapeutic arts to address mental, physical, and public health concerns. Advocacy groups (e.g., NeuroArts Blueprint, https://neuroartsblueprint.org/) recognize the importance of the arts in contributing to health outcomes and have developed core principles and recommendations to explore the translation of neuroscience evidence to arts-based healthcare and community practices. In a little less than a decade, ongoing advancements in neuroscience and physiology research have expanded consideration for how the Arts and Health (A&H) enhances well-being, promotes healing, and improves health outcomes (deWitte et al., 2021; Fancourt & Finn, 2019; Karkou et al., 2022). The Creative Arts Therapies (CATs) are considered within the broader scope of A&H, yet the specific distinctions are not always well understood (Vickhoff, 2023). CATs professionals (visual art, music, dance–movement, drama, psychodrama, expressive multimodal, and poetry/biblio) have specific education and training requirements and work within the therapeutic relationship capitalizing on both expressive and receptive creative engagement in the facilitation of client goals.[1]

A lack of definitional clarity is nothing new to CATs, and art therapists have become accustomed to defining what it is that we do and don't do in a way that makes sense for those outside of the profession. Although a range of stakeholders have amplified the conversations surrounding the impact of the arts and creativity on the human body and human experience, there is much work to be done. Fortunately, it seems society is paying more attention to how the neurosciences inform therapeutic arts, and how therapeutic arts are an important, if not integral, part of holistic care. However, there remains a lack of awareness at the national and global level of who the CATs are, what it is that we do, and how it is we contribute to the conversations taking place at the intersection of neuroscience, arts, and related therapeutics. Bolstering awareness of the CATs in contemporary healthcare requires cross-disciplinary, translational, and collaborative research-to-practice initiatives, and an understanding of what neuroscience can help us know, inform the understanding of what we don't know, and illuminate what it is that we are needing to learn (King, 2018). Neuroscience and psychotherapy present unique complex wicked problems involving understanding and integration, made even more complex when including the arts (King, 2016; Vickhoff, 2023). In addition to the multiple and intersecting factors that contribute to the reasons why and how people change in therapy, the therapeutic relationship remains the primary therapeutic factor across most psychotherapy disciplines (Czamanski-Cohen & Weihs, 2016; deWitte et al., 2021; Norcross & Lambert, 2019). We do not exist in isolation and while connection is central to human survival and thriving, it does make studying mechanisms of change more difficult.

DOI: 10.4324/9781003348207-11

Mechanisms of change in psychotherapy are considered the basis for effecting change. These include the processes and events that are responsible for the change, the reasons why the change occurs and how it comes about (Kazdin, 2007). Our profession is lacking in scientific evidence that articulates clearly how and why art therapy is effective and what mechanisms account for those changes (deWitte et al., 2021; King et al., 2019). Examining and challenging the theoretical foundations and applications of art therapy in the context of neuroscience and neurobiology is crucial to establish evidence for the profession, and different levels of analysis are required to bridge the gaps between nervous system function and psychological, emotional, and behavioral aspects of the human experience. It is a courageous scientist who dares to consider these questions in the context of experimental designs, and fortunately CATs researchers and practitioners alike are used to adopting a bold and expansive worldview when investigating how, and why, art therapy works.

11.1   BUILDING DEFINITIONAL CLARITY: PRINCIPLES OF CATS

A recent review of studies on change factors found three key factors that are theorized to be agents of change in the application of arts in the context of health: symbolism and metaphor, embodiment, and concretization (deWitte et al., 2021). These factors are termed joint *change factors*; namely, well-specified factors that are shared across all art forms and are theorized to produce therapeutic benefits in CATs. These factors utilize creative expression and interaction within the therapeutic relationship. This is an important distinction between art therapy and therapeutic arts and contributes to professional definition and scope of practice.

For example, Czamanski-Cohen and Weihs (2016) introduced a *Bodymind Model* that explores the mechanisms of art therapy and the positive effects it has for ameliorating both mental health and medical symptoms, strengthening relationships, and fostering resilience. This model approaches research in the domains related to four identified mechanisms of change: the triangular relationship, self-engagement, embodiment of self-expression through transition from implicit to explicit processing, and metacognitive processes. The triangular relationship between the therapist, the process of creating art, and the final product are understood to be the key factors to healing that are contingent upon the tactile experience of art making that takes place within the therapeutic relationship. The therapeutic relationship is often the first goal in psychotherapy and has been well established as a priority in trauma treatment (Cloitre et al., 2012; Flükiger et al., 2012; Norcross & Wampold, 2011; Siegel & Soloman, 2003).

Establishing a therapeutic alliance must also account for and consider the ethical responsibilities of therapists for self-assessment of their biases and countertransference reactions along with potential blind spots, necessary cross-cultural considerations, and ableism. Individual and group differences matter greatly in psychotherapy and are dependent upon factors including (but not limited to) current situation, life stage, personality, economic position, gender experience, racial and ethnic identity (McWilliams, 2021). Art therapists have additional responsibilities to be mindful of. It is essential that an art therapist creates and initiates "interventions and experiences that take into consideration their clients' diverse art traditions, preferences for art materials, and beliefs and practices related to the creation of imagery" (Stepney, 2022, p. 109). The art therapist is best served to attend to sensitivities regarding client material choice, subtleties regarding a therapist's preference for or disinclination toward specific art materials, and the role of the materials and art products as integral elements of the therapeutic relationship (Hilbuch et al., 2016).

We provide here a brief and in no way exhaustive overview of advances in neuroscience-informed art therapy research and practice and offer recommendations for the future based on King's (2016) *Three Tenets*. These Tenets intersect, overlap, and are used to guide the consideration for the integration of neuroscience with the dynamic nature of art therapy theory, practice, and research that are grounded within an experiential, emotional, and relational context.

Tenet One: The art-making process and the artwork itself are integral components of treatment that help to understand and elicit verbal and nonverbal communication, self-awareness, and reflection within the therapeutic relationship.

In Chapter 3 of this text, Lusebrink and Hinz provided us with a revitalized understanding of the Expressive Therapies Continuum (ETC) that has been bolstered with new knowledge on large scale brain networks (LSBN). New research foci have emerged exploring the neuroscience of the default mode network (DMN) regarding neural synchrony, mentalization, empathy, and "interbrain coupling through shared experiences" (Vaisvaser, 2021, p. 6). The evolving body of research on interpersonal resonance, neural systems involved in processing observed movements, embodied simulation, and the phenomena of and capacity for empathy expands the complexity of current-state research endeavors and opens the door for creating and bolstering fundamental knowledge of psychotherapy in general (Heyes & Catmur, 2021; Levy & Bader, 2020; Vaisvaser, 2021). It is posited that embodied simulation is a mechanism that enables individuals to resonate with the mental and emotional state of another and contributes to the understanding of empathy within psychotherapy (Gallese, 2017; Franklin, 2010; Vaisvaser, 2021). Implications from research into interbrain coupling, potentially possible through advancements in EEG hyperscanning methods and mobile brain/body imaging (MoBI) technology, may well impact CATs education and professional development at the core level (Dikker et al., 2017; King & Parada, 2021; Parada & Rossi, 2018; Vaisvaser, 2021).

This dynamic simulation process becomes intrinsic in person-centered treatment and involves the therapists' activation and identification of internal emotional, cognitive, and sensorimotor phenomena, or interoception (King & Parada, 2021; Vaisvaser, 2021). Art therapists must be able to allow room for awareness of themselves and the potential impact of internal processes involved in the therapeutic relationship but must also fully understand how to discern and distinguish our own unique affective and perceptive responses, intuitions, and insights within the interactive, therapeutic encounter. Neuroscience perspectives offer an opportunity to broaden the research scope and inch closer to extrapolating the phenomena of therapeutic experiences, potentially in real time, and to consider realms of true human experience and origins of dysfunction more deeply. Thus, the importance and the development of a healthy therapeutic relationship must be considered as a focus within neuro-art therapy research.

Tenet Two: The multi-directional processes of creativity are healing and life enhancing. The effects of art therapy take place in the embodied context of the relationship and rely on the creative process.

As previously noted, the *Three Tenets* are overlapping and intersecting when contextualized in the treatment context, similar to the change factors identified by deWitte et al. (2021). These factors help to understand more deeply the transformational mechanisms that elicit a shift from maladaptive to adaptive responses (deWitte et al., 2021; Kaimal, 2019). A goal for all CATs is to understand through examination how and why change occurs during therapy; therefore, fundamental questions drive the inquiry at the intersection of art therapy and neuroscience: *how* specifically does art making elicit or contribute to positive behavioral and emotional outcomes in psychotherapy; *what* specific mechanisms are influential to effect positive change on various diagnosed disorders, specifically, trauma; and *how* does art therapy change the brain? Like all theories, empirical testing will increase validity and utilization, supporting evidence-based practice.

The CATs are lacking randomized and controlled outcome studies, and empirically tested frameworks, standards, and sets of guidelines for best practice treatment within art therapy (Baker et al., 2018; Schouten et al., 2015; Bowen-Salter et al., 2022). However, Hass-Cohen (2008, 2016) and Hass-Cohen et al. (2018) have continued to weave research about relational neuroscience, memory processes including recall and reconsolidation, and art therapy practice together with current approaches to trauma treatment into an informed art therapy relational neuroscience approach (ATR-N). This work has resulted in the development of a protocol designed to facilitate memory reconsolidation (Hass-Cohen & Clyde Findlay, 2019), offered a promising framework for development of empirical research using this protocol, and contributed to the development of the Bodymind Model (Czamanski-Cohen & Weihs, 2016). You can read more about the ATR-N in Chapter 5 of this current text.

Tenet Three: The materials and methods used effect self-expression, assist in emotional self-regulation, and are applied in specialized ways.

In this context, the materials and art-making processes are change agents that are integral to the therapeutic relationship. Art therapy research appears to be moving toward an expanded neurological and physiological approach using research-based rationale for informed application of art processes and materials within art therapy.

Neuroscience of Art Therapy, ETC Theory, and the Tools of the Trade

In the United States, the most well-known theory for this application is the Expressive Therapies Continuum (ETC) developed by Kagin and Lusebrink in 1978. Expanded discourse into this theory integrated art therapy and neurobiology by building upon what has been learned about human information processing into a framework which also categorizes the materials and tasks involved in making art in art therapy (Hinz, 2019; Hinz et al., 2022; Lusebrink, 2004, 2010, 2014; Lusebrink et al., 2013; Lusebrink & Hinz, 2016, 2020). The ETC incorporates a set of contrasts in art making between kinesthetic and sensory processing, perceptual and affective depictions, and symbolic representations and cognitive processes along a continuum of creativity (Hinz, 2019; Hinz et al., 2022; Lusebrink, 2004, 2010; Lusebrink & Hinz, 2020). The ETC outlines the various ways art making offers a window into neural functioning which can then be applied to theory development and neurologically informed protocols.

Current and emerging research has been focused on a line of inquiry to continue to build foundational evidence to further understand the mechanics of the ETC theory: (1) What happens in the brain, and what mechanisms and structures are involved or impacted, during or because of art making? (2) What is the impact on the body and the mind because of art making? (3) What are the differences or the variation in mechanisms activated when using specific art materials? (4) What is the effect of the use of specific art materials in art therapy by a specific group of people (e.g., similar diagnoses and conditions)? (5) Are there ideal protocols and materials depending on the presenting or underlying issues? (6) Can art therapists be mechanics for the underlying neural and physiological structures that elicit negative emotions, perceptions, and behavioral patterns to facilitate greater functioning and improved perceptions of quality of life? Answering these questions will likely require technology such as neuroimaging, along with mixed methods designs that capture the phenomenological experience of the participants involved.

Neural Mechanisms and Structures Involved During Art Making

Primarily, it is significant to understand the underlying neural mechanisms involved in the art making of art therapy (Lusebrink, 2004). Much like neural networks and systems, the ETC is organized in ascending levels of complexity from the bottom up and in an interconnected fashion. Here, the aim is to evaluate cognitive and emotional functioning and to encourage improved information processing as indicated by "uninterrupted connections between levels" (Lusebrink & Hinz, 2020, p. 113) (Figure 11.1). The components of the ETC have been associated with brain structures (Lusebrink,

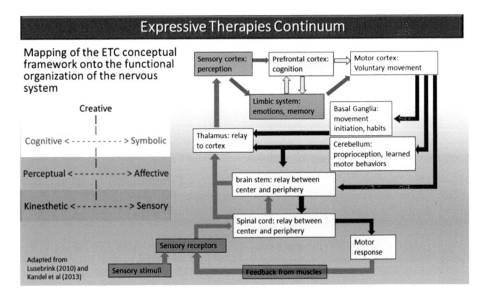

FIGURE 11.1 The Expressive Therapies Continuum & Human Information Processing (Strang, 2021, used with permission)

2010) and with the functions of large-scale brain networks (Lusebrink & Hinz, 2020), as shown in Table 11.1, providing testable hypotheses to begin identifying potential mechanisms for the impact of art and art making.

We have taken the liberty of expanding the conceptual framework of the ETC to incorporate multimodal inputs in the kinesthetic–sensory level of the ETC (Figure 11.1; Table 11.1). The kinesthetic–sensory reflects basic sensory processing. It is pre-verbal and requires minimal cognitive involvement (Rastogi et al., 2022). In a hierarchical conceptualization of nervous system functioning, visual, tactile, olfactory, and motor feedback inputs necessarily inform higher level perceptual–affective and cognitive–symbolic processes. For example, art therapy involves seeing (visual processing), but also creating (fine and gross motor control), and sensory input when someone is fully engaged in the sensory kinesthetics of art making (e.g., broad brush strokes, the feel of clay in their hands), and visual inputs are coordinated with the behavior. In fact, intact visuo-spatial inputs are not strictly necessary for successful art therapy interventions (Herrmann, 1995; Weiss 1990; Bitondo & Vaccaro, 2019; Cucca et al., 2021).

TABLE 11.1 Hypothesized parallels of ETC levels and neural pathways

ETC Level	Theorized Brain Network (Lusebrink, 2004, 2010; Lusebrink & Hinz, 2020)
Kinesthetic (K) / Sensory (S)	*Primary Visual Association Cortex*
	Stimuli from spine → Occipital Lobe → Striate and Extrastriate Cortices
	(K) Primary Motor Cortex and pathways to Basal Ganglia / Hippocampus
	(S) Primary Somatosensory Cortex
Perceptual (P) / Affective (A)	*Secondary Visual Association Cortex*
	(P) Ventral Visual Pathway (lower) "What" pathway in the Inferior Temporal Lobe
	(Shapes, Color, Form)
	Dorsal Visual Pathway (upper) "Where" pathway, Parietal Lobe, Multimodal Association Processes
	(Spatial Relationships)
	(A) Ventral Visual Pathway which is connected through the Thalamus to the Prefrontal and Limbic System (Anterior cingulate cortex, Anterior insula, Amygdala, Hippocampus)
	(Emotional Regulation)
	Salience network (SN)
Cognitive (C) / Symbolic (S)	*Frontal Cortex*
	(C) Prefrontal and Anterior Cingulate Cortices
	Central executive network (CEN)
	(Attention, Cognition, Action)
	(S) Orbitofrontal and Posterior Cingulate Cortices and pathways to Sensorimotor cortex
	Default Mode Network (DMN)
	(Meaning)

The perceptual–affective level of the ETC balances the perception of sensory information, such as form, color, texture, and temperature with the experience and expression of emotion. Perception can be mapped to higher-level cortical sensory integration areas, while the affective level can be mapped to connections between the limbic system and cortex (Rastogi et al., 2022). Affect can be influenced by sensory information. The direct connections from the olfactory system to limbic and memory systems (Kandel, 2001) mean that scents of materials and spaces can create and activate emotional memories. Together these processes are thought to involve the salience network (SN) (dynamic switching) (Lusebrink & Hinz, 2020).

Processes at the cognitive–symbolic level are mediated by regions of the prefrontal cortex, which integrates the lower levels of the ETC hierarchy and underlies the planning and ability to make deliberate and conscious expressive and symbolic choices for communication (Rastogi et al., 2022) and appear to involve switching between the central executive network (CEN) (cognition) and the default mode network (DMN) (meaning) (Lusebrink & Hinz, 2020).

An expanding number of studies in cognitive neuroscience and art therapy literature have shown some preliminary results while utilizing qEEG and fMRI technology for measuring brain activity in response to art making (Belkofer & Konopka, 2008; Belkofer et al., 2014; Bolwerk et al., 2014; Kaimal et al., 2017; King et al., 2017; Kruk et al., 2014; Pénzes et al., 2023). Such research, focused to examine the neural mechanisms involved in art-making tasks, has provided important empirical data to further bolster Lusebrink's (2004, 2010) working correlation between the ETC theory of differentiated art-making processes and neural mechanisms and involved brain areas. It is important to note that these data do not yet provide mechanistic information for the role of the therapeutic relationship, the influence of art making on that relationship, and the processes by which art making within a therapeutic relationship bolsters health and well-being.

Drawing and the Brain. Drawing tasks have been at the forefront of cognitive neuroscience explorations since the early 20th century with the introduction of the Goodenough Draw-a-Person test (DAP) (Goodenough, 1926) and the mid-20th century dating back to the introduction of the Clock Drawing Test (CDT) to assess for constructional apraxia (Aprahamian et al., 2009; Critchley, 1953; Freedman et al., 1994). Since that time, drawing tasks have been utilized throughout neuropsychology, psychiatry, and clinical psychology to assess for cognitive, developmental, and emotional impairments as indicated by characteristics or qualities of the drawn product. Those early assessments insinuated a window into the brain's functioning and broadened the inquiry about the specific neural mechanisms involved in drawing tasks (Raimo et al., 2021). The approaches to examining drawing have included fMRI and qEEG, both with limitations particular to their operation; both require limited movement to some degree in order not to obfuscate the recordings. In most neuroscience research, to be able to focus inquiry about the impact of a specific stimulus, (e.g. the phenomena of art making) on corresponding brain activation and functioning, requires that other variables must be considered and attempts to isolate those experiences belie the real-world situations this research is intended for. For instance, human perception, relative to functions of the DMN, would likely be activated during a course of scientific research so that the subject may have additional trains of thought related to that experience in and of itself. The aspect of reductionism must be contemplated in the attempt to invoke simultaneously occurring experiences and phenomena in targeted research methods.

Moving beyond reductionism, the collective findings from meta-analysis and a systematic review of collected research demonstrate evidence and support that the activity of drawing involves activation of the bilateral parieto-frontal network in which the posterior parietal lobe, left inferior parietal lobe, premotor cortex, inferior temporal gyrus, precuneus are consistently identified (Chechlacz et al., 2014; Griffith & Bingman, 2020; Ino et al., 2003; Trojano et al., 2009; Raimo et al., 2021). This information when applied to the framework of the ETC will require collaborative efforts to fully incorporate aspects of therapeutic art making to translate knowledge into practice.

Clay and the Brain. While there have been significantly fewer studies involving clay work related to art therapy and therapeutic interventions, the studies have shown incredible positive benefits with implications for targeting clay work to address specific dysregulation or dysfunction. We have learned activation patterns of clay work align with theta/delta wave activity, which can provide relaxation in line with positive therapeutic effect (Elkis-Abuhoff & Gaydos, 2016; Kruk et al., 2014; Pénzes et al., 2023). Specifically, clay art making has been found to be correlated with elevated theta waves in the frontal lobe, possibly indicative of invocation of a meditative state (Kruk et al., 2014), and, similarly, induced soothing calming states (Chong, 2015; van Lith et al., 2020), and stress reduction (Beerse et al., 2019, 2020). Clay work, particularly, involved in therapeutic art making with adults has shown general benefits for enhanced mood and decreased stress; specifically, toward remarkable symptom reduction for adults with Parkinson's disease and their caregivers (Elkis-Abuhoff et al., 2008), and adults with depression (Nan, 2015; Nan & Ho, 2017; Nan et al., 2021). Clay work decreases stress and induces calming, most likely activating the sensorimotor cortex and along the ventral visual association pathway with linkage to the thalamus; much like the ETC transition from K/S level to P/A level (Nan et al., 2021). Lusebrink (2004) stated the two most important aspects of the sensory functions for art therapists are of touch and haptic sense and described how touch "activates the cutaneous senses that respond to pressure, vibration, cooling and heating" (p. 127), which is certainly involved in clay work. The thoughtful use of clay in art therapy may allow a client to transition through the ETC levels with increasingly improved processing as results have shown symptom-reducing effects along with stress reduction (Nan et al., 2021). These initial theories imperatively fuel further investigation in the neural mechanisms and physiological effects involved in clay work.

Impact on the Body and Mind Because of Art Making

Beyond the brain, art therapists have traditionally viewed and conceptualized the role of art making from a holistic standpoint; that is, the art making itself is therapeutic affecting inner thoughts and feelings of the creator that are reflected in behavioral changes, and the act of reviewing artistic content has allowed for greater client insights, growth, and perceptual changes. Therefore, a focus on and isolation of areas of the brain involved in each step of art making provides neither a subjective sense of what art creation is like for the creator emotionally nor information about their opinions or beliefs.

Recently there has been a definitive shift in art therapy studies toward investigation of physiological effects and impact of specific art materials involved in art making. To seek a deeper understanding, art therapy researchers have examined cortisol levels, emotional response, and heart rate variability (HRV) during art making. These are particularly compelling physiological measures allowing assessment of various states of arousal, stress responses, and physical reactions to art making and that tap into a view of the autonomic nervous system and emotional regulation processes. In fact, promising research about the physiological effects of art making with various art media has contributed preliminary empirical evidence to broaden the conceptualization of art making as a holistic phenomenon, such as reduction in cortisol levels (Kaimal et al., 2016), anxiety reduction and emotional regulation (Beerse et al., 2019, 2020; Loudon & Deininger, 2017), and the effect on HRV to indicate arousal, modulation, or mediation of emotional response while art making (Haiblum-Itskovitch et al., 2018; Loudon & Deininger, 2017; Rankanen et al., 2022). For instance, Haiblum-Itskovitch et al. (2018) explored HRV and emotional response between pencil drawing, oil pastels, and gouache painting. They found that specific art materials elicited "unique emotional and physiological responses," as "art-making with gouache paint and oil-pastels resulted in improved positive mood, while pencil did not" and that comparatively, oil pastels evoked the most activation of the sympathetic nervous system (Haiblum-Itskovitch et al., 2018, p. 1). In another study, Rankanen et al. (2022) measured HRV, sleepiness, and mood states during different fast and slow drawing and clay activities. While clay forming was found to be the more physically demanding between the types of art making, fast drawing appeared "to be the most effective manner to free up mental resources and yield a relaxed mental state"; however, participants noted that forming clay was "the most inspiring, creativity enhancing and emotionally positive process" (p. 79). These findings have incredible implications for developing responsible and "safe" art therapy protocols in trauma-informed treatment!

Combining information that has been gained through physiological and neurological research during art making can build on the emerging neurobiological framework of art therapy and may illuminate the mechanics of the therapeutic effect of art making (Czamanski-Cohen & Weihs, 2016; Griffith & Bingman, 2020; Gu et al., 2018; King & Kaimal, 2019; King & Parada, 2021; Lusebrink, 2010; Rankanen et al., 2022; Vaisvaser, 2021). Further research is necessary to examine these initial findings further, potentially with other clinical populations to demonstrate positive and/or potentially reparative effects.

11.2 ADVANCING SCIENTIFIC INQUIRY INTO ART MAKING AND THE MATERIALS OF ART THERAPY

There have been a few efforts to expand what has been learned in replication studies of some of the work here. Pénzes et al. (2023) replicated the qEEG methodology from Kruk et al. (2014) with a larger participant group, and examined the differences in neural activation during art making between three different conditions: drawing freely with pencil on paper, drawing following instructions to draw a map, and working freely with clay. Results specific to the clay condition were found in-line with Kruk et al. (2014) and further support evidence that clay work elicits relaxation (Pénzes et al.,

2023). Beerse et al. (2020) expanded their own study (2019) which provided intriguing results indicating potential benefits for stress reduction amongst college students through mindfulness-based art therapy with clay and utilization of an online resource. As we gain more empirical evidence about both the impact of art making on the brain, and the characteristics of psychological disorders in the brain, we may be able to synthesize these findings to inform treatment approaches. Due to enhanced theoretical knowledge about sensory-based art therapy approaches, the potential for art therapy to underscore effective treatment for trauma continues to grow.

Art therapy research focused on trauma continues to produce compelling outcomes and considerations for further investigation into art therapy protocols developed from a neurologically informed approach (Hass-Cohen & Clyde Findlay, 2019). Considering what has been learned about the neural activation of various art-making processes, neuroplasticity (Sasmita et al., 2018), the visual cortex (Likova, 2012), structural patterns involved in dysfunction and brain areas involved in the trauma stress response (amygdala, hippocampus, prefrontal cortex) (Bremner, 2007), and the various brain areas involved in creative thinking and problem-solving, it appears emerging theories could be tested to apply specifically designed art tasks aimed to improve functioning and enhance outcomes (King et al., 2019).

CATs allow for therapists to "tap into the brain's potential for change and mobilize plasticity in the process of therapeutic development," and require an "emotionally attuned experiential practice, enriched in multisensory and expressive tools, which provides a safe space for self and self-other explorations" (Vaisvaser, 2021, p. 8). Additionally, expressive arts practices have become increasingly indicated as necessary and relevant treatment interventions (see for example Malchiodi, 2020; 2022). As such, CATs, and specifically art therapy, are uniquely qualified for the treatment of trauma as these integral and necessary components are heralded. Art therapy research studies addressing art therapy treatment for post-traumatic stress disorder (PTSD) purport several benefits to include symptom reduction, improved memory processing, and treatment adherence (Baker et al., 2018; Campbell et al., 2016; Schnitzer et al., 2021; Schouten et al., 2015; Walker et al., 2018). Additionally, as a treatment approach for trauma, art therapy has been shown to be a helpful adjunct to standardized forms of treatment and may provide benefit by modulating avoidant responses and intense or intrusive feelings of guilt and shame (Campbell et al., 2016; Schnitzer et al., 2021). Bolstering future research with investigations that explore mechanisms of action or change is a necessary endeavor that is made more possible with translational, collaborative, and transdisciplinary efforts (Baker et al., 2018; King, 2018). Further, amalgamation of the emerging and growing body of evidence of the impact of art making on the human experience, and how this impact can be channeled therapeutically, is another responsibility facing art therapists in the development of neuro-informed theory and practice.

11.3   LOOKING FORWARD

The American Art Therapy Association (AATA) has shown ongoing support for its membership interest in neuroscience and art therapy. For example, the AATA has initiated and maintained the Neuroscience Special Interest Group (Neuro SIG) since 2015, and has peppered its programming with several plenary panels, papers, and poster presentations over the years. The Neuro SIG gathers each year to discuss neuroscience in art therapy, how the Neuro SIG can transform into initiatives and drive research interests, and how neuroscience may be integrated into art therapy education. A common inquiry is how art therapy students, educational and graduate programs, and practicing art therapists can access and incorporate a neuroscience framework into the education and practice environment. We believe this is the next question to be addressed as collective conversations in research and current practice applications emerge.

Gathering perspectives from artists, students, neuroscientists, other physiological researchers, physicians, psychiatrists, psychologists, counselors, and art therapists can be the impetus for developing a community in which everyone has a seat at the table. Ultimately, all are gathered due to a collective and similar interest in the transformative power of the arts, across all art forms involving and imbuing creation, creativity, and curiosity to enhance our human quality of life. These conversations will lead us beyond reductionism inherent in isolating and focusing solely on areas of brain activation and toward a better understanding about the connection between neurobiological mechanisms involved in art making and subjective experiences of the individual, and further, how together they lead to and facilitate change and healing.

Truly, our world is adapting and changing rapidly; so too, are the methods and mechanisms involved in providing therapy. Recently, a pronounced shift in service delivery required CATs therapists to explore virtual platforms to provide therapy services. While telehealth and telemedicine practice are not new (Collie & Čubranić, 1999), CAT may have additional considerations for the execution of quality and effective experiences that lack some of the sensory and interpersonal aspects of traditional therapy settings. New emerging research explored the impact and realities of such a pervasive shift toward tele-CAT services (Feniger-Schaal et al., 2022) which art therapists have shown to be effective in theory and practice taking place in our increasingly virtual world (Winkel, 2022). Certainly, art therapists embrace flexibility and adaptability as characteristics intrinsic in successful practice due to the nature of art making; these qualities will need to be tested in the development of an ideal virtual, telehealth platform for CAT engagement.

Because there is such variability in human experience, true understanding of what mechanisms and interventions are generalizable requires the correlation of ephemeral, powerful, qualitative experiences with those that can be measured at the current level of physiological and neurological research. Understanding the mechanisms by which art therapy exerts its effects can lead us to more effective generalizable approaches that still honor the individual and their lived experiences. We aim for the perspectives, voices, science, and stories in this text to build upon our valuable history as we work together towards positive change and healing for all involved.

NOTE

1 For a detailed and accessible description of Arts & Health professions, including CAT, see Davies, C. R., & Clift, S. (2022). Arts and health glossary: A summary of definitions for use in research, policy and practice. *Frontiers in Psychology, 13*, 949685.

REFERENCES

Aprahamian, I., Martinelli, J. E., Neri, A. L., & Yassuda, M. S. (2009). The clock drawing test: A review of its accuracy in screening for dementia. *Dementia & Neuropsychologia*, 3(2), 74–81. https://doi.org/10.1590/S1980-57642009DN30200002

Baker, F. A., Metcalf, O., Varker, T., & O'Donnell, M. (2018). A systematic review of the efficacy of creative arts therapies in the treatment of adults with PTSD. *Psychological Trauma: Theory, Research, Practice, and Policy*, 10(6), 643–651. https://doi.org/10.1037/tra0000353

Beerse, M. E, Van Lith, T., & Stanwood, G. D. (2019). Is there a biofeedback response to art therapy? A technology-assisted approach for reducing anxiety and stress in college students. *SAGE Open*, 9(2), pp. 1–12. https://doi.org/10.1177/2158244019854646

Beerse, M. E., Van Lith, T., Pickett, S. M, & Stanwood, G. D. (2020). Biobehavioral utility of mindfulness-based art therapy: Neurobiological underpinnings and mental health impacts. *Experimental Biology and Medicine*, 245(2), 122–130. https://doi.org/10.1177/1535370219883634

Belkofer, C. M., & Konopka, L. M. (2008). Conducting art therapy research using quantitative EEG measures. *Art Therapy: Journal of the American Art Therapy Association*, 25(2), 56–63. https://doi.org/10.1080/07421656.2008.10129412

Belkofer, C. M., Van Hecke, A. V., & Konopka, L. M. (2014). Effects of drawing on alpha activity: A quantitative EEG study with implications for art therapy. *Art Therapy: Journal of the American Art Therapy Association*, 31(2), pp. 61–68. https://doi.org/10.1080/07421656.2014.903821

Bitondo, T., & Vaccaro, A. (2019). Art therapy with individuals with vision loss [Documents]. *JSTOR*. https://jstor.org/stable/community.24927962

Bolwerk, A., Mack-Andrick, J., Lang, F. R., Dörfler, A., & Maihöfner, C. (2014). How art changes your brain: Differential effects of visual art production and cognitive art evaluation on functional brain connectivity. *PLOS ONE*, 9(7), e101035. https://doi.org/10.1371/journal.pone.0101035

Bowen-Salter, H., Whitehorn, A., Pritchard, R., Kernot, J., Baker, A., Posselt, M., Price, E., Jordan-Hall, J., & Boshoff, K. (2022). Towards a description of the elements of art therapy practice for trauma: A systematic review. *International Journal of Art Therapy*, 27(1), 3–16. https://doi.org/10.1080/17454832.2021.1957959

Bremner, J. D. (2007). Neuroimaging in posttraumatic stress disorder and other stress-related disorders. *Neuroimaging Clinics of North America*, 17(4), 523–538. https://doi.org/10.1016/j.nic.2007.07.003

Campbell, M., Decker, K. P., Kruk, K., & Deaver, S. P. (2016). Art therapy and cognitive processing therapy for combat-related PTSD: A randomized controlled trial. *Art Therapy: Journal of the American Art Therapy Association*, 33(4), 169–177. https://doi.org/10.1080/07421656.2016.1226643

Chechlacz, M., Novick, A., Rotshtein, P., Bickerton, W., Humphreys, G. W., & Demeyere, N. (2014). The neural substrates of drawing: A voxel-based morphometry analysis of constructional, hierarchical, and spatial representation deficits. *Journal of Cognitive Neuroscience*, 26(12), 2701–2715. https://doi.org/10.1162/jocn_a_00664

Chong, C. Y. J. (2015). Why art psychotherapy? Through the lens of interpersonal neurobiology: The distinctive role of art psychotherapy intervention for clients with early relational trauma. *International Journal of Art Therapy*, 20(3), 118126. https://doi.org/10.1080/17454832.2015.1079727

Cloitre, M., Courtois, C. A., Ford, J. D., Green, B. L., Alexander, P., Briere, J., & Van der Hart, O. (2012). The ISTSS expert consensus treatment guidelines for complex PTSD in adults. www.istss.org/

Collie, K., & Čubranić, D. (1999) An art therapy solution to a telehealth problem. *Art Therapy: Journal of the American Art Therapy Association*, 16(4), 186–193. https://doi.org/10.1080/07421656.1999.10129481

Critchley, M. (1953). *The parietal lobes*. Williams & Wilkins.

Cucca, A., Di Rocco, A., Acosta, I., Beheshti, M., Berberian, M., Bertisch, H. C., Droby, A., Ettinger, T., Hudson, T. E., Inglese, M., Jung, Y. J., Mania, D. F., Quartarone, A., Rizzo, J.-R., Sharma, K., Feigin, A., Biagioni, M. C., & Ghilardi, M. F. (2021). Art therapy for Parkinson's disease. *Parkinsonism & Related Disorders*, 84, 148–154. https://doi.org/10.1016/j.parkreldis.2021.01.013

Czamanski-Cohen, J., & Weihs, K. L. (2016). The bodymind model: A platform for studying the mechanisms of change induced by art therapy. *The Arts in Psychotherapy, 51,* 63–71. https://doi.org/10.1016/j.aip.2016.08.006

deWitte, M., Orkibi, H., Zarate, R., Karkou, V., Sajnani, N., Malhotra, B., Ho, R. T. H., Kaimal, G., Baker, F. A., & Koch, S. C. (2021). From therapeutic factors to mechanisms of change in the creative arts therapies: A scoping review. *Frontiers in Psychology, 12,* 1–12. https://doi.org/10.3389/fpsyg.2021.678397

Dikker, S., Wan, L., Davidesco, I., Kaggen, L., Oostrik, M., McClintock, J., Rowland, J., Michalareas, G., Bavel, J. J., Ding, M., & Poeppel, D. (2017). Brain-to-brain synchrony tracks real-world dynamic group interactions in the classroom. *Current Biology: CB, 27*(9), 1375–1380. https://doi.org/10.1016/j.cub.2017.04.002

Elkis-Abuhoff, D. L., & Gaydos, M. (2016). Medical art therapy applied to the trauma experienced by those diagnosed with Parkinson's disease. In J. King (Ed.). *Art therapy, trauma, and neuroscience: Theoretical and practical perspectives* (pp. 195–210). Routledge.

Elkis-Abuhoff, D. L., Goldblatt, R. B., Gaydos, M. & Corrato, S. (2008). Effects of clay manipulation on somatic dysfunction and emotional distress in patients with Parkinson's disease. *Art Therapy: Journal of the American Art Therapy Association, 25*(3), 122–128. https://doi.org/10.1080/07421656.2008.10129596

Fancourt, D., & Finn, S. (2019). What is the evidence on the role of the arts in improving health and well-being? A scoping review. *World Health Organization Health Evidence Network synthesis report, 67.* www.ncbi.nlm.nih.gov/books/NBK553773/?report=classic

Feniger-Schaal, R., Orkibi, H., Keisari, S., Sajnani, N. L., & Butler, J. D. (2022). Shifting to tele-creative arts therapies during the COVID-19 pandemic: An international study on helpful and challenging factors. *The Arts in Psychotherapy, 78,* 101898. https://doi.org/10.1016/j.aip.2022.101898

Flückiger, C., Del Re, A. C., Wampold, B. E., & Symonds, D. (2012). How central is the alliance in psychotherapy? A multilevel longitudinal meta-analysis. *Journal of Counseling Psychology, 50*(1), 10–17. https://doi.org/10.1037/a0025749

Franklin, M. (2010). Affect regulation, mirror neurons, and the third hand: Formulating Mindful empathic art interventions. *Art Therapy, 27*(4), 160–167. https://doi.org/10.1080/07421656.2010.10129385

Freedman, M., Leach, L., Kaplan, E., Winocur, G., Shulman, K., & Delis, D. C. (1994). *Clock drawing: A neuropsychological analysis.* Oxford University Press.

Gallese, V. (2017). Visions of the body: Embodied simulation and aesthetic experience. *Aisthesis. Pratiche, linguaggi e saperi dell'estetico, 10*(1), 41–50. https://doi.org/10.13128/Aisthesis-20902

Goodenough, F. L. (1926). *Measurement of intelligence by drawings.* World Book Company.

Griffith, F. J., & Bingman, V. P. (2020). Drawing on the brain: An ALE meta-analysis of functional brain activation during drawing. *The Arts in Psychotherapy, 71,* 101690. https://doi.org/10.1016/j.aip.2020.101690

Gu, S., Gao, M., Yan, Y., Wang, F., Tang, Y., & Huang, J. H. (2018). The neural mechanism underlying cognitive and emotional processes in creativity. *Frontiers in Psychology, 9,* Article 1924. https://doi.org/10.3389/fpsyg.2018.01924

Haiblum-Itskovitch, S., Czamanski-Cohen, J., & Galili, G. (2018). Emotional response and changes in heart rate variability following art-making with three different art materials. *Frontiers in Psychology, 9,* Article 968. https://doi.org/10.3389/fpsyg.2018.00968

Hass-Cohen, N. (2008). CREATE: Art therapy relational neuroscience principles (ATR-N). In N. Hass-Cohen & R. Carr (Eds.), *Art therapy and clinical neuroscience* (pp. 283–309). Jessica Kingsley.

Hass-Cohen, N. (2016). Secure resiliency: Art therapy relational neuroscience trauma treatment principles and guidelines. In *Art therapy, trauma, and neuroscience* (1st ed.). Routledge.

Hass-Cohen, N., Bokoch, R., Findlay, J. C., & Witting, A. B. (2018). A four-drawing art therapy trauma and resiliency protocol study. *The Arts in Psychotherapy, 61,* 44–56. https://doi.org/10.1016/j.aip.2018.032.003

Hass-Cohen, N., & Clyde Findlay, J. M. A. (2019). The art therapy relational neuroscience and memory reconsolidation four drawing protocol. *The Arts in Psychotherapy, 63,* 51–59. https://doi.org/10.1016/j.aip.2019.03.002

Herrmann, U. (1995). A trojan horse of clay: Art therapy in a residential school for the blind. *The Arts in Psychotherapy, 22*(3), 229–234. https://doi.org/10.1016/0197-4556(95)00023-X

Heyes, C., & Catmur, C. (2021). What happened to mirror neurons? *Perspectives on Psychological Science, 17*(1), 153–168. https://doi.org/10.1177/1745691621990638

Hilbuch, A., Snir, S., Regev, D., & Orkibi, H. (2016). The role of art materials in the transferential relationship: Art psychotherapists' perspective. *The Arts in Psychotherapy, 49,* 19–26. https://doi.org/10.1016/j.aip.2016.05.011

Hinz, L. (2019). *Expressive therapies continuum: A framework for using art in therapy* (2nd ed.). Routledge. https://doi.org/10.4324/9780429299339

Hinz, L. D., Rim, S., & Lusebrink, V. B. (2022). Clarifying the creative level of the expressive therapies continuum: A different dimension. *The Arts in Psychotherapy, 78,* 101896. https://doi.org/10.1016/j.aip.2022.101896

Ino T., Asada, T., Ito, J., Kimura, T., Fukuyama, H. (2003) Parieto-frontal networks for clock drawing revealed with fMRI. *Neuroscience Research, 45*(1), 71–77. https://doi.org/10.1016/S0168-0101(02)00194-3

Kagin, S. L., & Lusebrink, V. B. (1978). The expressive therapies continuum. *Art Psychotherapy, 5,* 171–180. https://doi.org/10.1016/0090-9092(78)90031-5

Kaimal, G. (2019). Adaptive response theory (ART): A clinical research framework for art therapy. *Art Therapy: Journal of the American Art Therapy Association, 36*(4), 215–219. https://doi.org/10.1080/07421656.2019.1667670

Kaimal, G., Ray, K., & Muniz, J. (2016). Reduction of cortisol levels and participants' responses following art making. *Art Therapy: Journal of the American Art Therapy Association, 33*(2), 74–80. https://doi.org/10.1080/07421656.2016.1166832

Kaimal, G., Ayaz, H., Herres, J., Dieterich-Hartwell, R., Makwana, B., Kaiser, D. H., & Nasser, J. A. (2017). Functional near-infrared spectroscopy assessment of reward perception based on visual self-expression: Coloring, doodling, and free drawing. *The Arts in Psychotherapy, 55,* 85–92. https://doi.org/10.1016/j.aip2017.05.004

Kandel, E. R. (2001). The molecular biology of memory storage: A dialogue between genes and synapses. *Science, 294*(5544), 1030–038.

Karkou, V., Sajnani, N., Orkibi, H., Groarke, J. M., Czamanski-Cohen, J., Panero, M. E., Drake, J., Jola, C., & Baker, F. A. (2022). Editorial: The psychological and physiological benefits of the arts. *Frontiers in Psychology, 13.* https://doi.org/10.3389/fpsyg.2022.840089

Kazdin, A. (2007). Mediators and mechanisms of change in art therapy research. *Annual Review of Clinical Psychology, 3*(1), 1–27. https://doi.org/10.1146/annurev.clinpsy.3.022806.091432

King, J. (Ed.). (2016). *Art therapy, trauma, and neuroscience: Theoretical and practical perspectives* (1st ed.). Routledge.

King, J. (2018). Summary of twenty-first century great conversations in art, neuroscience and related therapeutics. *Frontiers in Psychology, 9,* 1428. https://doi.org/10.3389/fpsyg.2018.01428

King, J. L., & Kaimal, G. (2019). Approaches to research in art therapy using imaging techniques. *Frontiers in Human Neuroscience, 13,* 159. https://doi.org/10.3389/fnhum.2019.00159

King, J., Kaimal, G., Konopka, L., Belkofer, C., & Strang, C. E. (2019). Practical applications of neuroscience-informed art therapy. *Art Therapy: Journal of the American Art Therapy Association, 36*(3), 149–156. https://doi.org/10.1080/07421656.2019.1649549

King, J. L., Knapp, K. E., Shaikh, L. A., Li, F., Sabau, D., Pascuzzi, R. M., & Osburn, L. L. (2017). Cortical activity changes after art making and rote motor movement as measured by EEG: A preliminary study. *Biomedical Journal of Scientific and Technical Research, 1*(4), 1062–1075. https://doi.org/10.26717/BJSTR.2017.01.000366

King, J. L., & Parada, F. J. (2021). Using mobile brain/body imaging to advance research in arts, health, and related therapeutics. *European Journal of Neuroscience, 54*(12), 836–8380. https://doi.org/10.1111/ejn.15313

Kruk, K. A., Aravich, P. F., Deaver, S. P., & deBeus, R. (2014). Comparison of brain activity during drawing and clay sculpting: A preliminary qEEG study. *Art Therapy: Journal of the American Art Therapy Association, 31*(2), 52–60. https://doi.org/10.1080/07421656.2014.903826

Levy, J., & Bader, O. (2020). Graded empathy: A neuro-phenomenological hypothesis. *Frontiers in Psychiatry, 11.* https://doi.org/10.3389/fpsyt.2020.554848

Likova, L. T. (2012). Drawing enhances cross-modal memory plasticity in the human brain: A case study in a totally blind adult. *Frontiers in Human Neuroscience, 6.* https://doi.org/10.3389/fnhum.2012.00044

Loudon, G. H., & Deininger, G. M. (2017). The physiological response to drawing and its relation to attention and relaxation. *Journal of Behavioral and Brain Science, 7*(3), 111–124. https://doi.org/10.4236/jbbs.2017.73011

Lusebrink, V. B. (2004). Art therapy and the brain: An attempt to understand the underlying processes of art expression in therapy. *Art Therapy: Journal of the American Art Therapy Association, 21*(3), 125–135. https://doi.org/10.1080/07421656.2004.10129496

Lusebrink, V. B. (2010). Assessment and therapeutic application of the expressive therapies continuum: Implications for brain structures and functions. *Art Therapy: Journal of the American Art Therapy Association, 27*(4), 168–177. https://doi.org/10.1080/07421656.2010.10129380

Lusebrink, V. B. (2014). Art therapy and the neural basis of imagery: Another possible view. *Art Therapy: Journal of the American Art Therapy Association, 31*(2), 87–90. https://doi.org/10.1080/07421656.903828

Lusebrink, V. B., & Hinz, L. (2016). The expressive therapies continuum as a framework in the treatment of trauma. In J. King (Ed.)., *Art therapy, trauma, and neuroscience* (pp. 42–66). Routledge.

Lusebrink, V. B., & Hinz, L. (2020). Cognitive and symbolic aspects of art therapy and similarities with large scale brain networks. *Art Therapy: Journal of the American Art Therapy Association, 37*(3), 113–122. https://doi.org/10.1080/07421656.2019.1691869

Lusebrink, V. B., Mārtinsone, K., & Dzilna-Šilova, I. (2013). The expressive therapies continuum (ETC): Interdisciplinary bases of the ETC. *International Journal of Art Therapy, 18,* 75–85. https://doi.org/10.1080/17454832.2012.713370

Malchiodi, C. (2022). *Trauma-informed expressive arts therapy.* Guilford.

Malchiodi, C. A. (2020). *Trauma and expressive arts therapy: Brain, body, and imagination in the healing process.* Guilford.

McWilliams, N. (2021). Diagnosis and its discontents: Reflections on our current dilemma. *Psychoanalytic Inquiry, 41*(8), 565–579. https://doi.org/10.1080/07351690.2021.1983395

Nan, J. K. M. (2015). *Therapeutic effects of clay art therapy for patients with depression* [Doctoral dissertation, Hong Kong University]. *HKU Theses Online (HKUTO).* http://dx.doi.org/10.5353/th_b5570798

Nan, J. K. M., Hinz, L. D., & Lusebrink, V. B. (2021). Clay art therapy on emotion regulation: Research, theoretical underpinnings, and treatment mechanisms. In C. R. Martin, L. Hunter, V. B. Patel, V. R. Preedy, & R. Rajendram (Eds.). *The neuroscience of depression* (pp. 431–442). Academic Press. https://doi.org/10.1016/B978-0-12-817933-8.00009-8

Nan, J. K. M., & Ho, R. T. H. (2017). Effects of clay art therapy on adults outpatients [sic] with major depressive disorder: A randomized controlled trial. *Journal of Affective Disorders, 217*(1), 237–245. https://doi.org/10.1016/j.jad.2017.04.013

Norcross, J. C., & Lambert, M. J. (2019). Evidence-based psychotherapy relationships: The third task force. In J. C. Norcross & M. J. Lambert (Eds.), *Psychotherapy relationships that work* (3rd ed., Vol. 1, pp. 1–23). Oxford University Press.

Norcross, J. C., & Wampold, B. E. (2011) What works for whom: Tailoring psychotherapy to the person. *Journal of Clinical Psychology, 67*(2), 127–132. https://doi.org/10.1002/jclp.20764

Parada, F. J., & Rossi, A. (2018). If neuroscience needs behavior, what does psychology need? *Frontiers in Psychology, 9.* https://doi.org/10.3389/fpsyg.2018.00433

Pénzes, I., Engelbert, R., Heidendael, D., Oti, K., Jongen, E. M. M., & van Hooren, S. (2023). The influence of art material and instruction during art making on brain activity: *A quantitative electro-encephalogram study, 83,* 102024. https://doi.org/10.1016/j.aip.2023.102024

Raimo, S., Santangelo, G., & Trojano, L. (2021). The neural bases of drawing. A meta-analysis and a systematic literature review of neurofunctional studies in health individuals. *Neuropsychology Review, 31,* 689–702. https://doi.org/10.1007/s11065-021-09494-4

Rankanen, M., Leinikka, M., Groth, C., Seitamaa-Hakkarainen, P., Mäkelä, M., & Huotilainen, M. (2022). Physiological measurements and emotional experiences of drawing and clay. *The Arts in Psychotherapy, 79,* 101899. https://doi.org/10.1016/j.aip.2022.101899

Rastogi, M., Strang, C., Vilinsky, I., & Holland, K. (2022). Intersections of neuroscience and art therapy. In *Foundations of Art Therapy* (pp. 123–158). Academic Press. https://doi.org/10.1016/B978-0-12-824308-4.00014-4

Sasmita, A. O., Kuruvilla, J., & Ling, A. P. K. (2018). Harnessing neuroplasticity: Modern approaches and clinical future. *International Journal of Neuroscience, 128*(11), 1061–1077. https://doi.org/10.1080/00207454.2018.1466781

Schnitzer, G., Holttum, S., & Huet, V. (2021). A systematic literature review of the impact of art therapy upon post-traumatic stress disorder. *International Journal of Art Therapy, 26*(4), 147–160. https://doi.org/10.1080/17454832.2021.1910719

Schouten, K. A., de Niet, G. J., Knipscheer, J. W., Kleber, R. J., & Hutschemaekers, G. J. M. (2015). The effectiveness of art therapy in the treatment of traumatized adults: A systematic review on art therapy and trauma. *Trauma, Violence, & Abuse, 16*(2), 220–228. https://doi.org/10.1177/1524838014555032

Siegel, D. J., & Soloman, M. F. (Eds.). (2003). *Healing trauma: Attachment, mind, body, and brain* (Norton series on Interpersonal Neurobiology). W.W. Norton.

Stepney, S. A. (2022). Multicultural and diversity perspectives in art therapy: Transforming image into substance. In M. Rastogi, R. P. Feldwisch, M. Pate, & J. Scarce (Eds.), *Foundations of art therapy: Theory and applications* (pp. 81–122). Academic Press. https://doi.org/10.1016/B978-0-12-824308-4.00010-7

Strang, C. E. (2021). *Exploring art therapy assumptions through the lens of neuroscience.* The American Art Therapy Association.

Trojano, L., Grossi, D., & Flash, T. (2009). Cognitive neuroscience of drawing: Contributions of neuropsychological, experimental and neurofunctional studies. *Cortex, 45*(3), 269–277. https://doi.org/10.1016/j.cortex.2008.11.015

Vaisvaser, S. (2021). The embodied–enactive–interactive brain: Bridging neuroscience and creative arts therapies. *Frontiers in Psychology, 12.* https://doi.org/10.3389/fpsyg.2021.634079

Van Lith, T., Beerse, M., & Smalley, Q. (2020). A qualitative inquiry comparing mindfulness-based art therapy versus neutral clay tasks as a proactive mental health solution for college students. *Journal of American College Health, 70*(6), 1889–1897. https://doi.org/10.1080/07448481.2020.1841211

Vickhoff, B. (2023). Why art? The role of arts in arts and health. *Frontiers in Psychology, 14.* https://doi.org/10.3389/fpsyg.2023.765019

Walker, M. S., Stamper, A. M., Nathan, D. E., & Riedy, G. (2018). Art therapy and underlying fMRI brain patterns in military TBI: A case series. *International Journal of Art Therapy, 23*(4), 180–187. https://doi.org/10.1080/17454832.2018.1473453

Weiss, R. (1990). An art therapy curriculum in an early intervention program for visually impaired children. *Art Therapy, 7*(2), 79–85. https://doi.org/10.1080/07421656.1990.10758897

Winkel, M. (2022). *Virtual art therapy: Research and practice.* Routledge.

GLOSSARY

Abuse – an action that intentionally causes harm or injures another person.

Action Potential – the change in electrical potential that occurs between the inside and outside of a nerve or muscle fiber when it is stimulated, serving to transmit nerve signals.

Adaptive Responding – one of the six CREATE Framework principles; cognitive and behavioral efforts to manage stressful conditions or associated emotional distress.

Adlerian Psychology – a humanistic and goal oriented approach to psychology that emphasizes the individual's strivings for success, connectedness with others, and contributions to society as being hallmarks of mental health.

Allostatic – the body's ability to achieve stability through adaptive responses to stressors and change.

Allostatic Load – the cumulative burden of chronic stress and life events.

Amygdala – a subcortical brain structure that is part of the limbic system and involved with initiating the autonomic nervous system "fight or flight" response to perceived danger.

Anterior Cingulate Cortex – front-most portion of the cingulate cortex implicated in several complex cognitive functions such as emotional expression, attention allocation, and mood regulation.

Anterior Insula – a cortical center of visceral information processing also significantly involved with the processing and organization of interoceptive stimuli.

Aphasia – a disorder that results from damage to portions of the brain that are responsible for language.

Axon – the long threadlike part of a nerve cell along which impulses are conducted from the cell body to synapses with other cells.

Auxiliary Self – in psychodrama, a group member, other than the therapist, who assumes the role of a significant figure in the protagonist's life.

Basal Ganglia – a group of subcortical structures involved in the coordination of movement. Connects with the cortex via the thalamus.

Bilateral Lingual Gyrus – a brain structure that is part of the occipital lobe linked to processing visual stimuli, especially related to letters. It also plays a role in the analysis of the logical order of events and encoding visual memories.

Blood Oxygen Level Dependent Magnetic Resonance Imaging (BOLD MRI) – brain imaging technology that detects changes in deoxyhemoglobin driven by localized changes in brain blood flow and blood oxygenation.

Bottom-up Information Processing – refers to information processing that begins with sensory or subcortical processing and progresses to more sophisticated, cortical areas of the brain.

Catecholamines – a type of neurohormone that is important in stress responses.

Central Executive Network – a large scale brain network important for higher order executive functioning such as cognitive control of thought/rumination, emotion regulation, and working memory.

Central sulci – the sulcus separating the frontal lobe of the cerebral cortex from the parietal lobe.

Cerebellum – section of the brain involved in balance and posture, regulation of movement, and implicit, procedural learning, located just below and behind the cerebral hemispheres at the level of the pons.

Cerebrum – the largest part of the brain consisting of two cerebral hemispheres bridged by the corpus callosum.

Child abuse or neglect – according to the U.S. Department of Health and Human Services (2014), child abuse is defined as "Any recent act or failure to act on the part of a parent or caretaker which results in death, serious physical or emotional harm, sexual abuse or exploitation"; or "An act or failure to act which presents an imminent risk of serious harm."

Cingulate Cortex – an integral part of the limbic system involved with emotion formation and processing, learning, and memory. It is highly influential in motivating behavior.

Cognitive/Symbolic Level of the ETC – represents the most sophisticated form of information processing in which logical, linear, and linguistic operations are emphasized on the cognitive component and personal or universal symbols are represented by the symbolic component.

Collectivist Psychotherapy Theory – an orientation that reflects the values, attitudes, and behaviors of a person–group relationship in which family and group life is emphasized and the concept of the self is less essential.

Common Threads Project – an integrative trauma recovery program for victims of sexual violence that uses sewing circles to heal from the trauma.

Compassionate Relapse Prevention – a varied set of cognitive-behavioral techniques that are employed to maintain desirable addictive and impulsive behavioral changes.

Complicated Grief – a response to death (or, sometimes, to other significant loss or trauma) that deviates significantly from normal expectations.

Contextualized Representations – word vectors that are sensitive to the context in which they appear.

Corpus Callosum – a large tract of nerve fibers running across the longitudinal fissure of the brain and connecting the cerebral hemispheres.

Cortisol – a hormone made by the adrenal cortex that helps the body use glucose, protein, and fats.

CREATE Framework – the six principles (creative embodiment, relational resonating, expressive communicating, adaptive responding, transformative integrating, and empathizing and compassion) that compose the Art Therapy Relational Neuroscience (ATR-N) approach.

Creative Embodiment – one of the six CREATE Framework principles; represents the creative manifestation of human senses, experiences, and expression.

Creative Transition Area – an area of the ETC occurring in the central area of each level, at which it is hypothesized that information processing with both components of a level contribute to optimally creative and therapeutic experiences.

Cultural Competence – awareness of one's own culture and the ability to learn from and adapt to working effectively with other cultures.

Decolonization – to free a people or area from colonial status.

Decolonizing – a process of establishing inclusivity and honoring the practices and values of marginalized peoples through removing Western/Eurocentric ideologies of power and knowledge.

Default Mode Network – a large-scale brain network supporting emotional processing, autobiographical memory, and self-referential thought leading to a coherent sense of self. Associated with "mind wandering" and daydreaming.

Dendrite – a branching, threadlike extension of the cell body that receives synaptic signals from other neurons.

Dorsal Anterior Cingulate Cortex – part of the anterior cingulate cortex associated with executive control, learning, adjustment, economic choice, and self-control.

Dorsolateral Prefrontal Cortex – a region of the frontal lobes typically associated with executive functions including general executive control, working memory and selective attention.

Electroencephalography (EEG) – a test that measures electrical activity in the brain using small, metal discs, called electrodes, attached to the scalp.

Embodied Cognition – the body's interactions with the environment contribute to cognitive processing.

Embodiment – an effect where the body plays an instrumental role in information processing.

Empathic Resonance – a way of experiencing what the client expresses that elicits a bodily felt sense in the therapist.

Empathizing and Compassion – one of the six CREATE Framework principles; the development of insight and compassion towards oneself, and others, as well as the capacity to tolerate emotional frustration.

Empathy – the ability to respond to someone else's feelings or experiences by imagining what it would be like to be in that person's situation.

Engagement – the process through which a client begins to actively participate in their treatment.

Entrainment – the process that activates or provides a timing cue for a biological rhythm or synchronization with another behavior.

Episodic Memory – a part of long-term explicit memory, composed of each person's unique recollection of specific experiences, events and situations.

Evidence-based Practice – using the best available evidence for decision making and providing efficient and effective care for patients on a scientific basis.

Explicit memory – long-term memory available for conscious recall; includes memory for facts, events, and concepts

Expressive Communicating – one of the six CREATE Framework principles; the ability to communicate using verbal language and non-verbal cues, as well as the fluctuating unconscious and attentive conscious states.

Expressive Therapies Continuum (ETC) – a theoretical model developed in 1978 by art therapists Sandra Kagin and Vija Lusebrink that explains how clients take in, process and express information as they use expressive modalities to create artistic expressions.

Externalization – a defense mechanism in which one's thoughts, feelings, or perceptions are attributed to the external world and perceived as independent of oneself or one's own experiences.

Event-related Potentials – very small voltages generated in the brain structures in response to specific events or stimuli. Typically measured by EEG.

Fasciculations – involuntary rapid muscle twitches that are too weak to move a limb but are easily felt by patients and seen or palpated by clinicians.

Flow – a state of concentrated and sustain attention in which a person is challenged by a task but able to master it, resulting in altered time perception, feelings of great satisfaction of moments of peak joy.

Forebrain – the part of the brain that develops from the anterior section of the neural tube in the embryo, containing the cerebrum and the diencephalon.

Frontal Lobe – one of the four main lobes of each cerebral hemisphere of the brain, lying in front of the central sulcus. It is concerned with motor and higher order executive functions.

Functional Connectivity – the strength to which activity between a pair of brain regions covaries or correlates over time.

Functional magnetic resonance imaging (fMRI) – a procedure that uses MRI technology to measure and map brain activity by detecting changes in the brain's blood flow and oxygenation.

Functional near-infrared spectroscopy (fNIRS) – a non-invasive, brain imaging technology that uses low levels of non-ionizing light to record changes in cerebral blood flow.

Heart Rate Variability (HRV) – a measure of the variation in time between each heartbeat.

Hindbrain – region of the developing vertebrate brain that is composed of the medulla oblongata, the pons, and the cerebellum.

Hippocampus – a brain structure deep in the temporal lobes, an important part of the limbic system, helping to regulate motivation, emotion, learning, and memory.

Holistic – relating to or concerned with complete systems rather than with individual parts.

Hypothalamus – a region of the brain, between the thalamus and the midbrain, that functions as the main control center for the autonomic nervous system and that acts as an endocrine gland by producing hormones.

Imagery Rehearsal Therapy (IRT) – a short, CBT-based written exercise targeting the reduction of post traumatic nightmares.

Implicit Bias – a bias or prejudice that is present but not consciously held or recognized.

Implicit Memory – nonconscious memory of skills, procedures, and conditioned responses.

Interoception – the brain's representation of sensations from within the body.

Interoceptive Awareness – awareness of bodily information coming from sensation and emotion that informs the sense of self.

Intersubjectivity – the interchange of thoughts and feelings, both conscious and unconscious, between two persons, as facilitated by empathy.

Kinesthetic-Sensory Approach – the combination of body movements with touch, smell, and hearing activities in clinical interventions.

Kinesthetic/Sensory Level of the ETC – the first level of the ETC model corresponding to the movements made and sensations experienced during creative arts activities or interventions.

Large-scale Brain Networks (Intrinsic Brain Networks) – coordinated systems of brain structures that function together and are thought to underly complex actions and/or cognition.

Lateralization – localization, specialization, or asymmetry of function or activity on one side of the body or brain with respect to the other.

Ligand – a molecule that binds to a receptor to activate signaling within a cell and results in changes in electrical activity or cell structure.

Low Input–High Output – a mild stimulus (low input) evokes an extreme response (high output).

Low Resolution Brain Electromagnetic Tomography (LORETA) – a method of mathematically analyzing multiple EEG signals from across the scalp to determine their source from within the cortex.

Magnetic Resonance Imaging (MRI) – a medical imaging technique that uses a strong magnetic field and computer-generated radio waves to create images of organs and tissues.

Magnetoencephalography (MEG) – the measurement of the magnetic field generated by the electrical activity of neurons in the brain.

Maltreatment – the abuse or neglect of another person.

Manualized Approaches – treatment that follows a prescribed set of therapy directives over a pre-defined number of sessions.

Medial Prefrontal Cortex – a part of the prefrontal cortex that mediates decision making due to its role in reward processing. It also supports memory consolidation through the ability to recall the best action or emotional response to specific events.

Memory Reconsolidation – the process that serves to restabilize a memory that has been destabilized through memory retrieval.

Mentalizing – the ability to understand one's own and others' mental states, thereby comprehending one's own and others' intentions and affects.

Midbrain – the portion of the brain situation between the forebrain and hindbrain that includes the tectum, tegmentum, and substantia nigra.

Mindfulness Softening – maintaining a moment-by-moment awareness of your thoughts, feelings, bodily sensations, and surrounding environment, by relaxing the body, increasing flexibility, and exercising kindness and compassion.

Mirror Neuron – a class of neuron that modulates their activity when an individual executes a specific motor act and when they observe the same or similar act performed by another individual.

Mission Statement – something that states the purpose or goal of a business or organization.

Mobile Brain Body Imaging (MOBI) – a general research approach that embraces a variety of hardware and software solutions to record and analyze brain dynamics in actively behaving participants.

Moral Injury – the damage done to one's conscience or moral compass when that person perpetrates, witnesses, or fails to prevent acts that transgress one's own moral beliefs, values, or ethical codes of conduct.

Morphologies – the study of neuronal structure commonly used for identification and classification.

Motor Cortex – the region of the frontal lobe of the brain responsible for the control of voluntary movement.

Multimodal Association Cortex (Transmodal Cortex) – large areas of the cerebral cortex that receive sensory input from multiple different sensory modalities and various association areas and help make associations between various kinds of sensory information.

Myelin Sheath – the insulating covering that surrounds an axon with multiple layers of myelin, and that increases the speed at which a nerve impulse can travel along an axon.

Neglect – the state of not receiving enough care or attention.

Neuroaesthetics – the scientific study of the neural consequences of contemplating a creative work of art.

Neuroception – an automatic neural process of evaluating risk in the environment and adjusting our physiological response to deal with potential risks subconsciously.

Neurocounseling – the integration of neuroscience into the practice of counseling, by teaching and illustrating the physiological underpinnings of mental health concerns.

Neurodevelopment – the development of the nervous system.

Neurofeedback – a kind of biofeedback, which teaches self-control of brain functions to subjects by measuring brain waves and providing a feedback signal.

Neuron – a specialized, impulse-conducting cell that is the functional unit of the nervous system, consisting of the cell body and its processes, the axon and dendrites.

Neurophysiology – a branch of neuroscience that is concerned with the normal and abnormal functioning of the nervous system.

Neuroplasticity – a process that involves adaptive structural and functional changes to the brain.

Neurotransmitter – any of a group of chemical agents released by presynaptic neurons to stimulate neighboring cells allowing information to be transmitted from one cell to the next throughout the nervous system.

Orbitofrontal Cortex – an area of the prefrontal cortex found at the very front of the brain which has extensive connections with sensory and motor areas as well as limbic system structures involved in emotion and memory.

Occipital Cortex – one of the four major lobes of the cortex, involved with the reception and integration of visual stimuli.

Occipital Lobe – the posterior lobe of each cerebral hemisphere, includes the visual cortex.

Parietal Cortex – one of the four major lobes of the cortex. Includes somatosensory cortex responsible for processing sensations of touch, temperature and pain, and regions that associate touch, auditory, and visual stimuli.

Parietal Lobe – the middle part of each cerebral hemisphere behind the central sulcus that receives and manages sensory information.

Perceptual/Affective Level of the ETC – the middle level of the ETC model in which the formal art elements are emphasized on the perceptual side and the emotional aspects of artistic experiences are emphasized on the affective side.

Person-centered Approach – a non-authoritative approach that allows clients to take more of a lead in sessions such that, in the process, they discover their own solutions.

Person-centered art therapy – Emphasizes the therapist's role as being empathic, open, honest, congruent, and caring. This philosophy incorporates the belief that each individual has worth, dignity, and the capacity for self-direction.

Polyvagal Theory – theory positing that the autonomic nervous system contains 3 neural networks that are involved in social communication, mobilization, and immobilization.

Positive Emoting – an emotional response associated with positive affect.

Posterior Cingulate Cortex – the posterior part of the cingulate cortex, it is a central node of the Default Mode Network (DMN) implicated in human awareness, pain, and episodic memory retrieval.

Post Modern Psychotherapy Theory – focuses on deconstructing common beliefs and examining their value in an individual's life.

Post-traumatic Growth – the experience of a psychological growth following a traumatic experience characterized by a more positive and resilient view of the self, the world, and one's relationships.

Post-traumatic Nightmares – a re-experiencing of previous traumas that happened in real life during sleep.

Post-traumatic Stress (PTS) – an extended fight-or-flight or stress response due to experiencing a traumatic or stressful event. The associated symptoms do not reach a clinical level.

Post-traumatic Stress Disorder (PTSD) – a psychiatric diagnosis characterized by the individual undergoing a traumatic event followed by symptoms of hyperarousal and withdrawal from stimulation associated with the trauma.

Post-traumatic Stress Syndrome (PTSS) – symptoms consistent with post-traumatic stress disorder (PTSD), but that are within a short time of experiencing the traumatic event.

Prefrontal Cortex – a cortical structure that plays a central role in modulating emotions, cognitive control, influencing attention, impulse inhibition, prospective memory, and cognitive flexibility.

Primary Motor Cortex – a cortical structure that generates the efferent signals that result in the muscle contractions that underlie voluntary movement.

Pyramidal Cells – a type of neuron with a multipolar shape containing one axon and several dendrites.

Reconsolidation – the neurobiological stabilization of a reactivated memory.

Reflective Distance – the metacognitive process of viewing and reflecting on art.

Regulation – the ability of an individual to modulate an emotion or set of emotions.

Relational Resonating – occurs when a client communicates and presents narratives that evokes and/or activates the therapist's own personal and private experiences.

Resilience – the process and outcome of successfully adapting to difficult or challenging life experiences.

Safeness/safety – creating a secure environment to build a trusting therapeutic relationship.

Salience Network – a large-scale brain network involved in detecting, integrating, and prioritizing relevant interoceptive information and directing other networks to engage in goal-directed behavior.

Semantic Meaning – the study of meaning in language.

Semantic Memory – a type of long-term declarative memory that refers to facts, concepts, and ideas which an individual accumulates over the course of their life.

Social Prescribing – healthcare providers refer patients to art experiences to support their health and well-being.

Social Relational Psychotherapy Theory – a therapeutic approach based on the idea that mutually satisfying relationships with others are necessary for one's emotional well-being. This takes into account the ways in which social and familial factors relate to the relationships in a person's life.

Somatosensory Cortex – region of the postcentral gyrus that receives and processes somatosensory stimuli.

Storycloth – needlecraft on a flat textile surface depicting a scene, narrative, or culture.

Temporal Cortex – region of cortex in the temporal lobe primarily responsible for interpreting auditory stimuli and playing a significant role in recognizing and using language. It also facilitates object recognition and interacts with other structures to create new and long-term memories.

Temporal Lobe – a large lobe of each cerebral hemisphere that is situated in front of the occipital lobe and contains a sensory area associated with auditory processing, and subcortical structures associated with learning, memory, and emotions.

Thalamus – Subcortical structure in the diencephalon that conveys sensory inputs to cortex for processing for conscious perception and conveys inputs from cerebellum and basal ganglia to cortex for initiation of voluntary movement.

Therapeutic Attunement – a process encompassing therapist's ability to perceive and to respond to patient's inner state.

Theraplay – a short-term attachment-based intervention in which elements of play therapy are used to strengthen parent–child bonds and to promote secure attachments, self-regulation, and communication skills in children.

Third Culture Kid – a child who grows up in a culture different from the one in which his or her parents grew up.

Third Spaces – a public space outside of home and work that fosters civic engagement and democracy.

Top-down Information Processing – refers to processing which begins with the high level cortical areas that feed back to and influence subcortical structures and sensory processing.

Transformative Integration – one of the six CREATE Framework principles; combining cognitive functions with somatic experiences, tactile experiences, emoting, motivation, and motor control.

Trauma – distressing, disturbing, or life-threatening events, or a person's response to those events.

Trauma-focused Cognitive Behavioral Therapy (TF-CBT) – an evidence-based treatment for children and adolescents impacted by trauma and their parents or caregivers.

Traumatic Brain Injury (TBI) – an injury that occurs when external physical forces cause damage to the brain.

Traumatology – the evaluation and treatment of psychological trauma in individuals affected by severe mental or emotional stress or physical injury.

Universality – the character or state of being universal; existence or prevalence everywhere.

Vagus Nerve – a main component of the parasympathetic nervous system, serving both sensory and motor functions associated with digestion, heartrate, and breathing, and thought to be involved in mood and immune functions. The tenth and longest cranial nerve.

Visual Cortex – located in the occipital lobe, it receives information from the eyes and is responsible for the first stages of processing visual information.

INDEX

Note: Locators in *italic* indicate figures, in **bold** tables, and in ***italic-bold*** boxes

A New Kind of House (exhibit, Drexel University) 208, *209*
abuse 267; alcohol, drugs 29; sexual, physical 59, 77, 88, 132, 134–135, 136–137, 151, 157; *see also* maltreatment, childhood
action potential 17–18, 267
adaptive responding 107, *107*, 110–116, 267, 268; control 114–115; immobilization and engagement 111–112, *112*; mastery 115–116; relaxation, safeness, comfort 114; stress response, stress reduction 112–113, *113*
Adlerian psychology 220–221, 223, 267
adverse childhood experiences (ACEs) 3, 77
allostatic load 110, 112, 113, 267
Alzheimer's 22, 206
American Art Therapy Association (AATA) 2, 260–261
amorphous art, self-expression therapy project 233–236, *234–236*
amygdala (AMY) 267; activation, active coping area 26, 115; DMN (dys) regulation 22; emotion processing 53, 57, 100, 114, 120, 171, 176; instinctual trauma response (ITR) 81 (*see also under own heading*); memory, autobiographical self-referential processing 26, 100, *117*, 120, 171
Anderson, G. 198
Animal Strengths and Family Environment Directive intervention protocol 175–176
anterior cingulate cortex 176, **256**, 267
anterior insula (AI) 55, 267
aphasia 243, 267
Applied Educational Neuroscience **214**, 217–219, *217*
Armstrong, J. 197
art, functions 197
art therapists of color 2
art therapy: evidence based and integrative practice 5–6; neuroscience-based approaches 6–7; tenets, three 6, 197, 200, 213, 236, 253, 254
art therapy, concept, history: art as therapy vs art psychotherapy binary 1–2; culturally competent and culturally informed practice 2; defining 1; dual factor models 2; founders of color 2; holistic and embodied human engagement 2; interdisciplinarity 1; pluralistic worldview 1; as profession 1; social and human science 1
art therapy education, formed 220–224, *221–223*
art therapy relational neuroscience (ATR-N) approach 107–122, 254; adaptive responding 107, *107*, 110–116, *112–113*, 267; CREATE, memory reconsolidation principles 107, *107*; creative embodiment 107, *107*, 268; empathizing and compassion 107, *107*, 120–122, 268, 269; expressive communicating 107, *107*, 115–116, 116–118, 120, 268, 269; relational resonating 107, *107*, 108–109, 111–112, 162, 268, 274; transformative integration 107, *107*, 118–122, *119*, 268, 275
arts and health (A&H) 251
as foundation experiences; *see* preverbal traumas, foundation experiences
attachment, children: Cairns experiments 135; flawed/disrupted, caregiver failure 132–133, 134, 143; foster care 134, 135–136; neurobiology, brain development 80, 133–134; neuroplasticity, new attachment communication 134; secure, characteristics 133–134; SECURE, play therapy model 107, *107*, 134–135
attentional brain networks 23–24; dorsal 23–24, 85, 185–186; neural 24, 78, 80, 100, 172, 273
auxiliary self 108, 267
axon 17, 18, ***34***, ***40***, 267

Baker, F. A. 51
basal ganglia 17, 53, *119*, 267
Belkofer, C. M. 150–162
Berberian, M. 184
Berger, H. ***35***
bias 24, 37, 118, 150, 252, 270

bilateral lingual gyrus 57, 267
blood oxygen level dependent magnetic resonance imaging (BOLD MRI) *39*, 267
Bodymind Model 252, 254
BOLD (blood oxygenation dependent level) signals 171
bottom-up approach, trauma therapy: bottom-up information processing 267; case studies 61–66, *62–65*; ETC levels as action methods 58–59, 72–73; as nonverbal approach 76, 235; vs top-down (cognitive) approach 76
Bowlby, J. 133
brain: attentional brain networks 23–24; cellular function 17–18; communication within the brain 19, 20; functions 7; hemisphere model 7–8; hemispheric asymmetries, specialization, brain 26–28, 54, 80–82, 84, 85, 118, 120, 242; large-scale brain networks (LSBN) (*see under own heading*); mirror neurons and empathy model 7–8; neuroplasticity (*see under own heading*); sensory information processing 19–20, *21*; structure 17–18; traumatic brain injury (TBI) 21–22, 167, 170, 172–173, **179–181**, 181–183, 186, 243, 275
brain imaging studies and methods *35–40*; blood oxygen level dependent magnetic resonance imaging (BOLD MRI) *39*, 267; case studies 27–32, *28*, *30–31*; computed tomography (CT) *35*; diffusion tensor imaging (DTI) *40*; electroencephalography (EEG) *36*, *37*, 269; functional magnetic resonance imaging (fMRI) 171; low resolution brain electromagnetic tomography (LORETA) 29, *29*, *38*, 271; magnetic resonance imaging (MRI) *38–39*; magnetoencephalography (MEG) *40*, 182, 271; MRI spectroscopy (MRS) *39*; positron emission tomography (PET) 30, *30–31*, *38*, *40*; potential 25, 133; quantitative EEG (qEEG) 27–29, *28–30*, *36–38*, 257, 259; single photon computed tomography (SPECT) *40*
brain-to-behavior approach 32

Cairns, R. B. 135
Caribbean art therapy trauma practice 230–232
case studies: amorphous art *234–236*; body and trauma 154–161, *158–160*;

bottom-up approach, trauma therapy 61–66, *62–65*; brain imaging studies and methods 27–31, *28*, *30–31*; drawing 8, 59–61, *60*, *63*, 64, 66–71, 90–91, 130, *131*, 244–245; expressive therapies continuum (ETC) 59–61, *60*, 61–67, *62–65*, *67–71*, 71–72; externalization 243–244; Externalized Dialogue® (ED) 92–93, *93–98*; flow 64, 66, 69–70, 72; foundation traumas 99, 100, 101; Graphic Narrative® (GN) 90–91, 99; identity, new understanding through art therapy 243–245; Instinctual Trauma Response® (ITR) 86–101, 90–91, 99; narrative coherence and closure 61, 63, *64*, 66, 70–71; neuroplasticity 142, 143; post-traumatic nightmares (PTN) 240–242, *241–242*; preverbal traumas 61, 63, *64*, 66, 70–71, 90–92, 100–101, 154–161, *158–160*; resilience 59, 64, 66, 70, 72 ; severely traumatized children (neuroscience, art therapy) 130, *131*, 133, 134, 135, 136, 137–142, *139–141*, *143*, 144; top-down approach, trauma therapy 66–71, *67–71*
catecholamines 109–110, 267; *see also* stress response (short-/long-term)
cellular memory formation 26
cellular processes, brain 17–18
cellular structure / cellular learning 8, 18, 222, *222*
central executive network (CEN) 22–23, 55–57, 61, 70, 72–73, 171, 257, **257**, 267
central sulci 20, 268
cerebellum 30, *31*, 100, 116, 268
cerebrum 268
Chapman, L. 137, 142
Chatterjee, A. 239
childhood brain development, trauma effect *34–35*
children: abuse 59, 77, 88, 132, 134–135, 136–137, 151, 157, 267; attachment behaviour 135; as foundation experiences (*see* Instinctual Trauma Response® (ITR) model ; preverbal trauma); maltreatment, childhood 51, 77, 133, 137, 271; neglect 51, 77, 88, 130, 132, 136, 151, 272; preverbal traumas (*see under own heading*); severely traumatized children (neuroscience, art therapy) (*see under own heading*)
Chilton, G. 166–189

chronic trauma / chronic traumatic stress (CTS) 118, 120
Cincinnati Art Museum, Ohio 201
cingulate cortex 25, *30*, 53, 54, 268; anterior 55, 176, **256**, 267; posterior (PCC) 22, 55, *117*, **256**, 273
clay work 178, 258, 259–260; bottom-up approach, trauma therapy 61, 64–65; clay and the brain 258; ETC K/S level 153, 258; Parkinson's disease (PD) 213–215
Clyde Findlay, J. M. A. 162
cognitive behavioral therapy (CBT) 5, 115, 130, 275
cognitive processing therapy (CPT) 5, 184
cognitive restructuring 32, 54, 63, 64, 66, *67*, 68, 70
cognitive/symbolic (C/SY) level of ETC 53–54, *255*, 256, **256**, 268
Coles, A. 201
collectivist psychotherapy theory 221, 268
Common Threads Project 226–227, 268
compassionate relapse prevention 106, 268
complex wicked problem, term 4, 251
complicated grief 172, 174, 182, 268
computed tomography (CT) *35*, *40*
Conroy, J. 135
contextualized representations 106, 268
corpus callosum 7, 20, *35*, 80, 268
cortical/subcortical processing, development *21*, 26, *36*, 118, 137
cortical/subcortical structures, networks 20, 22, 23, *38*, 53, 55, 78, 118, 171
cortisol 108, 109–110, 112, *113*, 114, 230, 259, 268
Corwin, D. 135–136
Cowen, B. 207–208
Cox, A. 134
CREATE Framework 107, *107*, 122, 162, 268; adaptive responding 107, *107*, 110–116, *112–113*, 267, 268; creative embodiment 107, *107*, 268; empathizing and compassion 107, *107*, 120–122, 268, 269; expressive communicating 107, *107*, 115–116, 116–118, 120, 268, 269; relational resonating 107, *107*, 108–109, 111–112, 162, 268, 274; transformative integration 107, *107*, 118–122, *119*, 268, 275; *see also* Art therapy relational neuroscience (ATR-N) approach
creative arts therapies (CATs): awareness, raising 251; definitional clarity lack 251, 252–254; elements and key factors 5–6; ETC as framework 58 (*see also*

expressive therapies continuum (ETC)); future, tele-CAT services 261; principles, tenets 252–254; trauma treatment 260; treatment intervention potential 261
creative dimension (CR), ETC 54, 65, 66
creative embodiment 107, *107*, 268; *see also* CREATE Framework
Creative Forces®: NEA Military Healing Arts Network 167–170, 175; *The Animal Strengths and Family Environment Directive* 175; clinical practice: art therapy, family 175–176 / art therapy, individual vs group 182 / art therapy, service members 169–170 / art therapy, service members 172–175, *173–175*; clinical practice: interventions types 179, **179–181**; clinical sites *168*, 169, 170; community sites 169; complicated grief 172, *173–175*, 174, 182, 268; founding, concept, purpose 167; military culture, art therapy implication 167, **187–189**; moral injury 172, *173*, **188**, 272; network support 167; pillars 169, *169*; post-traumatic stress disorder (PTSD), symptoms, neuroimaging 170–173, 181, 183, 184, 186; research: clinical examples 172–175, *173–175*, 181 / engagement and flow state 176–177 / mask making 170, 172, *173*, 178, **181**, 182–184, 185–186 / material processes and therapy impact 177–179 / montage painting directive and behavioural outcome **180**, 185; therapy research and program evaluation 181–186; traumatic brain injury (TBI) 167, 170, 172–173, **179–181**, 181–183, 186
creative process 54, 176, 199, 238, 254
creative transition area (ETC) 56, 268
cultural competence 230–231, 268
culturally competent and culturally informed practice 2
CultureRx Initiative 197–198
Czamanski-Cohen, J. 177, 252

Damasio, A. 53
d'Aquili, E. G. 152
de Botton, A. 197
decolonizing / decolonization 230, 269
default mode network (DMN) 22, 55–57, 61, 72–73, 116, 171, 183, 185, 253, **257**, 269
Delima, J. F. 77
dementia 22, *40*, 206

dendrites 17–18, *34*, 222, *222*, 269
Department of Defense (DoD) 166, 167, 169, **187**; *see also* Creative Forces®: NEA Military Healing Arts Network
Department of Veterans Affairs (VA) 167, 169, 186
Desautels, L. 217–219
Diagnostic and Statistical Manual of Mental Disorders (DSM) 3, 83, 85
Dietrich, A. 176
diffusion tensor imaging (DTI) **40**
dissociation as trauma respond 81, 83, 85, 120
Donald, K. 230–232
dorsal attention network 23–24, 85, 185–186
dorsal vagal complex (DVC) 110, *111*, 112
dorsal-anterior cingulate cortex (dACC) 55, 269
dorsolateral prefrontal cortex (dlPFC) 22, 54, 55, 269
drawing 82, 100, 257–260; and brain, neural activity 257–258, 259–260; bridge with path drawing **180**; case studies 8, 59–61, *60*, *63*, 64, 66–71, 90–91, 130, *131*, 244–245; dual, dyadic 109; family drawing 136; Goodenough Draw-a-Person test (DAP) 257; Graphic Narrative® (GN) 84 (*see also under own heading*); kinetic 243–244; large gesture 115
Drexel University 208, *209*

electroencephalography (EEG) *36*, *37*, 269; case studies 27–29, *28–30*; quantitative EEG (qEEG) 27–29, *28–30*, *36–38*, 257, 259
Elkis-Abuhoff, D. L. 213–215
embodied cognition 197, 200, 269
embodiment, embodied experience 3, 6, 269; creative 107, *107*, 252, 253 (*see also* CREATE Framework); embodied context, art therapy 254; social 108
empathic resonance 108, 269
empathizing and compassion 107, *107*, 120–122, 268, 269; *see also* art therapy relational neuroscience (ATR-N); CREATE Framework
empathy 269; art therapy, therapeutic alliance 177, 237, 251; audio-visual transmitted inputs 237; bodily experience, art therapy 156; empathetic museum 198–199, 200; human mirror neuron system 7; mirror neurons (MN) 7

engagement, art therapy 64, 66, 69, 175, 237, 239, 269; brain processes 19, *21*, 22–23, 24, 29, 30; and flow 57, 176–177; immobilization and engagement 110–112, *111*; interpersonal social relationships, community/museum 109–110, 197–198, 199, 200, 206–210; kinesthetic art engagement 230–231; levels of engagement (ETC) 153 (*see also under expressive therapies continuum (ETC)*); neuroplasticity 215; SECURE, play therapy model 135; therapist 108
entrainment 156–157, 269
episodic memory 56, 82, 106, 116, 269
Eunice Kennedy Shriver National Institute of Child Health and Human Development 2
event-related potentials 270
evidence-based practice (EBP) 4–5, 130, 132, 269
executive control network; *see* central executive network (CEN)
explicit knowledge 6
explicit memory 81, 84, 86, 88, 99–100, 269
expressive communication 107, *107*, 115–118, 120, 268, 269; novelty and creativity 116–117, *117*; positivity 117–118; *see also* CREATE Framework; art therapy relational neuroscience (ATR-N) approach
Expressive Therapies Continuum (ETC): and brain functions 51–52, *52*; case studies 59–61, *60*, 61–67, *62–65*, *67–71*, 71–72, 154–161, *158–160*; concept, function 51–52, 153–154, 220, 223, *255*, 269; as conceptional art therapy framework 153–154, 223, 227, 254–257; creative dimension (CR) 54, 64, 66; creative transition area 269; creativity, flow, post-traumatic growth 51, 54, 59 (*see also* flow); levels and neural mechanism/pathways **256**; levels as top-down/bottom-up trauma therapy action methods 58–59, 72–73 (*see also* bottom-up approach, trauma therapy; top-down approach, trauma therapy); levels: cognitive/symbolic (C/SY) 53–54, *255*, 256, **256**, 268; levels: kinesthetic/sensory (K/S) 52–53, *255*, 256, **256**, 271 / perceptual/affective (P/A) 53, *255*, 256, **256**, 273 / polarities 52–54, *52*, 54; and LSBN similarities/differences 56; trauma treatment usage 58–59

externalization 8, 56, 78, 174, **179**,
181–182, 220, 240, 270; case studies
243–244
Externalized Dialogue® (ED) 78, 82, 84,
85–86; case studies 92–93, *93–98*

Fairbairn, W. R. D. 136
Farrell-Kirk, R. 197–210
fasciculations 270
Feldman, R. 133
fight or flight/flee response 81, 112, 115,
267, 273
Fitchburg Museum, Fitchburg Families
First program 206
flow: case studies 64, 66, 69–70, 72;
defining, mechanism 59, 138, 176;
engagement in, art therapy 176–177,
230; experience 51, 59, 69, 138, 176;
flow resilience 57–58
flow, blood; *see* blood oxygen level
dependent magnetic resonance
imaging (BOLD MRI)
forebrain 270
foundation traumas 76, 77, 80, 82–83,
84; case studies 99, 100, 101; *see also*
preverbal trauma
Fredrickson, B. L. 117
freeze response/state 81, 90, 110–112
freeze-or-faint response 110
frontal cortex 20, *35*, 52
frontal lobe 28, *28*, 81, *119*, 218, 219,
258, 270
functional connectivity *37*, 56, 57, 79,
171, 183, 185, 270
functional magnetic resonance imaging
(fMRI) 171, 186, 257, 270
functional near-infrared spectroscopy
(fNIRS) 270

Galili, G. 177
Gantt, L. 76–101
Garlock, L. 225–229
Gavron, T. 178
Gaydos, M. 213–215
genetic mapping 32
Graphic Narrative® (GN) 78, 79, 82,
84–85, 90; case studies 90–91, 99
Gruce, L. 233–236

Haiblum-Itskovitch, S. 177, 259
Harmon, A. 216–219
Hass-Cohen, N. 106–122, 231
Hayward, C. 201
"Healing Our Soldiers" (*National
Geographicl*) 170

health, defining 1
heart rate variability (HRV) 177–178,
259, 270
hemispheric asymmetries, specialization,
brain 26–28, 54, 80–82, 84, 85, 118,
120, 242
Herman, J. L. 89
Hill, A. 166
hindbrain 270
Hinz, L. D. 51–73
hippocampus 24, 53, 79, 100, 106, *117*,
171, 185, **256**, 270
holistic/whole person-centred approach
31–33, 52, 150–162, 270
Huntoon, M. 166
Huotilainen, M. 177
hurricane Katrina, New Orleans,
creativity and resilience 238
hypothalamic-pituitary-adrenal (HPA)
axis stress response 112, *113*
hypothalamus 270

identity understanding through art
therapy 243–245
imagery rehearsal therapy and art therapy
integration (IRT + AT) 240–242,
241–242
imagery rehearsal therapy (IRT) 240, 270
imaging methods; *see* brain imaging
studies and methods
implicit bias 252, 270
implicit knowledge 6
implicit memory 25, 77, 79, 81, 84–85,
100, 270
inferior parietal cortex (IPC) *117*
Instinctual Trauma Response® (ITR)
treatment approach 78–100; approach
84–86; case studies 86–101, 90–91,
99; concept, tenets, approach 78–79;
emotional self development, brain
structure/hemispheric asymmetries
79–80; Externalized Dialogue® (ED)
78, 82, 84, 85–86; foundation trauma,
symptoms and treatment need 83–84;
Graphic Narrative® (GN) 78, 79, 82,
84–85, 90; ITR clinic, Morgantown,
West Virginia 76, 92; as neuroplasticity
process 83; response components
81, 84, 90; training, assessments 101,
101; trauma processing 82–84; *see also*
foundation traumas; preverbal traumas
integrative potential/practice, art therapy
5–6, 157, 199, 213, 226, 237–239
Interior (Degas) *203–204*
interoception 80, 253, 270

interoceptive awareness 55, 69, 72, 80, 151, 270
interpersonal neurobiology 5, 80, 151
intersubjectivity 118, 177, 270
Ioannides, E. 207
ITR; *see* Instinctual Trauma Response® (ITR) model

Jernberg, A. 134–135
Johnson, D. R. 132, 152
Johnson, L. 170
Jones, J. P. 177, 182, 184
Jury, H. 201

Kaimal, G. 183, 184–185
Kaplan, J. 226
kinesthetic/sensory (K/S) level of ETC 52–53, 255, 256, **256**, 271
kinesthetic-sensory approach 230, 230–232, 256, **256**, 271
King, J. L. 1–9, 17–41, 251–260
Klorer, P. G. 130–146, 157
Konopka, L. M. 17–41
Konorski 18–19
Kramer, E. H. 172
Kruk, K. 259–260
Kruk-Borisov, K. 251–260

Laird, R. 207–208
large-scale brain networks (LSBN) 22, 51, 55–59, 271; central executive network (CEN) 22–23, 55–57, 61, 70, 72–73, 171, 257, **257**, 267; default mode network (DMN) 22, 55–57, 61, 72–73, 116, 171, 183, 185, 253, **257**; definition, concept 55; ETC similarities 56; flow stage 72 (*see also* flow); salience network (SN), 22, 23, 55–56, 171, 239, **256**, 257, 274; and trauma 56–59; *see also* triple network model
lateral prefrontal cortex 22
lateralization 27, 271
LeDoux, J. E. 77, 81
Legari, S. 201, 207
Leopold, K. 238
Lewis, T. 90
ligand 271
limbic regulation 90
LORETA; *see* low resolution brain electromagnetic tomography (LORETA)
low input–high output response 150, 271
low resolution brain electromagnetic tomography (LORETA) 28, 29, **38**, 271
Lusebrink, V. B. 51–73, 153, 227, 253–255, **256**, 257, 258

magnetic resonance imaging (MRI) 20, *38–39*, 271; art therapy response 186, 257; blood-oxygen level dependent (BOLD) MRI *39*, 267; case studies 30, *31*; functional magnetic resonance imaging (fMRI) 171, 186, 257, 270; MRI spectroscopy (MRS) *39*
magnetoencephalography (MEG) *40*, 182, 271
Malchiodi, C. A. 153, 161
maltreatment, childhood 51, 77, 133, 137, 271
Maltz, B. 184
manualized trauma protocol/approaches 132, 271
mask making 170, 172, *173*, 178, **181**, 182–184, 185–186, 241, *242*
McKeown, J. 207–208
Meares, R. 81
medial prefrontal cortex (mPFC) 55, 110, 116, *117*, *119*, 171, 271
Meltz, E. 237–239
memory reconsolidation 9, 79, 106–122, 271, 273; art therapy relational neuroscience (ATR-N) approach 107, *107*, 108, 254 (*see also under own heading*); guidelines 106; memory recall and processing 106; positive excitation, creativity, therapeutic art making 114, 115, 116, 120, 122; principles, guidelines 106–107; relational resonating 108; SAM response and 112
memory: autobiographical self-referential processing 26, 100, *117*, 120, 171; cellular memory formation 26; episodic 56, 82, 106, 116, 269; explicit 81, 84, 86, 88, 99–100, 269; implicit 25, 77, 79, 81, 84–85, 100, 270; positive memory retrieval 120; semantic 106, 122, 274; storage 100
mentalizing 108, 115, *117*, 118–119, 271
metaphor-based neuroscience teaching 220, 223–224, *223–224*
midbrain 137, 213, 271
mild traumatic brain index (mTBI) 38, 171, **179–181**
military cultural considerations for art therapist *187–189*
military-connected populations 166–189; amorphous art, self-expression therapy project 233–236; complicated grief 172, *173–175*, 174, 182, 268; Creative Forces®: NEA Military Healing Arts Network (*see under own heading*);

Department of Veterans Affairs (VA) 167, 169, 186; "Healing Our Soldiers" (*National Geographic*) 170; history of art therapy use 166–167; military culture, art therapy implication 167, **187–189**; moral injury 172, *173*, **188**, 272; National Endowment for the Arts (NEA) 167; National Intrepid Center of Excellence (NICoE) 167, 170, 181–182, 183, 184, 185, 186; *Operation Homecoming: Writing the Wartime Experience* initiative 167; post-traumatic nightmares (PTN) 240–242; post-traumatic stress disorder (PTSD) 170–173, 181, 183, 184, 186; traumatic brain injury (TBI) 167, 170, 172–173, **179–181**, 181–183, 186

Mindful Artists Club 218–219

mindfulness practice 80, 106, 114, 121, 206, 228, 260

mindfulness self-compassion (MSC) interventions 121–122

mindfulness softening 106–107, 271

mirror neurons (MN) 7, 108, 121, 122, 156, 271

mission statement 198, 271

mobile brain body imaging (MOBI) 253, 271

Molendijk, T. 172

montage paintings 5, **180**, 185

Montreal Museum of Fine Arts 201, 207

moral injury 172, *173*, **188**, 272

morphologies 17, 272

motor/sensory cortex 30, 81, 156, **256**, 258, 272

MRI; *see* magnetic resonance imaging (MRI)

MRI spectroscopy (MRS) *39*

Mrs. Peale Lamenting the Death of Her Child/ Rachel Weeping (Wilson) 203, *204*

multimodal association cortex (transmodal cortex) 52, 53, 272

multimodal cortex 53, 54

museums as art therapy settings 197–210; art therapy practice 201–206, *202–204*; art, functions 197; best practice recommendations 207–209; challenging subject matters 202–204; Cincinnati Art Museum, Ohio 201; collaboration, staff-therapy professionals 197, 199, 201–203, *202–203*, 205, 208–209; community trauma response: Coral Springs Museum of Art / Florida Art Therapy Association (FATA)

203, 205; CultureRx Initiative, pilot program 197–198; definition, framework, concepts 198–201, 207–209; Drexel University 208, *209*; Fitchburg Museum, Fitchburg Families First program 206; International Council of Museums (ICOM) 198; Montreal Museum of Fine Arts 201, 207; museum educator training 201–203, *202–203*; museum setting as therapeutic factor 200, 201; neuroscience foundation, embodied cognition 197, 200, 269; Philadelphia Museum of Art 202; Studio Museum of Harlem New York 201

myelin sheath 272

Nadal, M. 239

narrative coherence and closure 6, 54, 78–79, 82, 85, 132; case studies 61, 63, *64*, 66, 70–71; *see also* Graphic Narrative®

National Endowment for the Arts (NEA) 167

National Institutes of Health (Bethesda) 167

National Intrepid Center of Excellence (NICoE) 167, 170, 181–182, 183, 184, 185, 186

neglect 51, 77, 88, 130, 132, 136, 151, 272; *see also* abuse; maltreatment, childhood

neocortex 34

neural attention network 24, 78, 80, 100, 172, 273

neuroaesthetics 272

neuroception 222, 272

neurocounseling 220, 221, 223, 272

neurodegenerative disorders 22

neuro-developmental art therapy model 137, 142, 150, 272

neuroeducation 220, 221–222, *221–222*

neurofeedback 220, 222, *222–223*, 272

neuro-informed art therapy training approach 220–224, *221–223*

neuronal electrical activity *39*

neurons 17–18, 272; action potential 18; brain development, trauma effect *34*, 220; brain functioning 2, 17–18; brain structure 17; magnetoencephalography (MEG) *40*, 182, 271; *Mindful Artists Club* 218–219; mirror neurons (MN) 7, 108, 121, 122, 156, 271; morphologies 272; neuronal networks 18, 24, 33, 220; pyramidal cells 273;

rewiring, neuroplasticity 7, 18 (*see also* neuroplasticity); upper/lower motor neurons xvi
neurophysiology 28, *38*, 150, 186, 272
neuroplasticity 33, 133–134, 162; art therapy as promoter 162, 186, 215, 218–219; art therapy/creative processes and 8; case studies 142, 143; cellular learning, synaptic plasticity 18–19; cellular structure / cellular learning 18; definition, concept 8, 18–19, 215, 272; disruption, mood/anxiety disorders 8; enhancing treatment 8; ITR, Externalized Dialogue® 82; neural remodeling 18; neuroeducation 220, 221–222, *221–222*; and resilient adaptation 238; social neural plasticity 133; synaptic plasticity, synaptic contact pruning 18; trauma effect on brain development *34–35*; vs two-hemisphere brain concept 8, 27
Neuroplasticity is My Superpower project 219
neuroscience 2–3; categories 2; defining 2; interdisciplinarity 2; research/study limitations 2–3
neuroscience concepts 17–41; attentional brain networks 23–24; brain cellular processes 17–18; communication within the brain 19; large-scale brain networks (LSBN) / triple network model (*see* triple network model); neuroplasticity and learning 18–19 (*see also* neuroplasticity); sensory networks, sensory processing 19–21, *21*; traumatic memories 24–25
Neuroscience Special Interest Group (Neuro SIG) 260–261
neurosequential model of therapeutics (NMT) 137, 142
neuroscience-based approaches 6–7; brain plasticity approaches 8; knowledge transfer 6; model simplification 7–8
neurotransmitter 2, 17–18, 26, 27, *34*, *35*, *113*, *222*, 272
Newberg, A. B. 152
norepinephirne (NE) release *113*, 114

occipital cortex 54, 272
occipital lobe **256**, 272
Olafson, E. 135–136
Operation Homecoming: Writing the Wartime Experience initiative 167
orbitofrontal cortex (OFC) 53, 119, *119*, 272

Parkinson's disease (PD) 213–215
Palamara, A. 201
parietal cortex 20, 58, 272
parietal lobe 20, 52, 53, 54, **256**, 258, 273
Payano Sosa, J. 166–189
Pénzes, I. 259–260
perceptual/affective (P/A) level of ETC 53, *255*, 256, **256**, 273
Perry, B. D. 133, 134, 137, 142
person-centered art therapy approach 31, 33, 243, 245, 253, 273; *see also* holistic/ whole person-centred approach
Philadelphia Museum of Art 202
Polyvagal theory 5, 82, 222, *222–223*, 273
Porges, S. W. 5, 82, 177
positive emoting 8, 106, 116, 117–118, 120, 218, 273
positron emission tomography (PET) *38*, *40*; case studies 30, *30–31*
post-modern psychotherapy theory 273
posterior cingulate cortex (PCC) 22, 55, *117* **256**, 273
post-traumatic growth 51, 54, 59, 72, 273
post-traumatic nightmares (PTN) *241–242*, 273; post-traumatic nightmares (PTN) 240–242
post-traumatic stress disorder (PTSD): adverse childhood experience, correlation 77; art therapy, benefit research 51, 260; cognitive processing therapy (CPT) 184; DMN alteration 116; neuroimaging 170–171, 183; and traumatic brain injury (TBI) 172–173, 181, 183, 186
post-traumatic stress (PTS) 171, 172, 174, 183, 185, 186, 273
post-traumatic stress syndrome (PTSS) 24–26, *35*, 77, 273
prefrontal cortex (PFC) 26, 53, 57, 66, 72, 100, 120, 176, 216, 257, 273; dorsal anterior cingulate cortex 269; dorsolateral 22, 54, 55, 269; lateral 22; medial 55, 110, 116, *117*, *119*, 171, 271
preverbal traumas 76–101; awareness block 78; bottom-up (nonverbal) vs top-down (cognitive) approach 76; case studies 61, 63, *64*, 66, 70–71, 90, 90–92, 100–101, 154–161, *158–160*; dissociation 83; early trauma treatment, history 76–77; early trauma treatment, visual art (*see* Graphic Narrative® (GN)); ETC, K/S work 53; foundation trauma 76, 77, 80, 82–83, 84, 99, 100, 101; narrative closure lack 78–79, 132; nonverbal/emotional

brain 78, 80; tenets 78–79; treatment
    approach, instinctual trauma response
    (see Instinctual Trauma Response®
    (ITR) model)
primary motor cortex 53, **256**, 273
pyramidal cells 17–18, 273

quantitative EEG (qEEG) *36*, *37–38*, 257,
    259; case studies 27–29, *28–30*

Rafferty-Bugher, E. 220–224
reconsolidation, memory; see memory
    reconsolidation
reflective distance 63, 65, 230, 273
regulation, emotional 273; central-
    executive network (CEN), 55,
    57; dysregulation, childhood
    maltreatment/abuse 51; dysregulation,
    trauma 35; ETC levels 58, 61; *Three
    Tenets*, neuroscience-integrated art
    therapy 6
relational resonating 107, *107*, 108–109,
    111–112, 162, 268, 274; see also
    CREATE Framework
resilience 274; case studies 59, 64, 66,
    70, 72; flow resilience 57–58, 59;
    hurricane Katrina, New Orleans,
    creativity and resilience 238; military-
    connected people/families 172, 175,
    183; mother-child attachment 133, 134;
    neuroplasticity 133, 162, 238; positive
    emoting, positivity 117–118; resilience
    through creativity 51, 59, 238 (see also
    expressive therapies continuum
    (ETC)); resiliency and relapse
    prevention (ATR-N) 107, *107* (see also
    art therapy relational neuroscience
    (ATR-N)); salience network (SN) 57
Robson, S. 226

safeness/safety 114, 274; Art therapy
    relational neuroscience (ATR-N)
    model 107, *107*, 111; psychological /
    predictability, trust 145, *146*, 161, 166,
    209; SECURE, play therapy model 135;
    therapist role 134; three-phase trauma
    recovery model 89
salience network (SN), 22, 23, 55, 56,
    171, 239, **256**, 257, 274
Scaer, R. C. 77
Schore, A. N. 5, 80, 81, 135
SECURE, play therapy model 107,
    107, 135
secure remembrance model (SR-5)
    107, *107*

semantic meaning 200, 274
semantic memory 106, 122, 274
sensorimotor psychotherapy. 5
sensory networks, sensory processing
    19–21, *21*, *107*, 154
sensory/motor cortex 30, 81, 156,
    256, 258
service members and veterans; see
    military-connected populations
severely traumatized children
    (neuroscience-informed art therapy)
    130–146; attachment issues, complexity
    133–136, 143 (see also attachment,
    children); case studies 130, *131*, 133,
    134, 135, 136, 137–142, *139–141*,
    143, 144; neuroscience therapy
    approaches 143–145; neuroscientific
    understanding 133–135; practical
    applications 145–146, *146*; socio-
    emotional vs chronological age 143,
    145, *146*; treatment implications
    137–143
Sholt, M. 178
Siegel, D. J. 5, 79–80, 101, 156
single photon computed tomography
    (SPECT) *40*
Smithsonian Art Museum 225, *225*
Snyder, K. 197–210
social prescribing 197–198, 201, 274
social relational psychotherapy theory 274
somatosensory cortex 20, **256**, 274
Soo Hon, S. 230–232
Sours Rhodes, C. 166–189
Stamper, A. 240–242
Storycloths 225–229, *225*, *228–229*,
    244–245, *245*, 274
Strang, C. E. 1–9, 17–41, 251–260
stress response (short-/long-term)
    112–113, *113*, 114–115, 260
stress system *113*
structural dissociation theory 85
Studio Museum of Harlem New York 201
sympathetic-adreno-medullar (SAM) axis
    stress respond 112, *113*
synaptic plasticity, synaptic contact
    pruning 18

temporal cortex 54, 274
temporal lobe 53, 55, 81, 218, **256**, 274
textiles as art material/objects 138, 226;
    Common Threads Project 226–227,
    268; sewing 138, 144, 226, 228, *228*,
    239; stitching 225–226, *225*, 227, 228,
    228, 245; storycloths 225–229, *225*,
    228–229, 244–245, *245*, 274

thalamus 17, 53, 54, 81, 110, *117*, 183, 258, 274
therapeutic attunement 156, 274
therapeutic relationship/alliance 107, 109, 132, 222, 238, 243, 251, 252–253, 257
Theraplay (Jernberg) 134–135, 274
Third Culture Kid 244, 274
third spaces 208, 274
Three Tenets (King) xvii, 6, 197, 200, 213, 236, 253, 254
Tinnin, L. 76–101
top-down approach, trauma therapy: vs bottom-up (sensory) approach 76; case studies 66–71, *67–71*; ETC levels as action methods 58–59, 72–73; top-down information processing 274
transformative integration 107, *107*, 118–122, *119*, 268, 275; acceptance-incorporating therapies 121; autobiographical processing 118–121, *119*; empathizing and compassion 120–122; mindfulness self-compassion (MSC) interventions 121–122; neurogenesis 120–121; positive memory retrieval 120; social connectivity 121; *see also* art therapy relational neuroscience (ATR-N) approach; CREATE Framework
trauma 3–4, 275; a complex wicked problem 4; cumulative experiences 3–4; definitions, history and complications 3; DSM-5-TR description 3; etiology 4; large-scale brain networks (LSBN) and 56–59; response variety 3; symptoms 3; traumatic experiences as under layer of mental health disorders 3
trauma, and body 150–162; brain-based art therapy 152; brain-body linked art therapy 152; case studies 154–161, *158–160*; expressive art therapies (*see* Expressive Therapies Continuum (ETC)); interoceptive awareness loss 55, 69, 72, 80, 151, 270; low input–high output responses 150, 271; mental health and interpersonal relationships 151–152; physical and neurophysiological trauma manifestation 150–151; physical/physiological trauma manifestation 151; trauma effect on brain

development *34–35*, 151; *see also* body, and trauma
Trauma and Recovery (Herman) 89
trauma focused cognitive behavioral therapy (TF-CBT) 115, 130, 275
The Trauma Spectrum (Scaer) 77
traumatic brain injury (TBI) 21–22, 167, 170, 172–173, **179–181**, 181–183, 186, 243, 275
traumatic memories 24–25, 231; accessing, Graphic Narrative® 82; bottom-up vs top-down therapy approach 71, 76; brain structure alteration effects 100; establishment, encoding 25–26, 71; memory reconsolidation (*see under own heading*); as non-verbal, sensor-motor memories 8, 61, 71, 72, 76, 161; preverbal 77, 78–79; visual encoding 76
traumatology 107, 121, 275
triple network model 55; central executive network (CEN) 22–23, 55–57, 61, 70, 72–73, 171, 257, **257**, 267; default mode network (DMN) 22, 55–57, 61, 72–73, 116, 171, 183, 185, 253, **257**; salience network (SN) 22, 23, 55–56, 171, 239, **256**, 257, 274
Tripp, T. 76–101

universality 122, 220, 275

vagus nerve 110, 275
van der Kolk, B. A. 5, 85, 135, 152
van der Vossen, B. 243–245
Varutti, M. 198–199
Verweij, D. 172
Villinski, P. 225, *225*, 227
Vimpani, G. V. 77
visual association cortex 53, *117*, **256**, 260
visual cortex 20, *117*, 260, 272

Walker, I. F. 238
Walker, M. S. 166–189, 245
Walter Reed National Military Medical Center 167
Watson, E. 201
Weihs, K. L. 252
"Why our brains love arts and crafts" 177
wicked problem, term 4, 251
Wolf, D. 197–210